60 Q&A on bovine parasitology

A handbook of questions and answers

Revised by Dr Dwight D. Bowman

For this English edition:
60 Q&A on bovine parasitology

Plaza Antonio Beltrán Martínez nº 1, planta 8 - letra I
(Centro empresarial El Trovador)
50002 Zaragoza - Spain

First printing: July 2014

This book has been published originally in Spanish under the title:
60 Q&A sobre parasitología bovina. Libro de preguntas y respuestas
© 2013 Grupo Asís Biomedia, S.L.
ISBN Spanish edition: 978-84-941014-5-8

Translation:
AMR Scientific Translations S.L.

Revised by:
Dr. Dwight D. Bowman

ISBN: 978-84-942449-7-1
D.L.: Z 785-2014

Design, layout and printing:
Servet editorial - Grupo Asís Biomedia, S.L.
www.grupoasis.com
info@grupoasis.com

Warning:

Veterinary science is constantly evolving, as are pharmacology and the other sciences. Inevitably, it is therefore the responsibility of the veterinary clinician to determine and verify the dosage, the method of administration, the duration of treatment and any possible contraindications to the treatments given to each individual patient, based on his or her professional experience. Neither the publisher nor the author can be held liable for any damage or harm caused to people, animals or properties resulting from the correct or incorrect application of the information contained in this book.

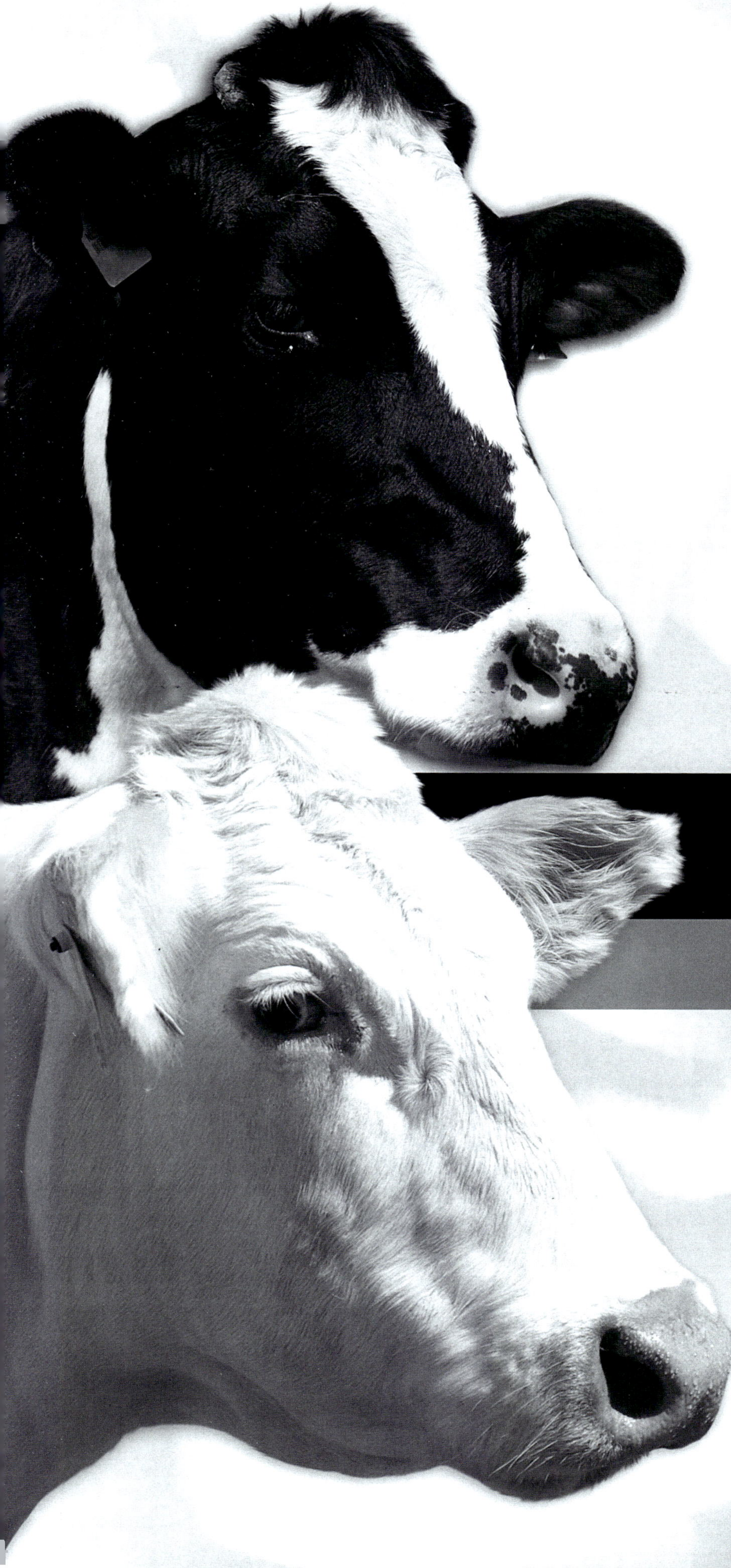

60 Q&A on bovine parasitology

A handbook of questions and answers

Aránzazu Meana Mañes
Francisco A. Rojo Vázquez

Revised by **Dr Dwight D. Bowman**

SERVET

"It is often said that Parasitology is a dreary subject, because of the emphasis placed on morphology and taxonomy neither of which is interesting or useful in an applied science. The knowledge of parasite morphology is as useful as the ability to recognised lethal and harmless snakes or, simply, the enemy."

A.M. Dunn

Acknowledgements

Although all works are the result of the study, experience and the efforts of their authors, this book could not have been written without the help of all those people who shared their knowledge and concerns in a purely selfless manner, prompting us to learn more and allowing us to discover new understandings and teaching options. The writing of this book is closely related to an "original" means of presenting parasitoses in cattle. The title contains the initials for questions and answers, in other words, a means of exposing clinical cases or practical examples (Q&A) that is, of course, not at all new.

We would like to thank the students involved in the teaching of parasitic diseases for having contributed to the search for new teaching methods and discussing the cases presented. We would also like to thank all our fellow vets specialising in parasitic diseases and bovine medicine, both clinicians and academics, for sharing their experiences, which have undoubtedly helped this work to be of a more practical nature.

Specifically, we would like to mention the following people who have collaborated with us: Alejandro Bohórquez, Nélida Fernández Pato, Miguel Llorens, Jorge Sangenis, Bernardino Prieto, Dr. G. Knubben-Schweizer, Dr. A. Gentile, Dr. A. Paz, Dr. A. Diaz Guerrier, Dr. J. V. Gónzalez, Dr. S. Astiz, Dr. P. García Palencia, Dr. A. S. Olmeda, Dr. F. Valcárcel, Dr. J. Pérez, Dr. C. Novoa, Dr. C. Botias, Dr. P. Jacquiet, Dr. Dubey, Dr. G. López, Dr. G. Militerno, Dr. J. Butler, Dr. R. Martin, Dr. K. Steininger, Dr. M. Castaño, Dr. M. Luzón, Dr. P. Morrondo, Dr. S. Hernández, Dr. S. Mitchel, Dr. T. Gómez, Dr. A. Encinas, Dr. I. González, Dr. J. Villalba and Dr. J. C. Domínguez F. de Tejerina.

Many of the photos are property of the authors, although others have been kindly provided by some of the people mentioned above or have been referenced in the text. We would therefore like to thank everyone who has provided us with photos or information. Above all, we ask that if you, the reader, have any comments, opinions or unique experiences with any of the topics covered in this book, you should contact us at one of the following email addresses.

Thank you to everyone for your help and we hope that you enjoy this book as much as we have enjoyed writing it.

Aránzazu Meana
ameana@ucm.es

Francisco A. Rojo-Vázquez
francisco.rojo@unileon.es

Authors

Aránzazu Meana Mañes

Holds a degree and doctorate in Veterinary Science from the Complutense University of Madrid (UCM) and is currently a lecturer in the Animal Health Department of the Faculty of Veterinary Medicine at the same university. She also holds a diploma from the European Veterinary Parasitology College (EVPC) and is the secretary of that institution.

She has worked as a companion animals vet in a private practice.

Her research work is centred on the pathophysiology and epidemiology of the most important parasitic diseases in domestic animals (gastrointestinal and hepatic helminths in herbivores, equine and bovine piroplasmosis) as well as methods for controlling parasitic diseases in both domestic animals and wildlife (chemoprophylaxis, anthelmintic resistance and genetic resistance to the infection by parasites).

She has published numerous research papers concerning parasitic animal diseases in international parasitology and veterinary science journals and has presented the results at numerous national and international parasitology conferences.

Furthermore, she has been a visiting researcher in the Departments of Veterinary Medicine of the Faculties of Veterinary Science at the Universities of Cambridge and Glasgow (UK).

She has been deputy head of the Animal Health Department of the Faculty of Veterinary Medicine (UCM), a member of the expert committees of the Ministries of Health, Education and Science and Agriculture, Fisheries and Food, a member of the Spanish Parasitology Society (SEP) and a member of the World Association for the Advancement of Veterinary Parasitology.

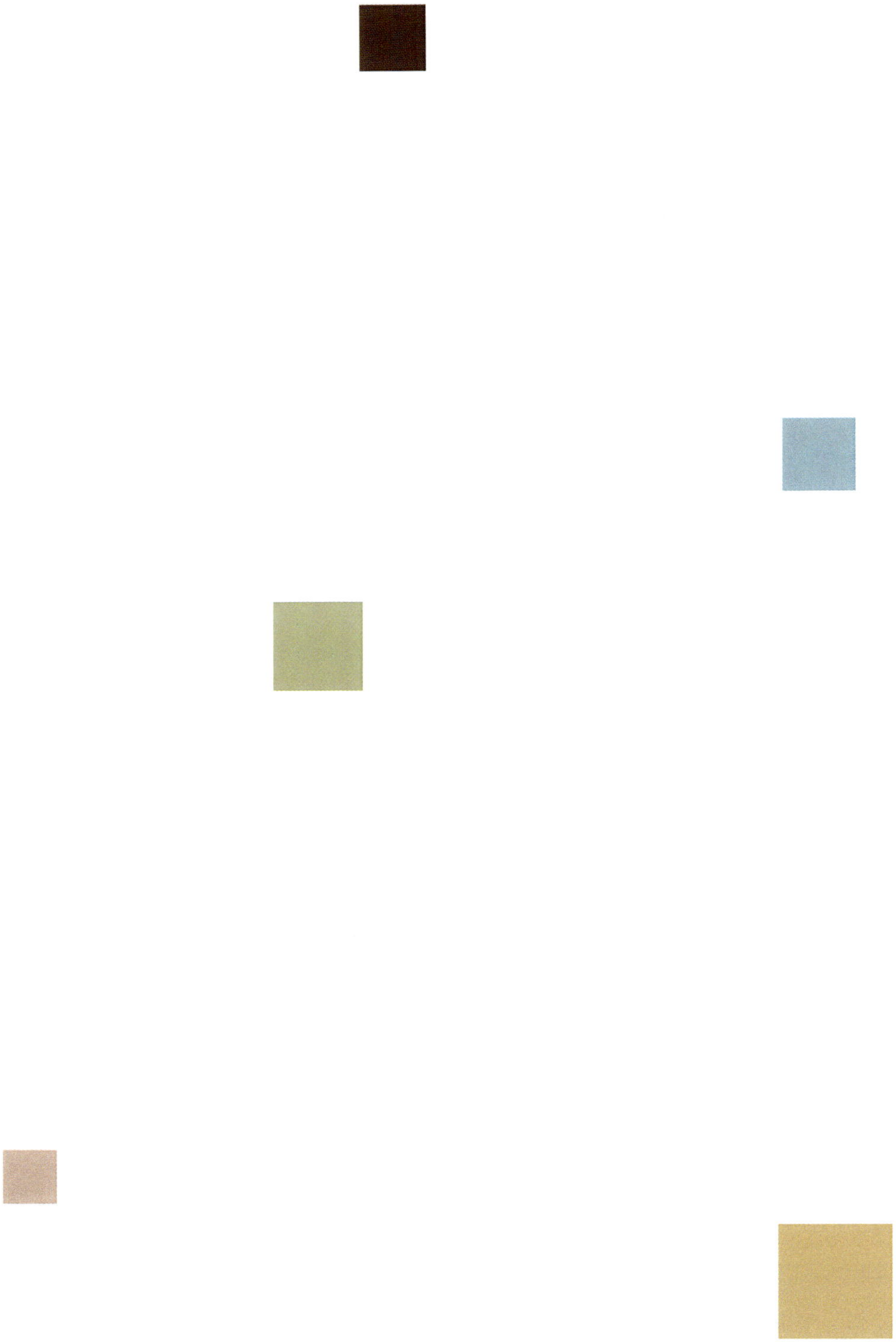

Francisco A. Rojo Vázquez

Holds a degree and a doctorate from the Faculty of Veterinary Medicine of León, University of Oviedo, and is a full professor at the Universities of Salamanca (Faculty of Pharmacy), Madrid (Faculty of Veterinary Medicine) and León (Faculty of Veterinary Medicine). He also holds a diploma from the European Veterinary Parasitology College and is Vice-President of the Spanish Royal Academy of Veterinary Science.

He has been a Scientist in the CSIC and as a visiting professor at the School of Veterinary Science in Philadelphia (USA), and has served as Head of the Animal Health Research Centre (CISA), Valdeolmos (Madrid), as Deputy General Manager for Research and Technology at the INIA, Ministry of Science and Innovation, and is currently a researcher at the Mixed Institute (CISC-ULE) of Highland Livestock Farming (IGM), in León.

His research activities are centred in the pathophysiology, epidemiology and immunology of parasitic diseases in domestic animals and in the control (chemoprophylaxis and anthelmintic resistance; genetic resistance to the infection by parasites) of parasitic diseases in these animals.

He has published numerous research papers concerning various aspects of parasitic animal and human diseases in international parasitology and veterinary science journals and has presented the results at national and international parasitology conferences.

He has been a visiting researcher in the Department of Parasitology, Central Veterinary Laboratory of the Ministry of Agriculture, Fisheries and Food (Weybridge, UK), the Department of Parasitology at the Moredun Research Institute (Edinburgh, UK) and in the Department of Large Animal Medicine, School of Veterinary Science, University of Pennsylvania (Philadelphia, USA).

He has held numerous university-based posts and is a member of the most important parasitology and veterinary science associations. He is a Founding Diplomate of the European Veterinary Parasitology College (EVPC).

Reviewer's foreword

It is exciting when one comes across a book that is fun, educational, and practical. This is exactly what happens when you pick up a copy of *60 Q&A on Bovine Parasitology*. This book presents the material in an excellent clinical-case format, and it is laid out beautifully with wonderful complementary photographs. The style, the clear and crisp look to the text, and the excellent line drawings that accompany the text, are all very expertly done. The authors and the editorial support staff at Servet are to be complimented on a job that is very well done and which has produced a very stylish volume.

Reading the text is a pleasure. I was able to sit down and read the text from beginning to end without pause. It was like picking up a great thriller. At the beginning of each case description, I wanted to see how things progressed, how the parasites were intertwined with the clinical signs, and how the diagnosis was reached. Then, there are the additional questions, or treatments, or what to do if no treatment for specific diseases. With the 60 questions, all the issues of importance in bovine parasitology have been covered. The book is ordered by systems, but it loses none of its basic parasitology as it presents the material on the different helminths, protozoa and arthropod parasites of each system. Also, it does not get boring the second or third time through a chapter; there is always a new little tidbit of information that can be teased from the material being discussed.

The scientific details within the text are up to date and the treatments are very clearly explained (it should not be forgotten that this is a Spanish text and that the treatments that are presented may not be available in all parts of the world). The basic science is all there, but it is presented in a format that gives it a true sense of importance. One really could not ask for much more than this from a textbook. It is wonderful that it has been translated into English so that it can be shared with a broader audience. This is a book that should be part of the collection of all those interested in bovine medicine and bovine parasitology in particular.

Dwight D. Bowman, MS, PhD

Professor of Parasitology, Department of Microbiology and Immunology
College of Veterinary Medicine, Cornell University, Ithaca, New York

Foreword

It is often stated that no one reads the introduction to a book. However, it is more important than it appears, as the introduction or foreword usually summarises the contents of the book and allows the authors, or someone close to them, to explain their intentions.

All books, and this one is no exception, are written to be read and, although it is said that there is no place for speculation in a text-book, they should always contain some. It is the authors' own view, or selection of scientific knowledge based on their own experience: a unique and unrepeatable selection. Furthermore, as scientific knowledge, the means of transmitting it and learning methods are highly dynamic, textbooks are always expected to offer something new. The most novel systems try to simplify the integration of information concerning specific phenomena or processes from an innovative and up-to-date point of view.

In veterinary science, parasitic diseases, and those with an infectious aetiology *sensu stricto*, form part of what has traditionally been known as "Special diseases in domestic animals", a speciality with a known and specific importance. Some treatises on the specialty, both classical and modern, are excellent exponents and often, an essential reading.

Ruminants, mainly bovines, stand out amongst domestic and useful animals in terms of veterinary practice. The breeding and farming of these animals using extensive or intensive systems requires various types of care. Indeed, disease plays a key role in daily activities and, although it is, by no means, the only facet to their activity, at some point all vets will have to handle the financial problems resulting from bovine diseases.

Although the best means of dealing with such parasite-related problems has been the subject of a great deal of debate, no consensus has yet been reached. In the opinion of many people, an opinion which is fully shared by us, a morphological and taxonomic approach to the study of parasites of veterinary importance is of little use from a practical viewpoint. However, such a structural basis is related to other characteristics, such as pathogenicity and sensitivity to the action of anti-parasitic agents.

In light of our work entitled *87 Q&A on equine parasitology*, which was published in 2010 and very well received, we decided to follow a similar structure to transmit our experience in a similar manner.

It was clear to us from the outset that the possible users of this work will mainly be veterinary science students. And this should not be any other way in light of our vocation as teachers whose audience comprises future veterinary science graduates. Consequently, we hope that the contents of this book and the way in which they are expressed, provide a stimulus to them while still in the classroom. Also, that the many questions that they will come across prompt them to broaden their understanding throughout their professional life irrespective of whether their work involves this, or any other, animal species.

Of course, student life comes to an end at a given point, and in the same way as this book is aimed at Veterinary Science students, we hope that practising vets may also find amongst its pages the answers to the many questions that arise day after day in their professional activity.

This book on bovine parasitic diseases (bovine parasitology in a colloquial and simplified manner) attempts to complement currently available information and present it in a somewhat different way whilst avoiding, as far as possible, unnecessary repetitions and selecting the most important processes.

This information is presented in an "original" manner by explaining the main problems in parasite aetiology by way of a questions and answers system. Indeed, the title itself (Q&A) alludes to this, although this is obviously by no means novel.

Indeed, the written transmission of veterinary knowledge by way of question-and-answer type publications concerning the breeding and diseases of domestic animals has occurred several times in history, in an attempt to ensure that the reader—the student in this case—reaches a sufficient level of understanding by way of this method, which has again come to the forefront in modern universities.

Perhaps one of the best known works to have used this format is a French publication by C. Daubenton, Professor of Natural History at the Paris Museum, which was "translated to the Spanish and supplemented by order of the King" by Francisco González, Professor of the Royal Veterinary School in Madrid, entitled *Instrucción para pastores y ganaderos (Instructions for shepherds and farmers)*, and published in Madrid by the Royal Printers in 1798.

It is difficult to find scientific publications (books or monographs) concerning bovine parasites and parasitoses in Spain. It is entirely possible that the magnitude of other problems may have eclipsed some parasitic diseases which, either *per se* or in co-existence with other diseases, have clinical and economic repercussions that are well known to vets. At certain times in history (second half of the 20th century), monographic works concerning some of the most important parasitic diseases have been published, although almost always with funding from the chemical/pharmaceutical industries responsible for manufacturing veterinary products. There has also been "official" interest at times, although this has been essentially anecdotal.

Herein we have included numerous parasite species belonging to the protozoa, helminths and arthropods that can infect bovines, causing discomfort, clinical symptoms of varying severity and, occasionally, death. In all cases they must be controlled by applying the epidemiological and clinical knowledge presented in the four chapters of this book, which comprises 60 clinical cases, and hence the title: *60 Q&A on bovine parasitology*.

The authors

Madrid–León, February 2013

Table of contents

1 Q&A on endoparasites of the digestive system

2 Q&A on endoparasites of the respiratory system

3 Q&A on systemic endoparasites

4 Q&A on cutaneous parasitoses

1

Q&A on endoparasites of the digestive system

Chapter 1

Q&A on endoparasites of the digestive system

Introduction

This first chapter is dedicated to understanding of some aspects of the most important parasites of the bovine digestive system.

Generally speaking, ruminants are host to numerous species. In most cases they are definitive hosts, although they may also play a role in the cycle of various parasitic species as intermediate hosts.

Helminths are the most important group of parasites amongst those living in the different parts of the bovine digestive apparatus. They are normally acquired by ingestion of infective forms that contaminate grass to a greater or lesser extent during grazing. However, some parasitic diseases can also be acquired in the stable, and the consequences of these infections are usually serious. In both cases the risk depends on factors closely related to management of the animals. Amongst these factors are the different grazing strategies and their duration, grazing systems (rotational, set-stocking, etc.), production methods (from extensive to semi-intensive or intensive), the season of the year and, therefore, climate conditions in each region.

Due to the unique aspects of their biological cycle in bovines *Toxocara* infections are included here, although gastrointestinal strongyles, mainly trichostrongylidae, are the important parasites of this section. Within this large group, special mention must be made of ostertagia which cause more or less severe symptoms that always require veterinary care. The various types of ostertagiosis, together with the enteric disorders caused by other genera of trichostrongylidae, fully justify the lenght of space dedicated to them here.

However, although other problems such as infections with adult cestodes do not normally require special care, they must nevertheless be taken into account when planning preventive measures for herds.

Although more restricted to certain areas, but of major importance in those regions where they are endemic, are the various clinical forms of *Fasciola* infection. This parasitosis is almost always chronic in bovines. Most probably as a result of the control measures aimed at fasciolosis, other parasite groups have become increasingly significant in recent years. The most important of these is possibly the trematode infections included amongst "Paramphistomidae", and deserve a specific section in this chapter.

As is in other animal species, irrespective of the taxonomic position occupied by the parasites responsible for digestive disorders, the diseases that appear in the first few days of life are the most important in bovines. The prevalence of most parasitoses during these early stages is very similar even when the production goal may not is be the same (meat or milk). Cryptosporidia, which are the causative agent of neonatal diarrhoeal syndrome and therefore the source of significant losses, are particularly common in this group of very young animals. Although clinically and economically much less important, giardia and strongyloid infections have also been included as they are often detected in very young animals.

However, other problems also arise at an early age. Thus, depending on the production system, coccidioses, which can have a severely negative effect to the farming enterprise, can be particularly important.

This chapter also includes unusual necropsy findings, which are more commonly detected during routine controls of wild bovines due to their much easier access to infective parasitic forms.

The most important parasites of the bovine digestive system

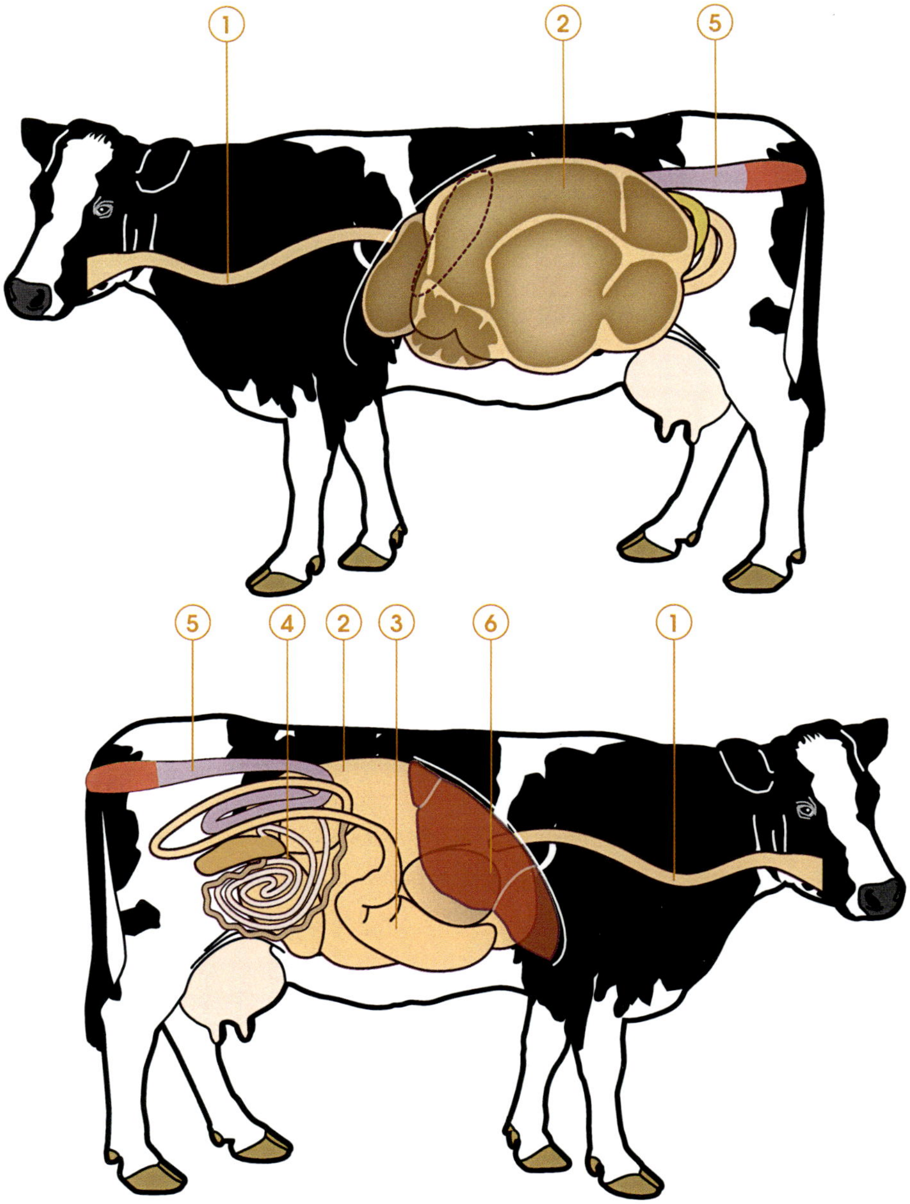

1. Oesophagus
Gongylonema
Hypoderma

2. Rumen
Paramphistomum
Callicophorum

3. Abomasum
Ostertagia
Trichostrongylus
Haemonchus

4. Small intestine
Toxocara
Trichostrongylus
Cooperia
Nematodirus
Strongyloides
Bunostomum
Moniezia
Eimeria
Cryptosporidium
Giardia

5. Large intestine
Oesophagostomum
Trichuris
Eimeria

6. Liver
Fasciola

How is *Strongyloides* transmitted to calves?

A calf found wandering along the road is caught and turned in at a veterinary clinic. The animal is in poor body condition, it barely responds to external stimuli, has breathing difficulties and presents acute haemorrhagic diarrhoea. Once located, the farmer tells us that it was weak at birth and had worsened over the past two weeks. It is so thin that it easily crosses through the fence. The vet informs the farmer that, as well as pneumonia, the calf has an enteritis compatible with colibacillosis and that a coprological analysis has detected embryonated eggs of some 50 µm lenght.

1. How can the clinical signs presented by the animal be explained?
2. How the calf become infected?
3. What other signs can be found on the farm from which the animal comes?

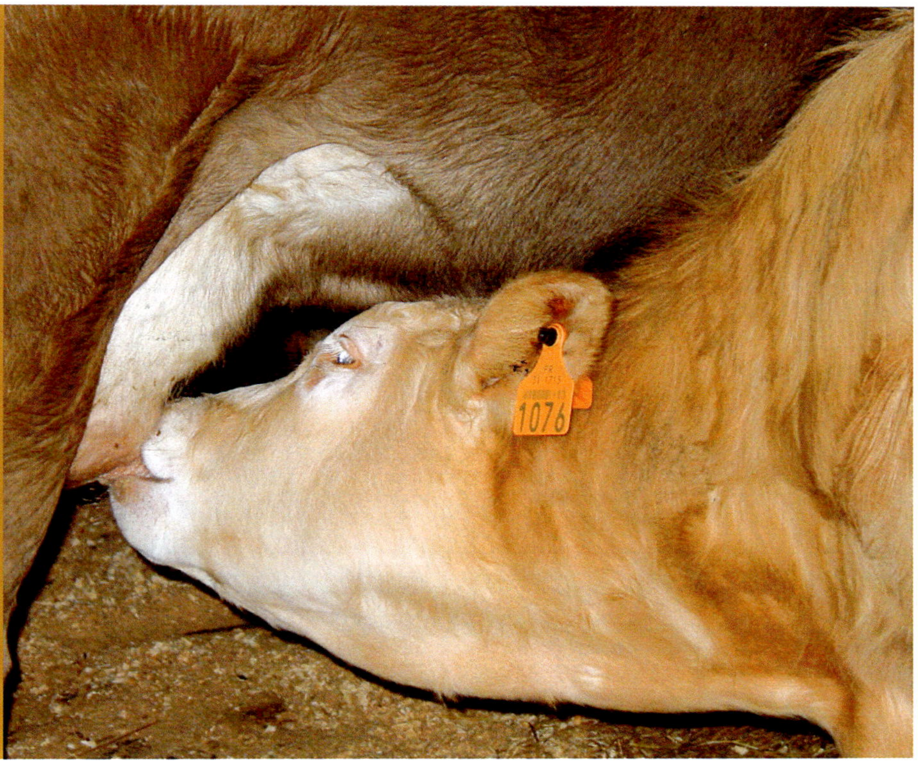

How can the clinical signs presented by the animal be explained?

Amongst the negative factors in feed-lots cattle are parasitoses, especially those caused by gastrointestinal nematodes.

Of the parasitic species found in bovines, *Strongyloides papillosus* is considered to be less pathogenic and dangerous than strongyles. However, this parasite can lead to sudden death syndrome in young animals in the event of very intense infections with no prior clinical manifestations. Indeed, fatal cases of strongyloidosis have been observed in calves under both experimental conditions and in natural infections. Under natural conditions, the disease is associated with damp sawdust bedding and favourable temperatures (between 20 and 35 °C). In other words, the management system may be a potential risk, with deficient hygiene conditions and overcrowding playing a key role.

In any case, infection occurs cutaneously, via undamaged skin, mainly in regions that have more contact with the floor (abdomen, udder and interdigital space). However, other possible infection pathways in these animals cannot be ruled out. Once infection has occurred, the larvae are transported to the lungs in the bloodstream and finally reach the intestine, where female parasites (2n chromosomes) develop some 10-15 days post-infection. Finally, eggs are excreted with the faeces. These eggs are around 40-60 µm long and 20-25 µm wide and contain a fully developed larva when they leave the body.

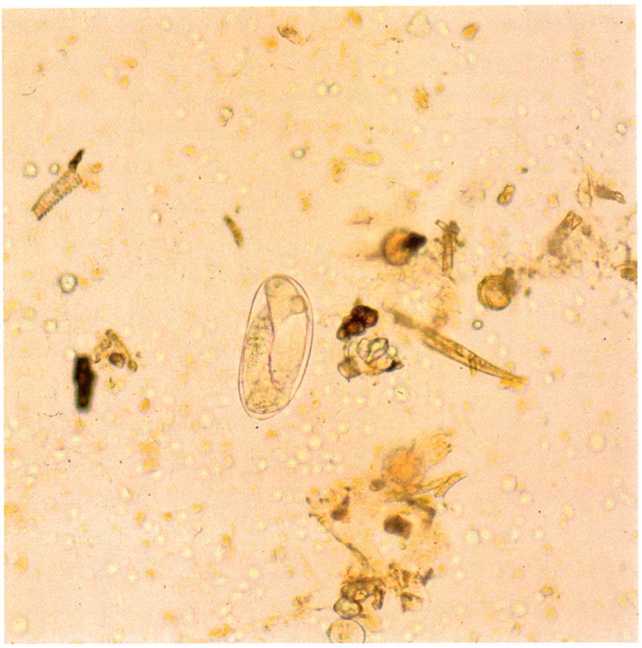

Strongyloides eggs contain larvae when eliminated in faeces. The L1 that hatches can develop and produce free-living males (n chromosomes) or females (2n chromosomes) after four moults (Maupas' Law: 1st moult to L2, 2nd moult to L3, 3rd moult to L4 and 4th moult to L5 or pre-adult) or continue as larva 3 (3n chromosomes), and mantain a parasitic phase after invading a new host.

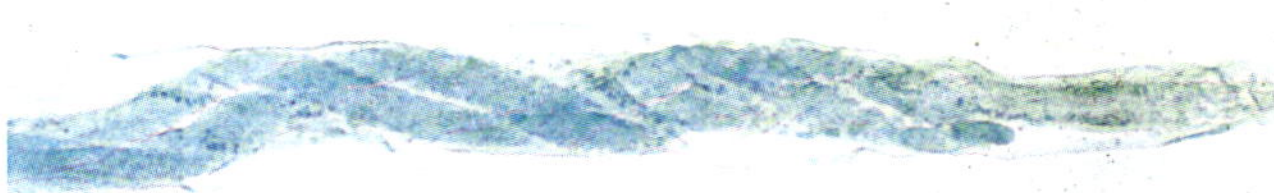

Strongyloides papillosus is a nematode that presents free and/or parasitic generations, in which the adult forms are only represented by parthenogenetic females, during its cycle. These females measure 3.5-6.0 mm and their body is long and filiform, being thinner in the cephalic region. The uterus has two branches, and the ovoid eggs measure between 42 and 48 µm and contain larvae when laid.

Penetration of larvae into the skin results in punctiform reddening together with mild pruritus. As infections tend to be mild, these skin lesions (which are also non-specific) often pass unnoticed.

The migration to the lung results in the appearance of cough and, occasionally, pneumonia, due to secondary infections. When this happens, respiratory function is partially annulled, possibly leading to death of the animals.

Finally, once they become established in the small intestine, adult parasites lead to digestive disorders that are most commonly expressed as intermittent diarrhoea with expulsion of bloody or mucous-containing stools accompanied by weight loss, occasionally tympanitis, growth impairment and even cachexia. Natural outbreaks are associated with catarrhal enteritis of the small intestine (duodenum and jejunum).

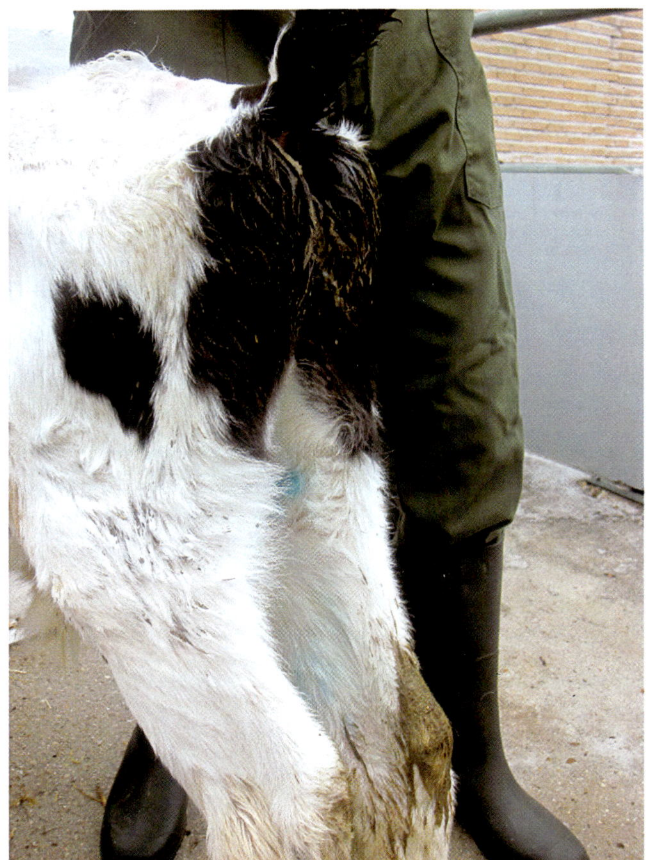

The most characteristic signs of strongyloidosis are diarrhoea, which on occasions is haemorrhagic, weight loss and emaciation. It is only observed in young animals in regions with a subtropical climate and under poorly hygienic conditions. Calves acquire immunity at 4 to 5 months.

2 How the calf become infected?

As previously stated, animals are mainly infected by penetration of strongyloid larvae into the skin, although oral infection is also possible. The larvae must cross the mucocutaneous coating (skin, buccal or oesophageal mucosa or forestomachs) directly as they die in the abomasum. Penetration occurs very rapidly, although skin thickness has an influence.

Infective *Strongyloides* larvae do not have a protective cuticle like that of strongyles, therefore they have very little resistance against adverse conditions, especially drying.

Transmammary infection has been observed in several parasite-host models, including *Strongyloides ransomi*-pig, *S. westeri*-horse and *S. papillosus*-cow and sheep, although all these species have other forms of infection.

The cycle of *S. papillosus* in cows and sheep appears to be similar to that of *S. ransomi*. In cows exposed to infection prior to giving birth, strongyloid larvae have been observed in milk samples at 7 and 19 days postpartum, and strongyloid eggs in calf faeces at 15 days after birth. Moreover, infection can occur by ingestion of maternal milk or colostrum, and thus, the prepatent period is shortened.

3 What other signs can be found on the farm from which the animal comes?

Under natural conditions, *Strongyloides papillosus* infections do not tend to be as severe and the pathogenic action is mild. However, mass infections result in more obvious alterations. For example, animals with a high parasite burden exhibit marked growth retardation and, as well as respiratory disorders, intraorgan migration of the larvae can favour the growth of other pathogens (viruses, bacteria), thereby worsening the clinical signs.

Repeated percutaneous infections in adult animals may also lead to the onset of marked cutaneous reactions such as pruritus, reddening and pain in thin-skinned regions characterised by an allergic reaction of the chorion (dermis) that is rarely observed in calves. More or less intense dermatitis is not uncommon in severe infections, and males may develop balanoposthitis. Mild lameness not easily explained from an aetiological viewpoint may also be observed.

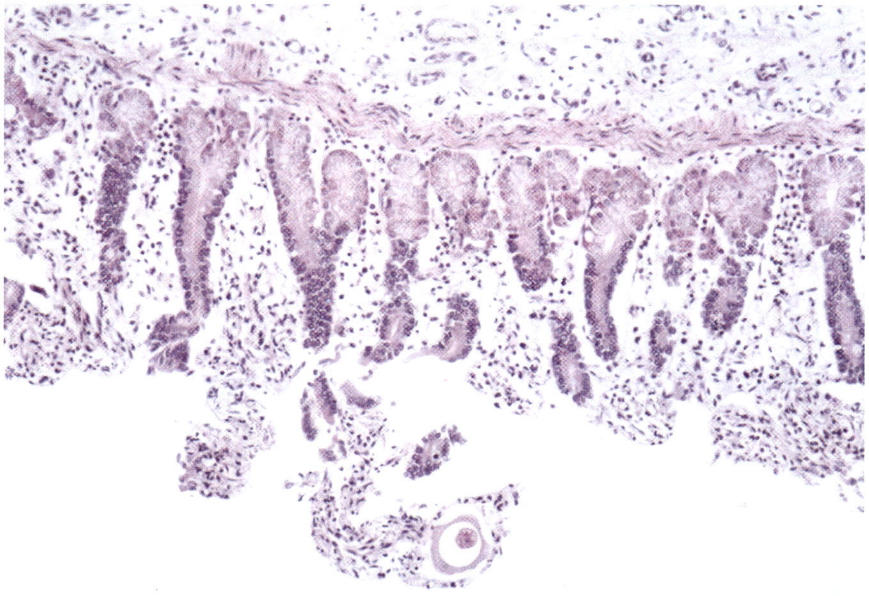

The parthenogenetic females live in the duodenum and jejunum, where they cause digestive and absorption alterations that lead to growth retardation and weight loss. The picture shows a dissected female in which the cuticle and digestive tube are stained bright blue surrounded by an inflammatory infiltrate containing macrophages and eosinophils.

2 Can calves be born with an ascarid infection?

When attending the birth of a dairy cow, the vet detects a very characteristic smell of rancid butter in the cowshed. He asks to inspect the calves and confirms his suspicions upon smelling butyric acid in exhaled air. The farmer confirms that animal growth is less than expected and that one calf with green diarrhoea died the previous month. The calves have not received deworming treatment, whereas the dry cows were treated with levamisole. Faeces are not regularly removed and the owner claims to have seen "worms) in the faeces of older calves. The vet returns the day after the birth and takes faecal samples from the newborn calf which, to his surprise, test positive for *Toxocara* eggs.

1. How are ascarids identified in cattle?
2. What do ascarids eat and why do infected animals smell rancid?
3. How are calves infected?
4. What conditions favour their transmission?
5. Can this be a common process on calf feedlots?
6. Can infected carcasses be impounded?

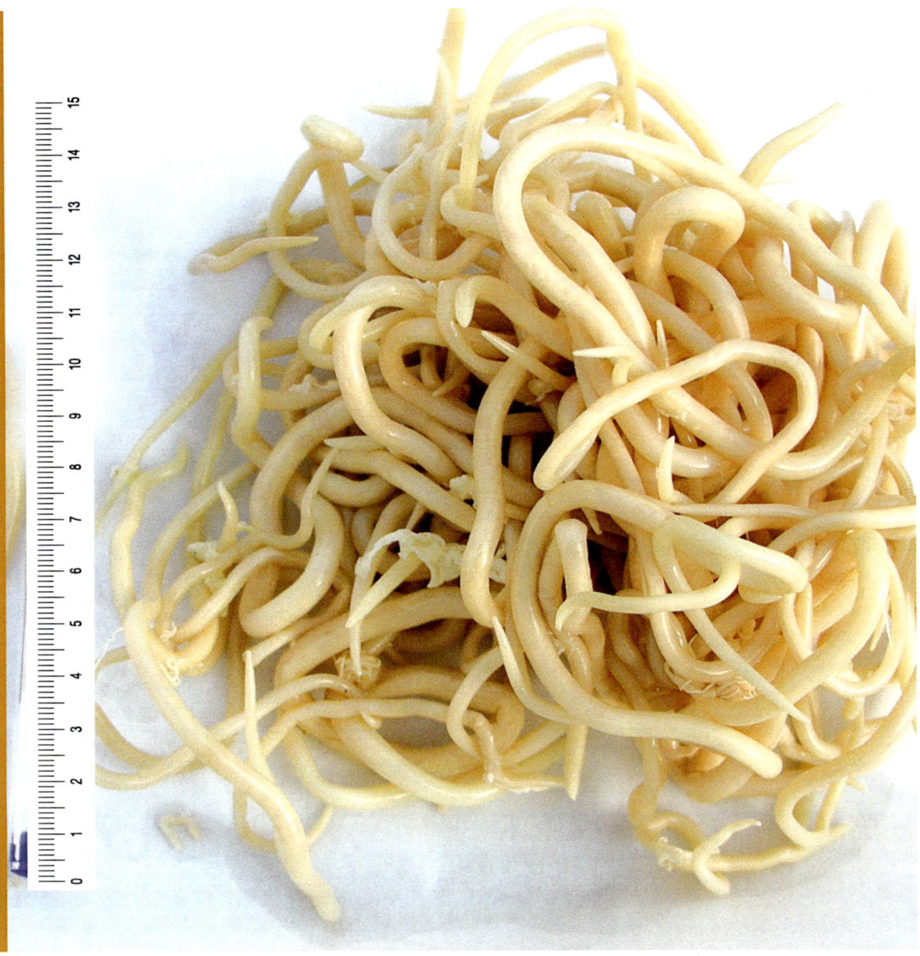

1 How are ascarids identified in cattle?

Calf worms are parasitic ascarids with a pinkish-white colour. Their cuticle is thin, almost translucent, and they have representatives in numerous animal species.

The parasitic species in bovines is *Toxocara vitulorum*, formally known as *Neoascaris vitulorum*, which is also found in the water buffalo and zebu. It is rarely parasitic in sheep, in which it does not always complete its biological cycle.

The adults live in the intestine and are large worms. Males measure up to 25 cm in length and 5 mm in width, with females reaching 30 cm × 6 mm. They have three broad-based but thin-edged lips at their anterior end and they lack cervical alae.

The females lay large numbers of sub-spherical, unicellular eggs (3-8 million/day), with a size of 69-93 × 62-77 μm and a relatively smooth (compared with that of *A. suum* eggs) speckled surface. These eggs have a thick wall that confers them a high resistance to adverse environmental factors and disinfectants.

2 What do ascarids eat and why do infected animals smell rancid?

Adults feed on the contents of the small intestine and larger numbers lead to more obvious disorders. They make particular use of carbohydrates, amino acids, minerals and vitamins. The production of valeric and caproic acids indicates that they may also use fatty acids. The toxic activity attributed to them is related to some of their metabolites and is one of the causes of disentery. These metabolites can be detected in exhaled air and urine, with a characteristic smell of rancid butter that can also be detected in enclosed spaces in the stables on intensive production farms. It even impregnates the meat, often meaning that the carcasses have to be impounded. The smell may even remain after cooking the joints of meat.

Two forms of infection have been described:

- In the mild form, it is almost exclusively detected by the breath and urine smelling like valeric or caproic acid, with some signs of nervous excitation (cough, grinding of the teeth).
- In the severe form, lack of appetite, constipation, foul-smelling diarrhoea, tympanitis, abdominal spasms, dysuria, clear watery urine and general disorders are also observed.

3 How are calves infected?

Calves acquire the infection orally, by ingestion of larvae directly in milk or larvae-containing eggs in contaminated feed, bedding or water. Nursing animals may also be infected via the mother's nipples. Rodents and fomites such as footwear or cleaning equipment may also help to spread the eggs. More favourable conditions for egg development increase the rate and intensity at which contagion occurs and therefore at which the infection spreads.

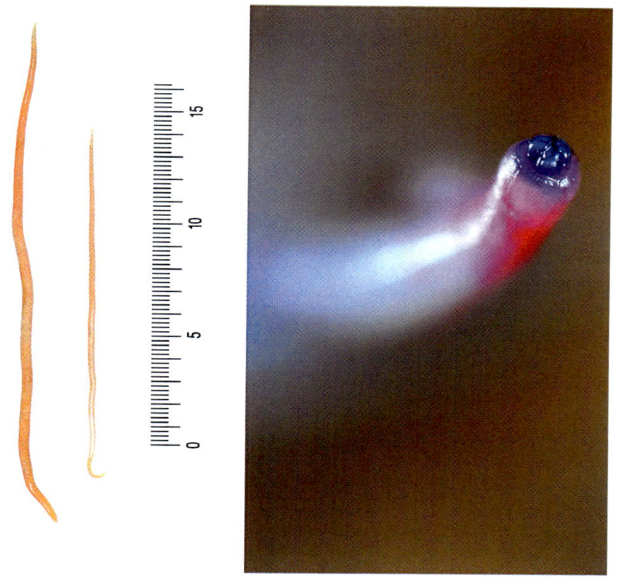

Adult *Toxocara vitulorum* are pinkish-white worms with a thin cuticle and the oral opening surrounded by three lips. Males measure 15-25 cm and have short spicules of equal length, with various papillae unevenly arranged in front of the anus together with a post-anal pair. Females are always larger and measure 20-32 cm (artistically coloured in red and blue to mark lips).

Stage 3 (L3) *Toxocara* larvae develop inside the egg after around 10 to 40 days, depending on the temperature and humidity. The optimal conditions are around 25 °C and a high humidity of 80 %.

Once the infective larva has developed inside the egg, its survival capacity is very high and has been estimated at around 2 years in a natural setting without exposure to drying or direct sunlight.

The eggs ingested by calves release their larvae, which migrate from the intestine to the liver, then the lung and finally the trachea, where they are swallowed to reach adulthood in the intestine.

The larvae ingested by weaned or adult animals migrate from the intestine to the liver and lung via the bloodstream but do not pass into the trachea. Instead, they return to the heart from the lungs and pass into general circulation, where they undergo somatic migration and are distributed throughout the body, remaining quiescent.

These quiescent larvae are mobilised in gestating females and can cross the placenta to infect the foetus prior to birth, with patency in cases of prenatal infection commencing from day 2 of life. However, they are much more commonly mobilised to the mammary gland and pass into newborn calves via the maternal colostrum, which contains numerous larvae in the first 2-5 days postpartum, and then via the milk, where their quantities increase up to around one month, when they subsequently disappear.

The larvae ingested with maternal milk or colostrum do not migrate and develop directly in the small intestine, where they reach sexual maturity after some 3 weeks. However, as self-healing occurs at around 4-5 months, patent infection is rare in animals aged more than 6 months.

4 What conditions favour their transmission?

Various epidemiological factors are involved in transmission of the infection. The factors that condition the intraorganic development times of the parasites and therefore, could facilitate contamination of the surroundings with *Toxocara* eggs, are related to the age of the animals when infected, their immune status and the infection pathway(s).

Moreover, the reproductive forms (eggs) eliminated with the faeces are able to survive outside the body for long periods of time, even under highly adverse environmental conditions. This means that the level of contamination in certain zones (for example corrals), and therefore the risk of a severe infection can be particularly high. They also remain viable in the depositions and other animal excretions that can subsequently be used to fertilise grazing zones, thus increasing environmental contamination and the likelihood that the animals will become infected.

5 Can this be a common process on calf feedlots?

This infection is considered to be endemic in tropical and sub-tropical regions and can become highly prevalent, thereby negatively affecting animal production.

The prevalence in temperate regions is related to intensive breeding and farming systems in which the likelihood of contagion is high due to the overcrowding experienced by the animals. It is therefore a very common parasitosis in calf feedlots, mainly those containing calves from various sources.

6 Can infected carcasses be impounded?

Generally speaking, all meat from animals suffering from infectious or parasitic processes falls within the category of unhealthy meats, namely those which can affect the health of anyone who handles or consumes them.

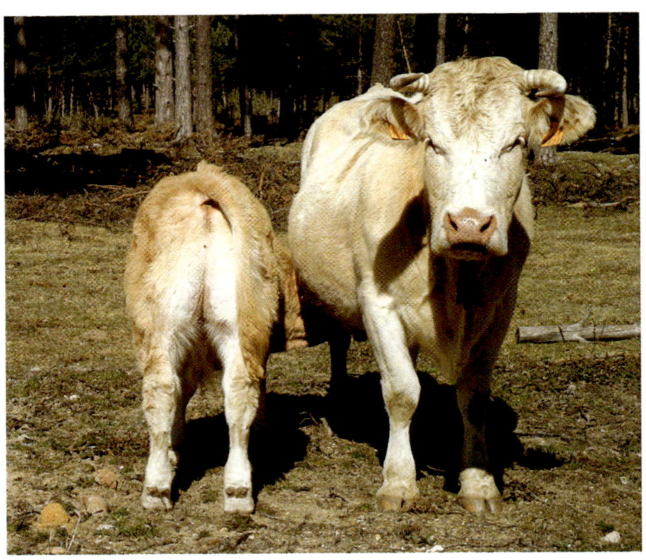

In nursing animals, the larvae reach the small intestine directly, where they reach sexual maturity after 20-30 days and commence patency which, in cases of prenatal infection, commences from the second day of life. Egg elimination by the calf peaks at an age of around 2 months and is maintained up to an age of 3 months. Adult parasites are thought to live for around 6 months.

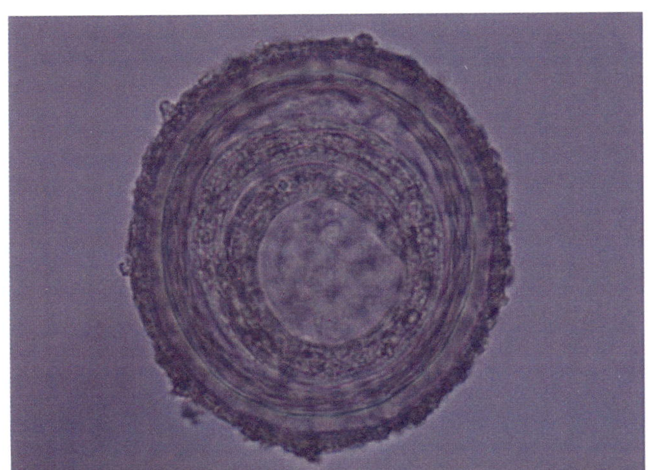

Infected animals can excrete millions of eggs a day during the few months that the infection remains patent. The eggs have a very thick wall that makes them highly resistant to adverse environmental conditions and disinfectants. The larva 3 (L3), which does not hatch outside the host, develops inside them under favourable conditions of temperature (11-13 days at 24-28 °C and 30-40 days at 18-20 °C) and relative humidity (80 %). It is thought to be able to remain infective for up to 2 years if external conditions are not extreme.

Unhealthy meats are unsuitable for consumption. So-called "febrile", "fatigued" or DFD meats, those impregnated with unsavoury of harmful substances, altered by putrefaction, or those presenting unpleasant tastes or smells, etc., in other words all meats whose quality decreases rapidly or with little nutritional value, have all traditionally been considered to fall within this category. As such, meats that "offend" the smell, sight or palate ("repugnant" or physically unpleasant meats) are given this name. Those considered unpleasant due to their smell include meats that are "repugnant" due to their abnormal smell. This is the case of bovines with toxocarosis, which give off a highly unpleasant smell that impregnates the entire muscle system, thus making the meat unsuitable for consumption.

Biological cycle of *Toxocara*

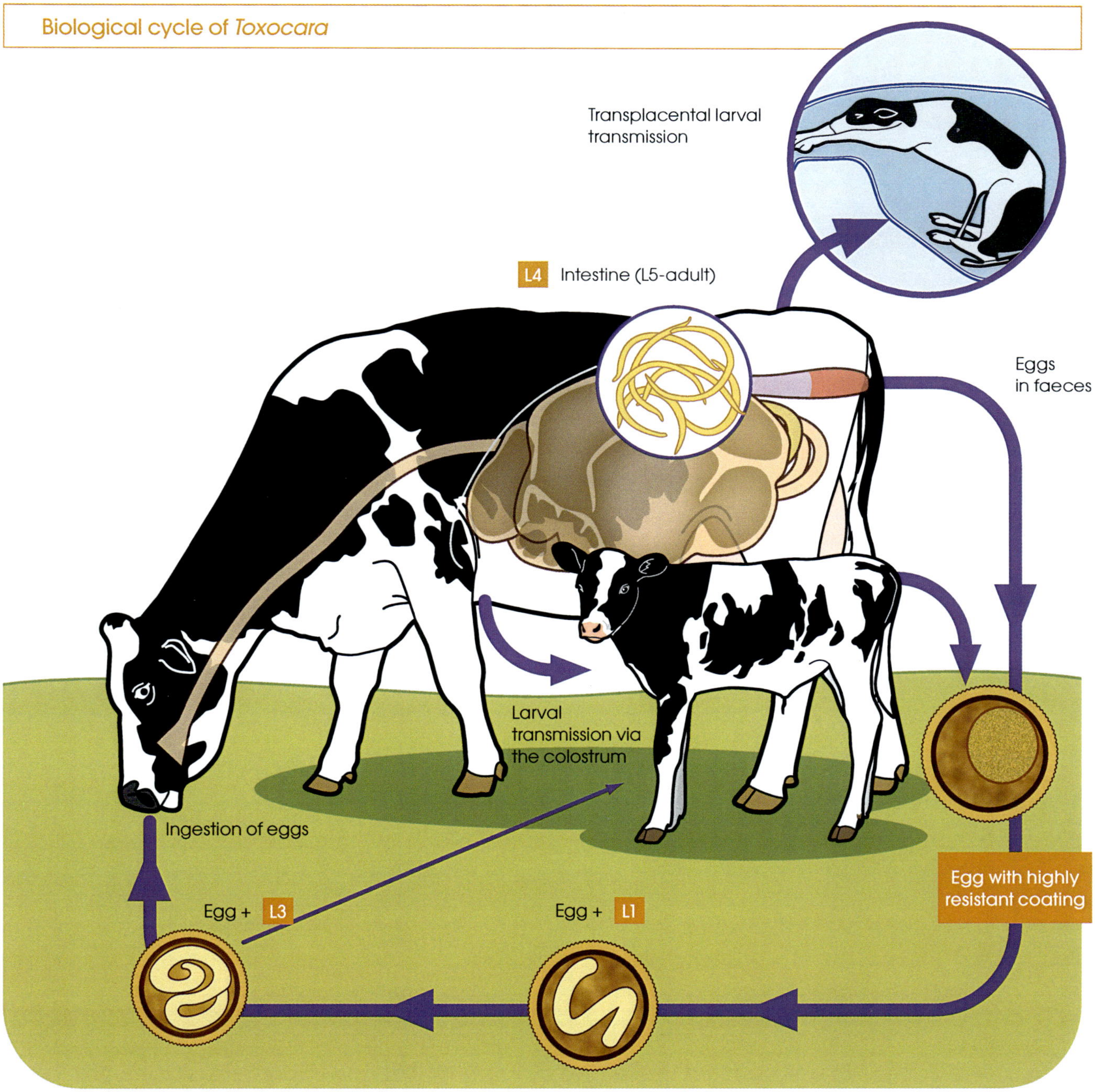

3 What are the repercussions of *Toxocara* infection in bovines?

On a beef cattle farm where manure from a nearby pig farm has recently begun to be used as fertiliser, the youngest animals have started to exhibit an acute respiratory problem. Two severely infected animals have been necropsied but only lesions compatible with the migration of helminth parasite larvae have been found. The owner would like to know whether the manure has caused this problem and what measures he can take to prevent it.

1. Which parasites present in pig manure can be transmitted to bovines?
2. What causes the respiratory disorders?
3. Can *Toxocara* block the intestine?
4. Is it possible to find milk spots in the liver?
5. How is it diagnosed in calves and adults?
6. How can *Toxocara* infection be controlled?

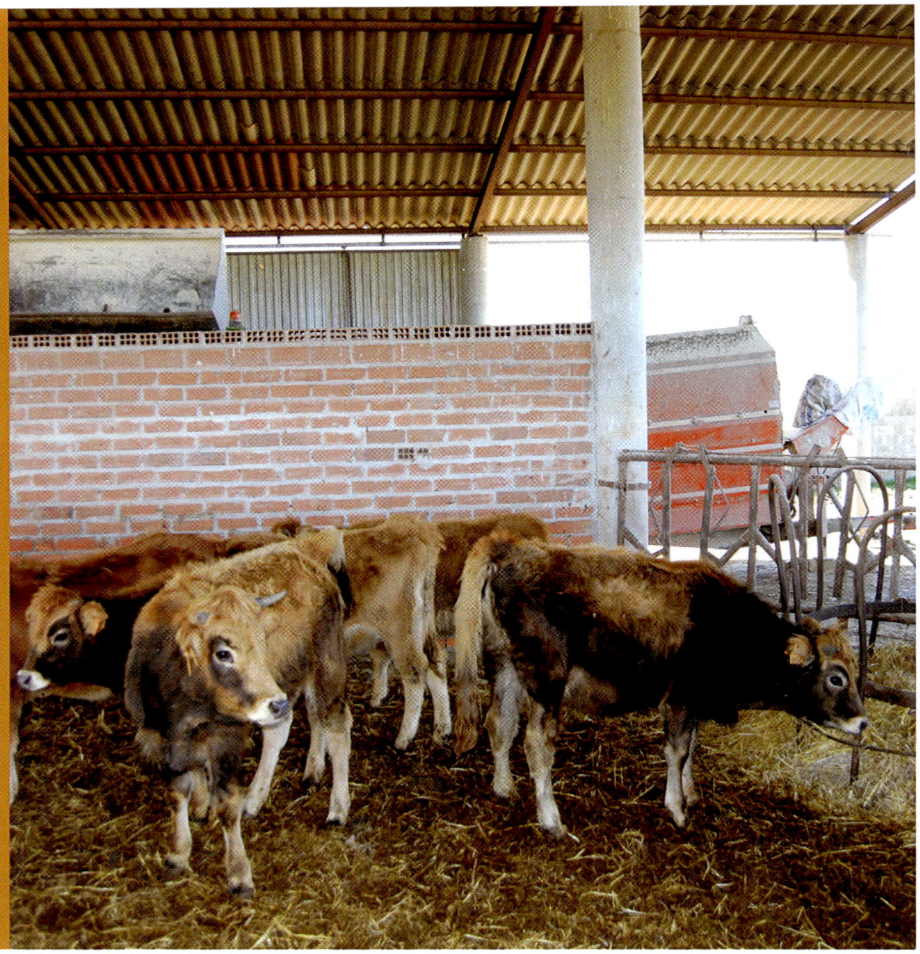

1 Which parasites present in pig manure can be transmitted to bovines?

It can be *Ascaris suum*, one of the most common parasites in pig herds. This species is known to be able to infect many other animal species by way of tissue migrations. The meadows used to raise ruminants, especially bovines, are occasionally fertilised using slurry or manure from pig farms, thus meaning that these animals can become infected with parasites specific to pigs and highly prevalent in them, such as ascaris.

When this occurs as a result of ingestion of eggs in the grass, the larvae hatch in the intestine and migrate to the lungs, where they cause respiratory disorders compatible with atypical interstitial pneumonia. These symptoms are more common when the calves remain in contaminated meadows, becoming infected again and again. This has been shown in calves aged 2-5 months sensitised with *Ascaris suum* eggs and subsequently reinfected. The clinical presentation shown by the animals under these circumstances is characterised by the onset of dyspnoea, cough, breathing difficulties, emphysema and tachycardia at 6-7 days post-infection.

In summary, amongst pig-specific parasites, calves can acquire *Ascaris* eggs present in the manure often used to fertilise meadows. As bovines do not normally host these parasites, their effects, which are mainly respiratory, are more marked.

2 What causes the respiratory disorders?

In the case of *Toxocara vitulorum*, there is also a migratory route through liver and lungs before making their way back to intestine to develop into adults. This can cause respiratory signs.

Eggs containing an infective larva (L3) hatch rapidly in the intestine, releasing the larvae. They migrate via the intestinal wall to the portal vein, from where they reach the lungs by venous circulation. Once present in the lungs, they ascend the bronchi to the trachea, where they are swallowed and again pass into the intestine, where they reach sexual maturity.

Symptoms tend to be more obvious in mass infections and younger animals. The signs in calves aged between 1.5 and 2 months are respiratory and digestive.

Passage of the larvae through the respiratory system results in lesions that manifest clinically as severe respiratory symptoms. As the larvae continue their migration towards the intestine, the respiratory signs may approximately coincide in time with digestive disorders characterised by foul-smelling diarrhoea, mucosal paleness and high body temperature together with a generally worsened state tof health that causes the animals to remain lying down.

3 Can *Toxocara* block the intestine?

Of course. The presence of ascarids in a calf's intestine can produce blockages of varying severity.

It should be remembered, for instance, that the size of these parasites —they can reach up to 30 cm in length— means that the presence of even a few in an animal's intestine can lead to at least a partial obstruction. The number of worms present in the digestive apparatus in severe infections can reach several dozen, thereby explaining, in light of their size, the obstructions frequently observed in heavily infected animals.

Chronic enteric catarrh, haemorrhage of the mucosa and ulcers may also occur in such cases, and the worms may also penetrate the pancreas, compress the bile duct and produce jaundice. They also occasionally perforate the intestine, thereby causing peritonitis.

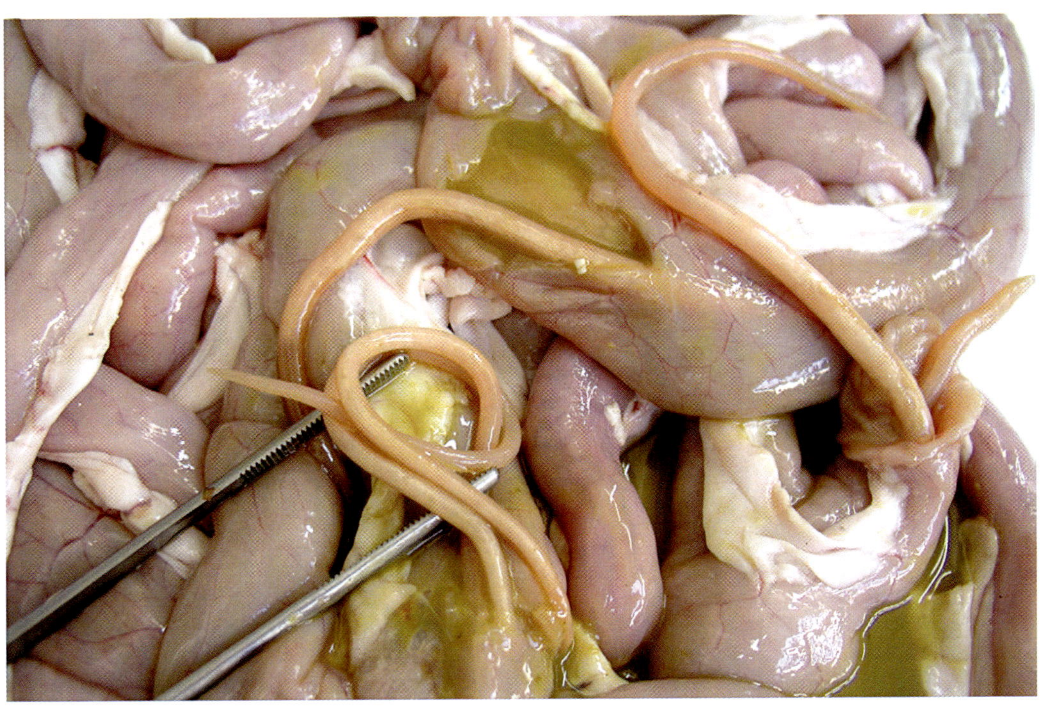

The effects of the parasitosis can be seen from an age of one month and are closely related to the parasite burden. The lesions caused by adults comprise enteritis. If the ascarids are abundant, they can cause an intestinal obstruction, which leads to colic pain, or block the bile duct as a result of erratic migration.

4 Is it possible to find milk spots in the liver?

The intraorgan journey of ascarids makes a stop in certain parts of the body, including the liver. Larvae reach this organ via the portal vein and cause mechanical tissue damage that leads to proliferations when penetrating the central veins of the lobules. Localised routes of hepatocellular necrosis accompanied by inflammation also occur. These routes are eventually replaced by connective tissue, which causes scarring. It is particularly notable on the surface of the liver.

5 How is it diagnosed in calves and adults?

It is important to consider the age of the affected animals when reaching a definitive diagnosis of *Toxocara vitulorum* infection. Only young animals show signs that could lead us to suspect the presence of an infection. Consequently, both age and the observation of respiratory and especially intestinal disorders, together with the characteristic butyric smell of the animals, are clinical signs that help the diagnosis. It can be confirmed by the presence of parasite eggs in the faeces (flotation methods).

Obviously, the presence of worms in the intestine, together with lesions (both enteric and pulmonary) and other findings, help to establish a definitive diagnosis so that appropriate prophylaxis and control measures can be initiated.

The detection of antibodies using techniques such as indirect hemagglutination assay and immunoenzymatic methods (indirect ELISA) can also be used, especially to detect the presence of larvae in tissues.

Other diseases should be ruled out, such as parasitic diseases like coccidiosis (*Eimeria* spp.), which is commonly associated with *Toxocara vitulorum* infection, and cryptosporidiosis, in younger animals.

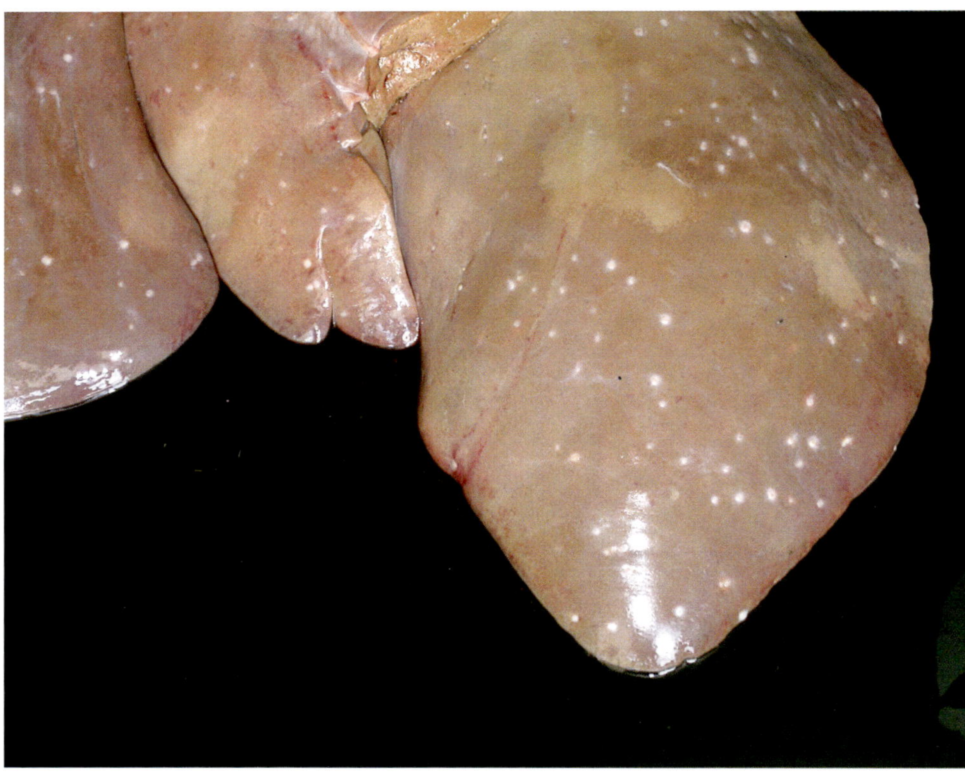

Larval migration leaves traces that initially comprise haemorrhagic petechiae, which subsequently transform into granulomas. These then become fibrotic ("milk spots", or "green spots"), especially in the liver, kidneys or ganglia.

6 How can *Toxocara* infection be controlled?

Classical drugs remain effective and recommended (and cheap), although they are currently not often used. These include piperazine salts, which are particularly effective against adult worms. However, drugs that also act against larvae are preferred. Some examples are imidazothiazoles (levamisole), tetrahydropyrimidines (pyrantel), benzimidazole carbamates such as fenbendazole and oxfendazole, and macrocyclic lactones, such as ivermectin, moxidectin and others, which are highly active against adults and probably also against larvae.

Control must obviously take various aspects into account, including the high resistance of the eggs of this parasite to a wide range of conditions. Control measures demand rigorous hygiene in calf feedlots, including the cleaning, disinfection and routine coprological analysis of any animal aged 4-6 weeks added to the farm. These animals must be dewormed if required, repeating this treatment at 2-3 weeks. A serological investigation of pregnant cows is also recommended, treating then positive animals.

If the area is highly contaminated, pastures should not be grazed. Instead, the fodder should be hayed or silaged.

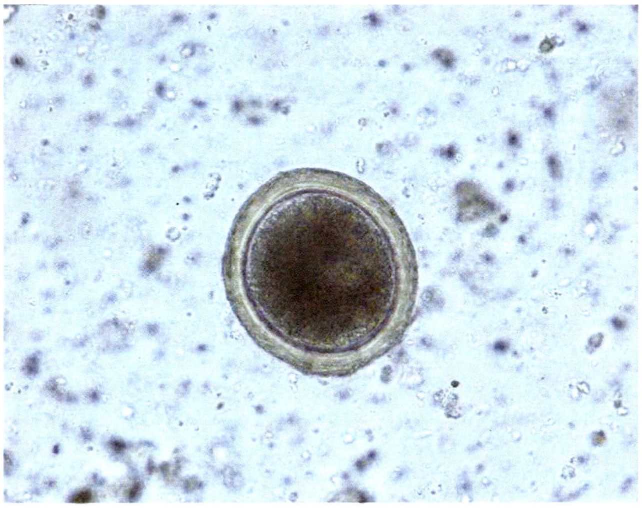

Female *Toxocara* eliminate millions of eggs every day (3-8 million/female). These eggs are rounded, 70-90 x 60-70 µm, dark brown in colour and have three coatings, the latter of which is slightly mamillated. Diarrhoea is normally associated with large-scale egg elimination. Patent infection is usually seen in animals younger than 3 months and it is rare in those older than 6 months. *Image courtesy of Dr. S. Mitchel.*

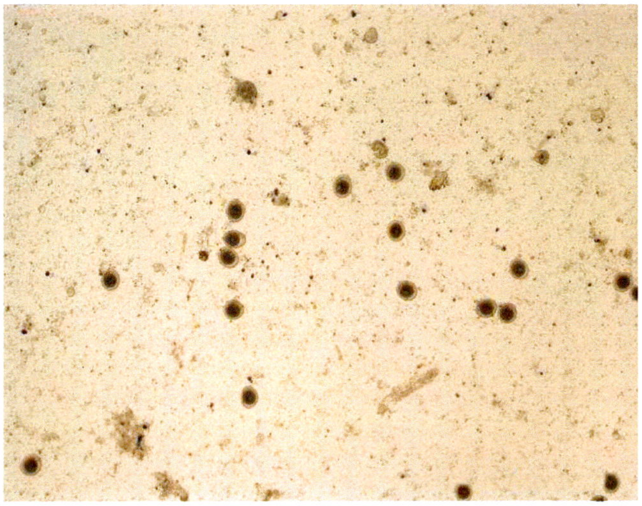

Numerous typical eggs, 70-90 x 60-70 µm in size, with a relatively smooth and speckled surface, a thick wall and brown in colour can be seen under the microscope. *Image courtesy of Dr. S. Mitchel.*

4 What is type II ostertagiosis?

In March, the services of a vet are requested on a meat farm in the Esla valley (León province, Spain). The calves born the previous spring are in poor condition and some present in an afebrile condition with unremitting diarrhoea despite the administration of injectable antibiotic therapy. The diarrhoea is watery, profuse and the stools are light brown in colour. The most affected animals present oedema in their lower regions, especially the limbs and submaxillary region. They have been stabled since mid November, as early autumn was very cold in the mountains. They receive a customised diet designed several years ago by the vet himself. Three calves have already died and the necropsy confirmed lesions typical of type II ostertagiosis (winter ostertagiosis in the northern hemisphere).

1. What types of lesions characterise this clinical presentation?
2. What blood parameters are likely to be altered?
3. What determining factor causes this symptomatology to occur?

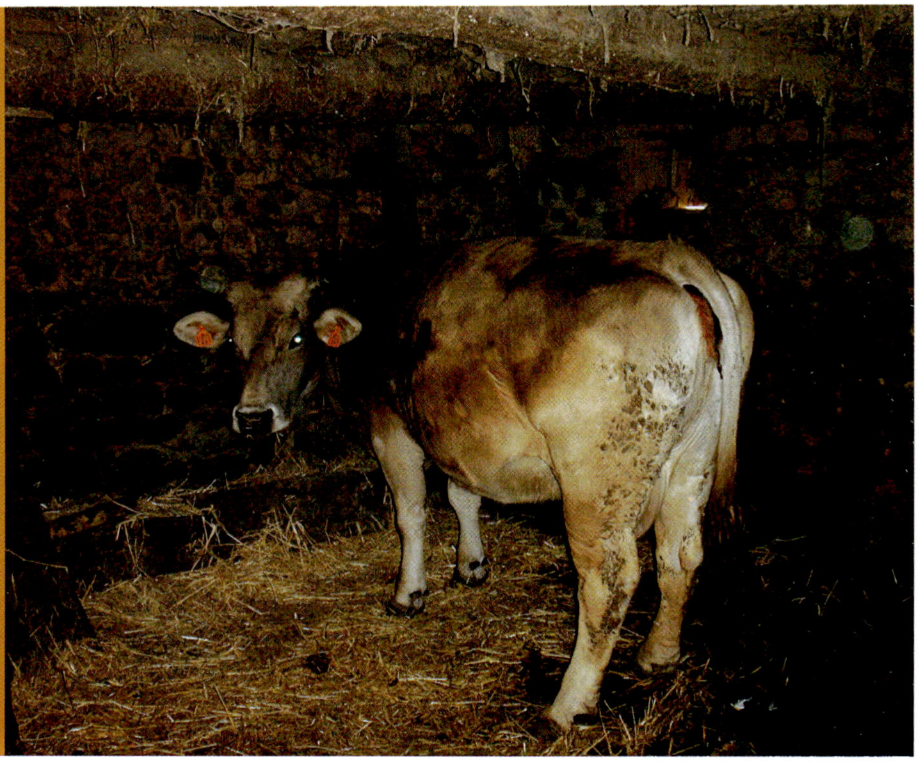

1 What types of lesions characterise this clinical presentation?

Necropsy shows extreme malnutrition and an absence of fat in the cadaver. The rumen, reticulum and omasum may be full of food, but the digestive apparatus is essentially empty after the cardia. The third-stage larvae (L3) of ostertagia (*Ostertagia ostertagi*) penetrate as far as the gastric submucosa, where they moult and can remain for several months. Gastric hyperplasia occurs as a result of active penetration of the larvae. The stomach appears to be covered with small raised nodules (up to the size of a lentil) or bleeding or inflamed regions 1-2 mm in diameter, with oedematous abomasal mucosa. During the histotropic phase, some larvae miss their chance to exit to the surface. If the larvae have already exited into the gastric lumen, a central orifice is observed in each small nodule. In intense infections, the nodular hyperplastic reaction means that the mucosa have a characteristic "embossed leather" look, which is pathognomonic.

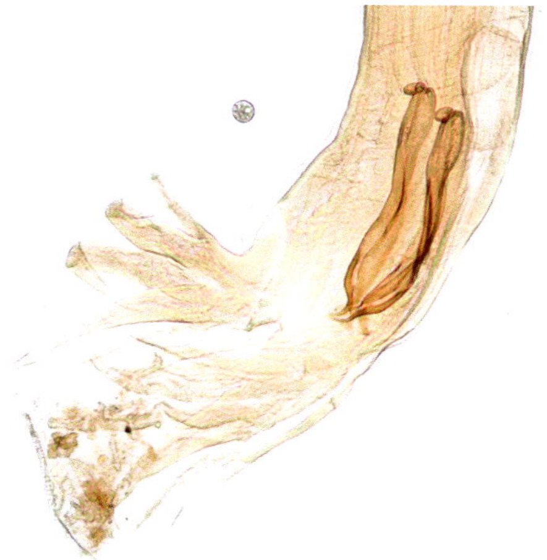

Male trichostrongylidae carry a copulatory bursa, with structures that allow specific identification, at their rear end. This is an extension of the cuticle in which finger-shaped support structures or bursal rays that grasp the female can be seen. During copulation other chitinous structures are used, such as spicules (which are inserted into the vagina) or the gubernaculum, which helps to guide the spicules. The copulatory bursa of *Ostertagia ostertagi* is formed by two lateral lobules and an additional dorsal lobule located symmetrically with respect to the former. In males, the spicules end in three hook-shaped protuberances.

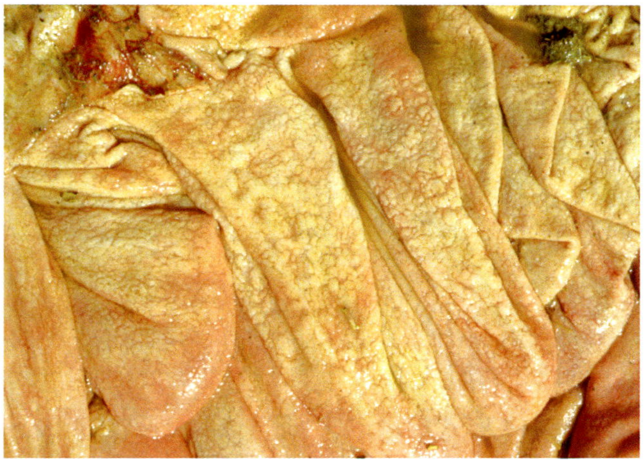

Macroscopically, the lesion produced in the mucosa by endogenous development of the parasites is a raised circular nodule, around 2-3 mm in size, with a central orifice if the larva has already left. In severe infections, this nodular reaction means that the mucosa acquire a characteristic "embossed leather) appearance.
Image courtesy of Dr. P. García Palencia.

Infection of the abomasum by ostertagia initially results in dilation of the affected gland and marked protrusion of that gland above the mucosal surface. The cells in its epithelium (mucosal, parietal and principal) are replaced by mucous secretion cells. Exit of the larvae from the glands leads to lysis of the epithelial cells in the upper edge of the glands, thus resulting in marked hyperplasia with mucosal thickening, submucosal oedema and increased plasma cell levels.

2 What blood parameters are likely to be altered?

The type and intensity of the anaemia in infected animals can be assessed by some blood constants (red blood cell count, haematocrit and haemoglobin rate). Thus, there is mild anaemia with a red blood cell count of around 5.6×10^6/ mm^3, a haemoglobin value of 8.4 g/100 ml and a haematocrit of 0.22-0.26. The determination of blood proteins and the albumin/globulin ratio may be of interest for diagnosis and prognosis, although decreased albumin and total protein levels are not exclusive to gastrointestinal nematode infections.

One of the most commonly performed enzymatic determinations in type II ostertagiosis is blood pepsinogen. In healthy animals, the blood pepsinogen value is 450 ± 150 milliunits (mUI) of tyrosine, whereas ostertagiosis results in values 6 or 7 times higher than baseline. However, the wide range of pepsinogen values for different animals means that this test cannot be used individually and is only applicable to groups of animals.

3 What determining factor causes this symptomatology to occur?

As is the case for type I, or summer (in the northern hemisphere) ostertagiosis, the direct cause of type II ostertagiosis is simultaneous maturation of a very high number of ostertagia, although clinical signs appear a long time post-infection rather than shortly after the ingestion of L3 with grass. The length of time required for development under normal conditions (type I ostertagiosis) is around three weeks, after which

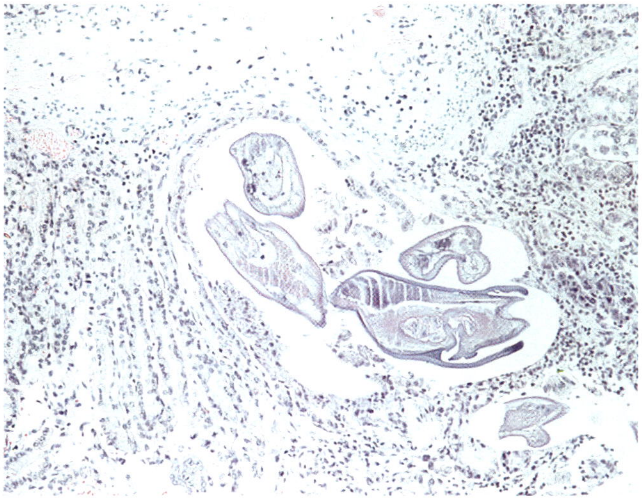

the parasites reach sexual maturity and commence patency. Under some circumstances, larval development in the host is halted and prepatency lasts for 4 or 5 months.

Several factors seem to be involved in this suspension of larval development in bovine gastric glands. Although the reasons for this slowdown in parasite development, known as hypobiosis, are not fully understood, inhibition occurs when the environmental conditions are adverse (cold months in European winters) such as, for example, when the L3 in grass are subjected to temperatures of around 4 °C for several weeks, in other words in Autumn/Winter. Moreover, some strains appear to be genetically predisposed to inhibition, thus meaning that this is a hereditary feature which, according to some authors, could be an adaptation of the parasite to host resistance, adverse environmental factors, or both. The host's age and prior exposure also have an effect.

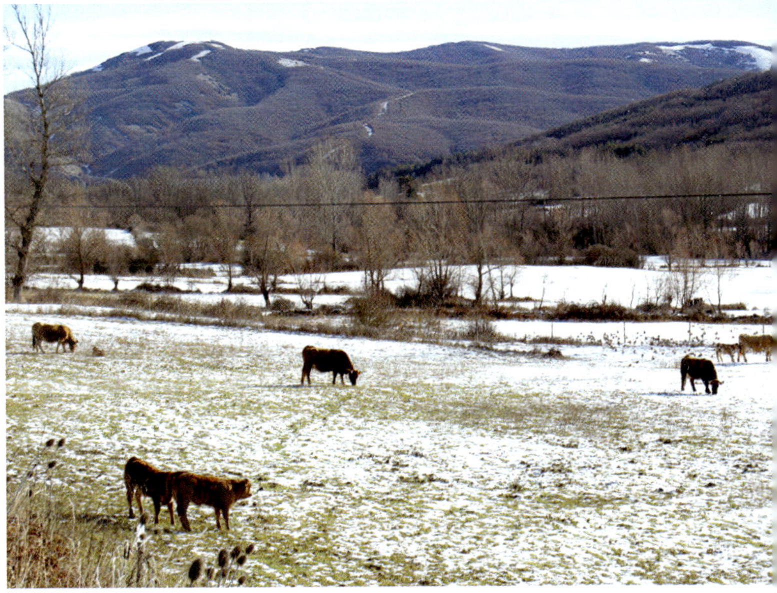

The inhibited larval development typical of winter ostertagiosis is a similar process to dormancy in insects and is the response of a parasite population that needs to survive under adverse environmental conditions. This response allows the parasite to remain in a region in which weather conditions are periodically adverse, recommencing development once environmental conditions are more suitable for biological cycle completion.

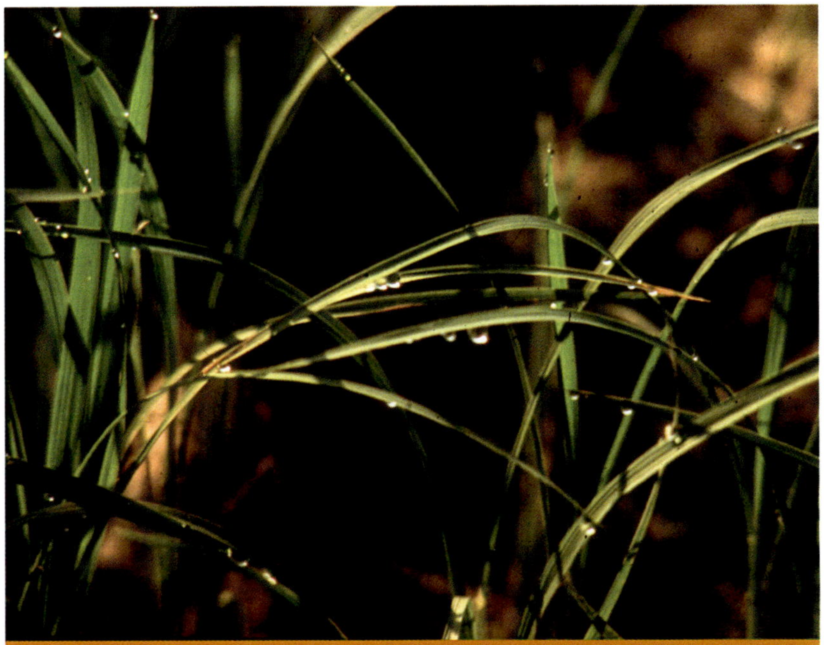

Animals ingest infective larvae when grazing. The exogenous phase of the biological cycle commences when infected animals excrete parasite eggs in faeces. The first larval stage, which hatches and leaves the egg, forms in the environment over a relatively longer period of time. This stage remains in the faecal mass, where it moults and transforms into a stage 2 larva which, after a further moult, leads to the infective phase or third stage (L3) larva.

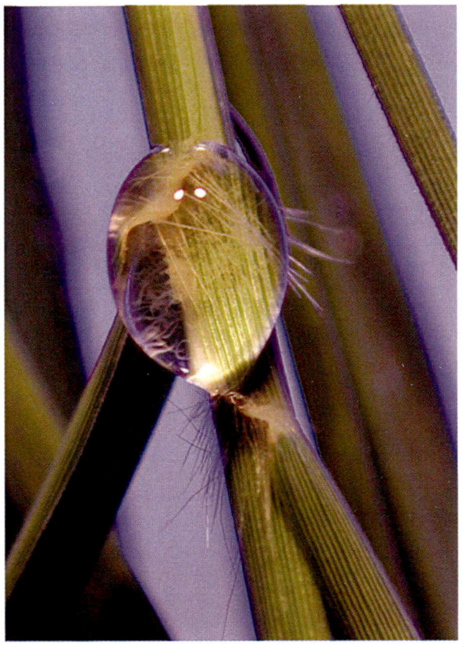

Under suitable conditions of temperature and humidity, third stage larvae leave their eggs and emigrate to the grass, attaching themselves to it in the hope of being ingested by the definitive host in order to continue the evolutionary cycle.

5 Can *Ostertagia* infection be detected in milk tanks?

In August, on a dairy farm in the north-west of Spain with 60 Friesian cows and 26 heifers with access to pasture, the assistance of a vet is requested as one heifer remains lying down and is unable to stand. This heifer was found in sternal recumbency with its head bent to one side and its hind third stained with faeces. The animal was one of a group of 9, aged between 11 and 14 months. The following day, the farmer found a further three heifers to be listless and inactive with an acute attack of diarrhoea. At the vet's insistence, the farmer admitted that this group had not been dewormed in spring despite the vet having informed him, after undertaking a stool analysis, of the elimination of large quantities of eggs in faeces during the peripartum of adult cows.

1. How can the need for treatment in this type of animal be assessed?
2. What is periparturient rise?
3. When does immunity to *Ostertagia* develop?

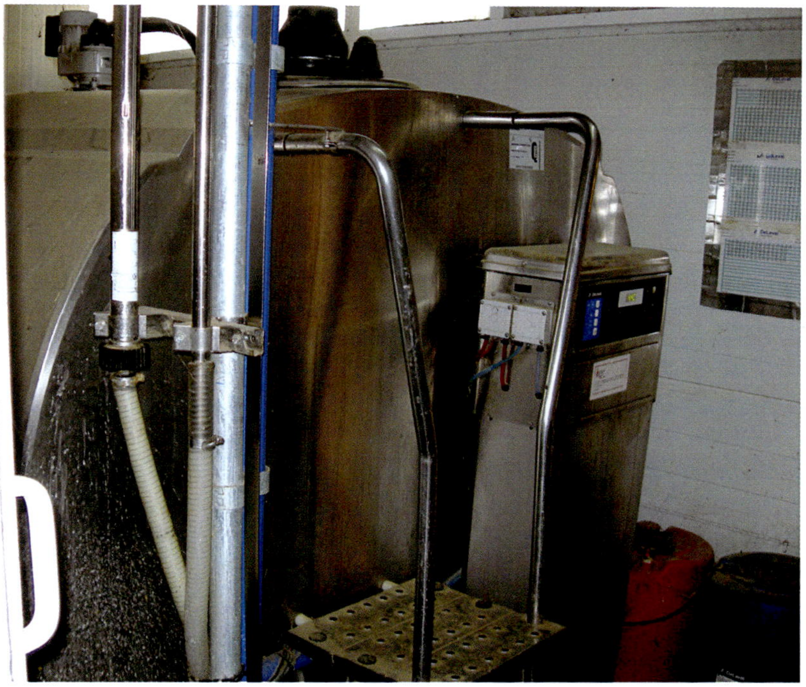

1 How can the need for treatment in this type of animal be assessed?

Although the clinical signs of *Ostertagia* infection may not be sufficiently clear to identify the problem, there is no doubt that they are useful when considered together with other, mainly epidemiological, findings. Thus, alongside the diarrhoea, zootechnical parameters that highlight a negative factor in the herd are also useful. Production yield is therefore very important when considering the possibility of a gastrointestinal parasitosis and establishing appropriate control measures.

Faecal analysis is obviously useful but it has limitations. Various aspects limit the benefits of a conventional coprological analysis as regards establishing a diagnosis prior to a deworming treatment. However, irrespective of this, it is vital to interpret the coprological findings correctly.

In almost all host-parasite systems, *Ostertagia* being no exception, the minimum parasite burden required to produce alterations in animals is not well defined, therefore its clinical value is limited. Attempts should always be made to confirm the species responsible for the problem, therefore faeces should be cultured in order to obtain L3s that can be easily identified. It should also be noted that, despite making the final diagnosis easier, faecal culture is not standard practice.

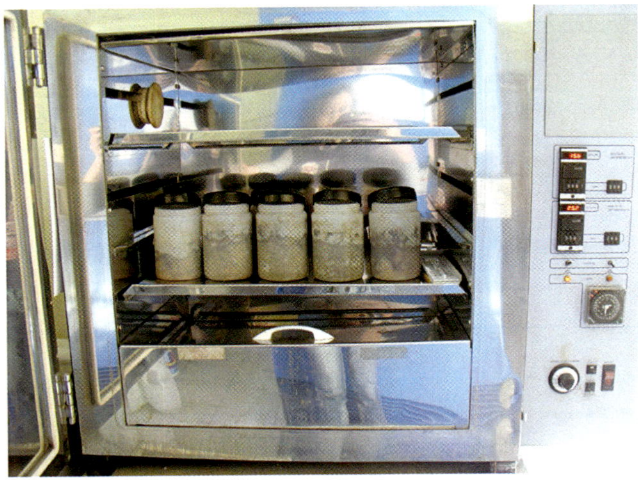

Faecal analyses must be performed on the group rather than individually and quantitative methods that allow the degree of infection to be estimated should be used. Identification of the species present is based on the morphometric characteristics of the infective larvae. Therefore, eggs must be grown under suitable conditions of temperature and humidity during faecal culture (coproculture). This involves placing the eggs in a recipient with a moist atmosphere at a temperature of 23-25 °C for 7-8 days. The larvae are subsequently collected using the Baermann-Wetzel technique, which is based on their positive hydrotropism.

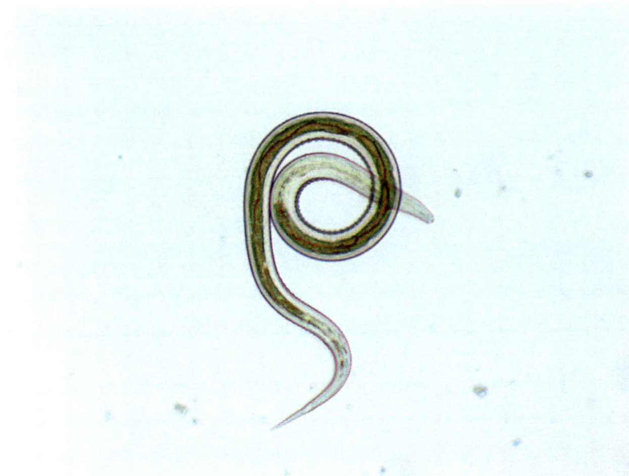

Third stage larvae are specific and can be identified, amongst other characteristics, by the space between the distal end of the larva and the terminal region of the cuticle. This region forms the "tail", which is used to classify larvae as short-tailed (20-40 µm), medium-tailed (40-80 µm) or long-tailed (>80 µm). Another important characteristic is the number and shape of the intestinal cells, which are imperceptible in some species (*Bunostomum*), whereas others contain eight such cells (*Nematodirus*) and yet others 16 (*Ostertagia, Cooperia, Haemonchus and Trichostrongylus*). Finally, some species present 32 (*Oesophagostomum*).

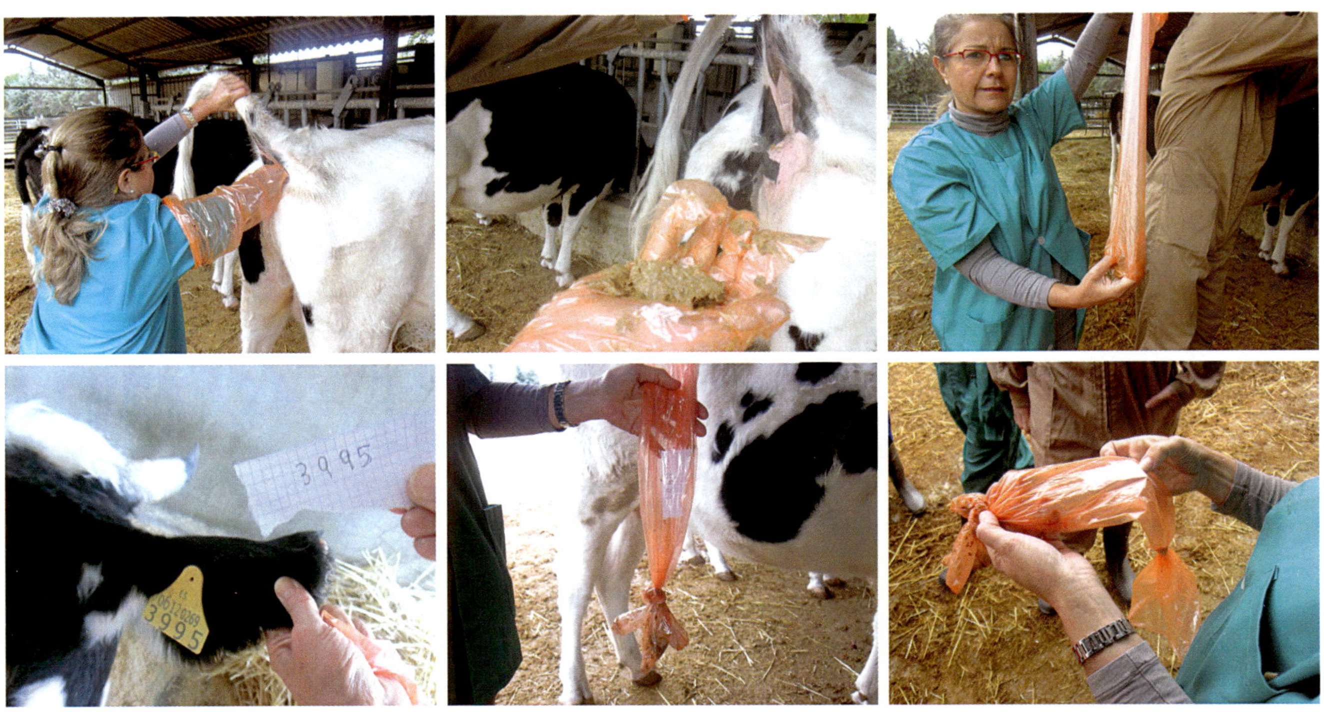

Stool samples should be taken directly from the animal's rectum in order to avoid contamination with nematode larvae living freely in the soil. It is recommended to use plastic rectal examination gloves, which allow more than 50 g of stools to easily be removed. This amount is sufficient for a complete coprological analysis. The square root of the number of animals in the herd appears to be the most suitable sample size.

Generally speaking, however, increased egg elimination in faeces is the first finding that should be taken into account, either due to the fact that this is a consequence of the sexual maturity of larvae that are no longer inhibited or because it reflects high levels of contamination of the environment in which the animals are grazing. In primary infections, the possibility that the coprology results are negative simply because the problem is caused by immature phases in ostertagia's cycle that have not reached sexual maturity must also be considered.

Detection of host-parasite contact also allows a diagnosis to be established, provided that certain aspects are taken into account. Immunoglobulin levels (in both serum and milk) also fluctuate markedly and are mainly affected by the parasite species, the animals' immune status and the phase of infection.

ELISA-based determination of the immunoglobulin levels in milk tanks is a method receiving considerable interest. Firstly, it should be noted that the analysis from individual cows milk provide more information regarding the level of infection in the herd than analysis of a milk tank. It is also important to determine in what lactation is the animal in order to interpret ELISA results for a milk sample. In any case, use of the level of antibodies in an isolated milk sample to determine the degree of protection of an animal after being dewormed remains uncertain. Despite this, the existence of a significant and positive relationship between the mean optical density for an individual animal and that for samples from milk tanks has been noted.

There also appears to be a relationship between the level of antibodies and various other parameters (farm size, production types, grazing and deworming treatments). Moreover, a correlation between high antibody levels and a decrease in milk production has also been found.

It is also obviously possible to confirm a problem if the final result of application of a specific treatment is an improvement in the animals. However, it must be remembered that this method has little scientific validity.

Guidelines for possible treatment of the animals, especially in their first grazing season, can be established. From a therapeutic viewpoint, the clinical signs, individual coprology results and pepsinogen levels have an estimative value. As regards productions, it would be interesting to determine the pepsinogen and antibody levels in the milk tanks. And, finally, coprological analysis at the onset of grazing and the pepsinogen levels when stabling commences are of interest for prevention purposes.

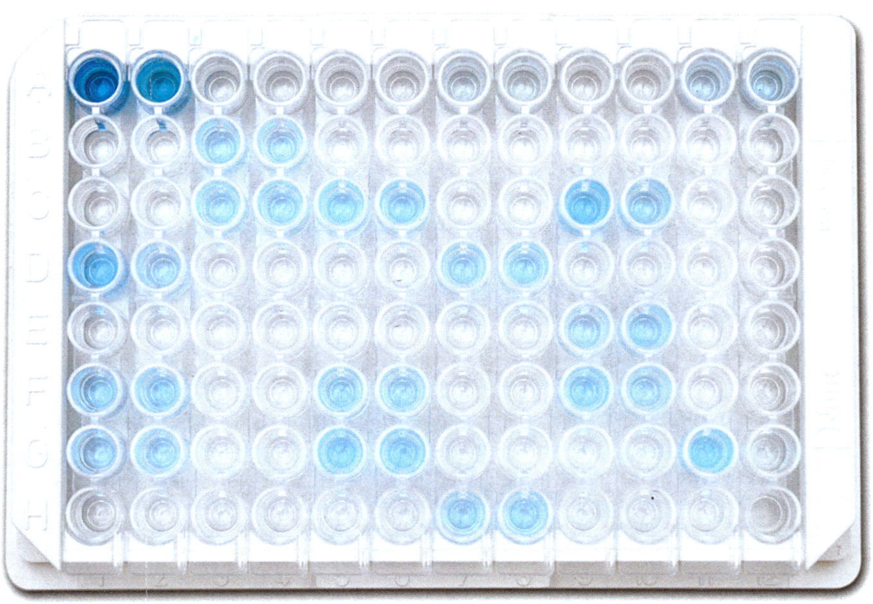

In bovines, both blood pepsinogen levels and the ELISA result for the milk tank can be used to retrospectively assess the degree of exposure of animals to ostertagia larvae, thus allowing anthelmintic administration to be optimised. The type of farming system concerned and the use of drugs have a more direct effect on antibody levels in the milk tank than variations due to the environment on the farm or weather conditions.

2 What is periparturient rise?

The intensity of infections is governed by various factors. First of all, the quantity of eggs excreted in the faeces of infected animals, which varies markedly, is of importance. As the host's age increases the degree of egg eliminations decreases, with higher elimination rates being found in calves, followed by heifers and, finally, adult cows, in which the quantity of eggs per gramme of faeces is particularly low. Obviously, this is related to the infections and re-infections throughout the productive life of the animals and, consequently, with acquired resistance.

The host's physiological status also affects the quantity of eggs excreted. An increase in the number of eggs excreted in faeces occurs in the period leading up to delivery (normally very close to giving birth). This increase usually lasts for around four weeks and varies in intensity. It was initially described in the spring and, as such, was termed spring rise. Later, it was shown to occur close to delivery and to be associated with endocrine changes during that period and during lactation, especially increased prolactin, corticosteroid and adrenocorticotropic hormone levels.

Periparturient rise is one of the most important factors in the epidemiology of trichostrongylida infections in general, and ostertargia in particular, as it is an important source of animal contamination.

3 When does immunity to *Ostertagia* develop?

There is a wide degree of variability in the development of protective immunity against parasitic gastrointestinal nematode species in cows. Thus, immunity against some species develops very rapidly, whereas against others it takes somewhat longer. Indeed, immunity against *Ostertagia* spp. tends to develop very slowly to such an extent that animals remain susceptible up to two years of age. As a result, *O. ostertagi* causes production losses in animals over very long periods of time, which is why it is considered to be the most important species in cattle worldwide.

In contrast to other host-parasite models, repeated reinfection with *O. ostertagi* leads to a decrease in IL-4 expression, which is not typical of the classic Th2 response, although it has been noted that infection induces a similar response to Th2 in the gastric lymph nodes. However, this response does not appear to be related to increased IL-4 expression or mechanisms in the abomasal mucosa. One of the explanations for the limited protection of animals against *O. ostertagi* infection is immunomodulation of the parasite's protective response.

The development of immunity affects infection dynamics in various ways. L3s can inhibit their development in the L4 phase, a phenomenon which appears to have a partial immune basis, or can be eliminated or displaced to most likely less favourable (more hostile) regions of the gastrointestinal tract if the animals have some degree of immunity.

The initial effect of the development of immunity against adult parasites is a reduction in the size and fecundity of the females, which translates into a reduction in faecal egg elimination. Another of the consequences of the development of protective immunity is a change to the female/male ratio in favour of the latter, possibly due to a higher mortality rate in females as a result of their increased metabolic needs and ingestion of higher amounts of "immune compounds". It has been demonstrated in *O. ostertagi* that the mortality rate for adult worms in reinfected animals increases with immunity.

6

What factors affect the onset of clinical ostertagiosis?

In January, the cows and calves from a Morucha herd on an extensive farm in Salamanca (Spain) are brought in. The low number of animals to be ear tagged is confirmed, even though the farmer had expected many more due to the number of pregnant cows observed during the summer. Indeed, the summer had been very wet, with high and very green pastures. As the farm is large, with steep areas, it was not easy to verify how many calves had died. It was clear that the calves were sick as they appeared cachetic and the hind third of many of them was stained with faeces.

1. Could summer rain have affected the onset of type I ostertagiosis?
2. What effect does temperature have? And humidity?
3. How can it be determined whether a pasture is heavily contaminated?

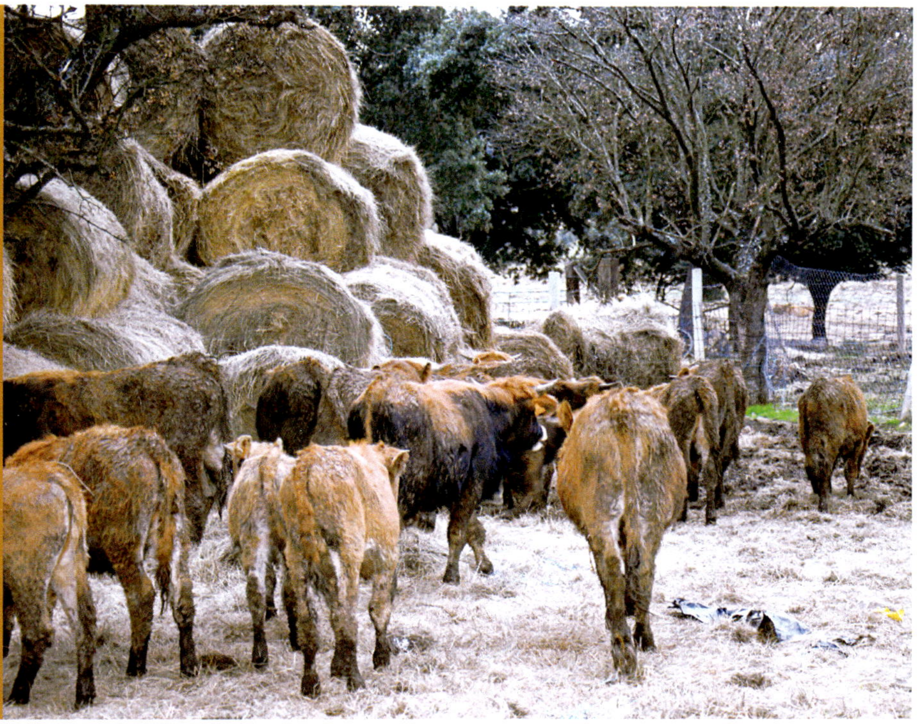

1 Could summer rain affect the onset of type I ostertagiosis?

Although the biological cycle of gastrointestinal nematodes is direct and could be considered to be a "simple" or "straightforward" cycle, it is clear that the epidemiology of any infections that occur is anything but "simple".

Indeed, summer rains favour the onset of clinical entities, such as so-called summer ostertagiosis in the northern hemisphere, more correctly known as type I ostertagiosis.

Under natural conditions, the development of *Ostertagia* eggs up to L3 occurs over long time periods (up to 5-7 months). All pre-parasite phases develop and survive outdoors depending on the temperature and humidity. Low temperatures delay development and lead to a high mortality. *Ostertagia* does not develop below 5 °C. Development increases with temperature, although mortality is once again high at temperatures above 26-27 °C. Humidity is more limiting than temperature, with a relative humidity of between 70 % and 100 % being considered appropriate.

All pre-parasite phases (from egg to L3) develop in the faecal mass which, under unfavourable conditions, comprises a major larval reservoir. Migration of the the L3s from faeces to grass occurs in the event of sufficient humidity, although a light stimulus is also important. Thus, the humidity provided by summer rainstorms is sufficient for L3s "retained" in the faecal mass to actively migrate to the grass and contaminate the environment in a more or less synchronous fashion. This poses a risk to grazing animals, which can ingest a large quantity of infective larvae in just a short space of time.

Climate changes can also play a key role in the onset of clinical outbreaks which, in the case of ostertagia, would produce an infection immediately after the grass has become contaminated, in other words a type I ostertagiosis.

2 What effect does temperature have? And humidity?

Embryo formation and egg hatching are temperature-dependent and reflect adaptive differences in different regions. For example, the ability of eggs to resist low temperatures limits their geographical distribution, or implies a restriction to certain microclimates, to such an extent that ostertagia eggs hatch at temperatures which are lethal for other genera of the trichostrongylidae. Thus, they can hatch at 4 °C and develop at 5 °C and, moreover, the temperature range is from 5 °C to 37.5 °C. Similarly, the sufficient humidity is crucial for embryo formation and egg hatching.

The rate of development from eggs to L3 is also temperature- and humidity-dependent. L3 can be obtained in the laboratory by culturing the eggs in faeces at around 25-27 °C whilst maintaining sufficient humidity to prevent the faeces from drying out.

3 How can it be determined whether a pasture is heavily contaminated?

The main factor governing the transmission of trichostrongylidae infection is the contamination of grass with infective larvae (L3). An understanding of the infection levels, and especially, their fluctuations with time, is the first step in determining the scale of the risks and putting into place the appropriate prophylactic and control measures.

As would appear logical, the degree of contamination of pastures can be deduced from the occurrence of gastrointestinal symptoms, and their scale, after several weeks of grazing in pastures that have been grazed previously.

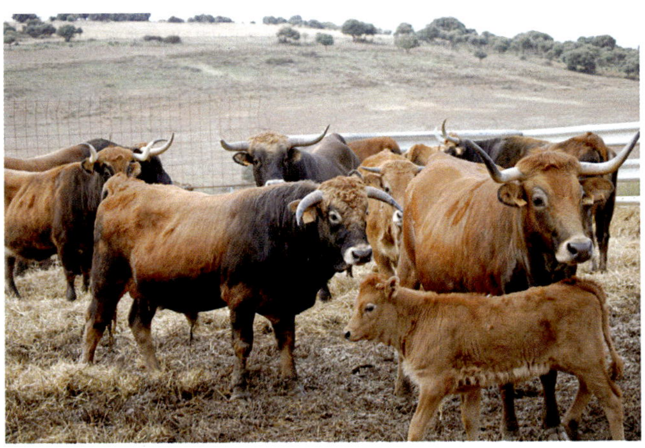

Resistance mechanisms depend on the immune response acquired after contact with the parasites and on the innate physiological ability of the animals to adapt to an infection. Immunity to gastrointestinal nematodes depends directly on the T-cell response and is also promoted by the presence of specific antibodies against the parasites. In primary infections, the humoral antibody response is greater in adult than in young animals (there is no lymphocytic response in ruminants at birth —it develops during the first 5 months of life).

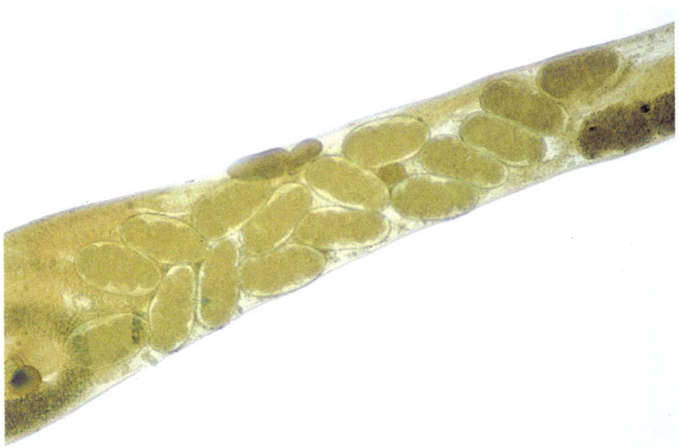

The host's immune response prevents the parasite from feeding properly, thereby affecting its growth and reproductive capacity. In resistant animals, female parasites lay a lower number of eggs and develop less.

However, it is preferable to be aware of the potential risk of any particular zone that is to be used by animals, especially in their first grazing season, *a priori*. As such, attempts should be made to determine the quantity of L3s in the grass.

Of the many techniques described for this purpose, Taylor's remains particularly useful. This technique, which has been modified on numerous occasions, basically comprises randomly sampling a variable number of points (around a hundred) separated by about 10 steps. Four grass samples are collected at each point (front, back, left and right) using scissors and following two *W* shapes (one of which is inverted) such that a total of around 400 samples are collected in a plastic bag.

The grass collection frequency and inter-sampling time periods vary but, if possible, samples should be collected throughout the grazing season, at the same time, and with a frequency of once or twice per month.

Samples should be refrigerated for transport to the laboratory to prevent drying and destruction of the larvae. Once in the laboratory, the samples are placed in containers of warm water until the grass is completely covered and a detergent is added to release the larvae. The grass is stirred and left to soak, stirring occasionally. The following morning the grass is washed and drained, then dried in an oven and weighed to determine the quantity of dry grass.

The water from the container and the wash water are filtered through two consecutive sieves, the first with a mesh size of 150 µm and the second, in which the L3s are retained, with a mesh size of 20 µm. The filtrate retained by the second sieve is transferred into a receptacle, labelled and stored cold. The volume of the supernatant is reduced to 20-30 mL, then homogenised and an aliquot taken, which is then concentrated by centrifugation. Afterwards, a solution with a higher density than water is added (optimal density: 1.25-1.30) to form a slightly convex meniscus placing then a cover-slip without spilling liquid. This cover-slip is then placed on a microscope slide with one drop of Lugol solution to immobilise the larvae and facilitate their identification. Finally, the larvae are examined under a microscope and the L3s present identified and counted. A simple calculation allows the number of L3s per kilogram of dry grass, and therefore the contamination/infection risk for the animals, to be estimated.

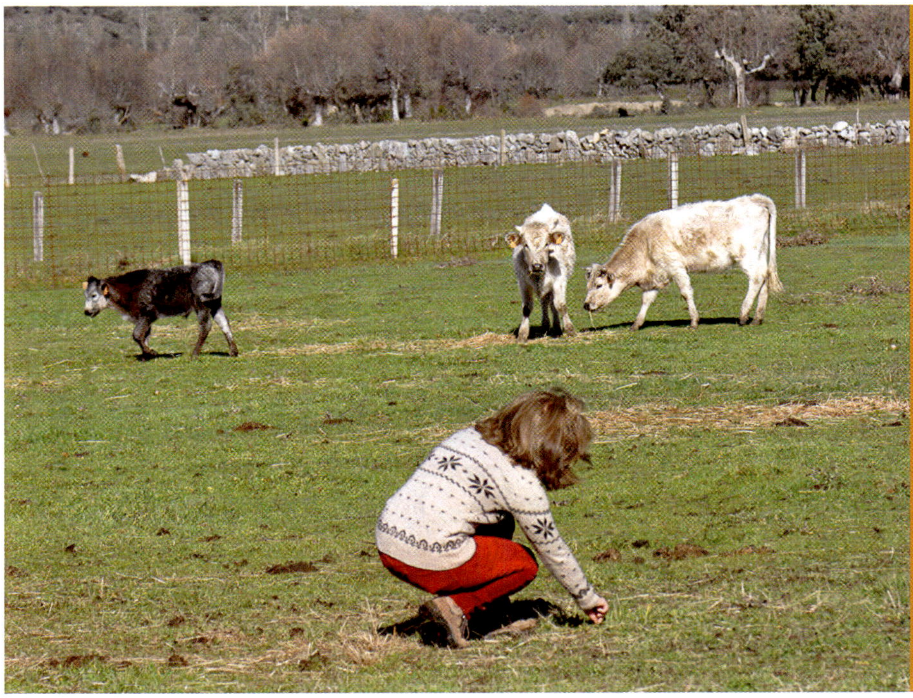

It is easy to assess the parasite burden of a pasture by taking samples in a systematic manner in order to collect and quantify the infective larvae present. This is the most direct means of determining the infection risk to which animals are exposed at different times of year and to assess the need to administer anthelmintics at the appropriate time.

7 How can ostertagiosis-related financial losses be avoided?

In a herd of 200 Limousin cattle destined for beef production, maintained using a semi-extensive system on an irrigated farm in Cáceres province (Spain), diarrhoeal symptoms recur in animals in their first grazing season. The farm is well managed, animals feed on fresh grass, as well as hay or silage produced on the farm itself, with mineral blocks. The first clinical cases were detected at least four years previously, after installation of the irrigation system in the pastures. The cases first start in early spring and are characterised by dark green diarrhoea and marked weight loss in animals that sometimes present with dehydration-related polydipsia. Almost all have shaggy hair and sunken eyes. Mortality is low but the effects on their subsequent development are clear.

1. What causes the diarrhoea and loss of physical condition in ostertagiosis?
2. Why does the hair become dull and brittle?
3. What control measures exist?

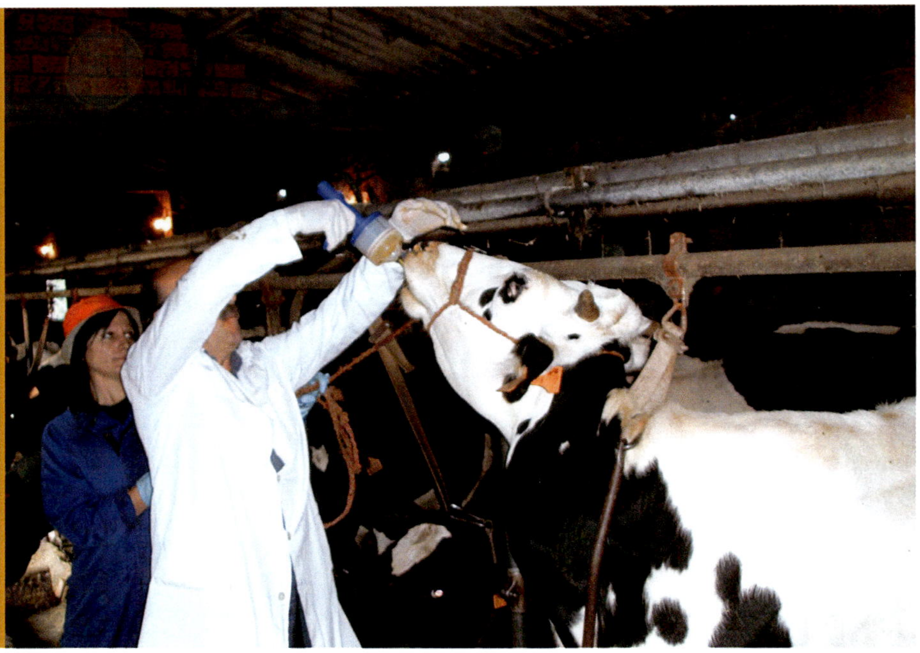

Image courtesy of Dr. A. Paz.

1 What causes the diarrhoea and loss of physical condition in ostertagiosis?

The main lesions and biochemical changes associated with this disease occur immediately after the parasites leave the gastric glands. The changes related to prior invasion of the gastric glands by the larvae post-infection are limited to the glands affected.

At approximately 18-21 days post-infection, *Ostertagia* begin to exit the gastric glands and marked changes occurr, including hyperplasia and loss of cell differentiation, especially in the HCl-producing parietal cells, which affects both infected and neighbouring cells. Although some cells can be observed ultrastructurally, they are no longer functional. In intense infections some of these lesions combine with others and, as a consequence of the damage produced, gastric pH increases (from 2 to 7), pepsinogen does not transform into pepsin, protein denaturation fails and the bacteriostatic effect is lost, thus resulting in an increase in the number of bacteria in the abomasum. The permeability of the wall to macromolecules also increases due to alterations to the intercellular junctions, plasma pepsinogen levels increase and a marked hypoalbuminaemia occurs due to the passage of albumin from circulation into the gastric lumen. The clinical effects of these changes are altered digestion and diarrhoea.

As a result, the animals' physical condition may be seriously compromised to the extent that it may be difficult for them to remain upright. Appetite may be diminished and the animals often lose considerable amounts of weight.

2 Why does the hair become dull and brittle?

Ostertagiosis appears insidiously. In mild and moderate infections the signs are often unclear and comprise weakness and delayed growth. More severe infections lead to somewhat clearer symptoms, although many of these are not pathognomonic. Generally speaking, young animals lose weight and present marked growth retardation. They produce softer stools, which are often dark green or yellow in colour, and present other signs such as curling of the hair, which appears dull and sometimes brittle, mainly due to changes to plasma protein levels. Their eyes often appear sunken, especially in the final phases of the disease.

Alterations to mineral metabolism and imbalances in some amino acids mean that the hair of infected animals becomes brittle, with regions of shaggy, fragile and unequal hair occasionally appearing, thus meaning that these animals appear to be in poor health.

As well as the lack of pepsin, which directly affects protein digestion, ostertagiosis also results in increased deamination due to higher bacterial levels in the gastrointestinal tract. These factors lead to lower amino acid absorption, which has direct consequences for protein metabolism and can be seen in all appendages.

3 What control measures exist?

In light of the complex factors that play a part in the epidemiology of infections with ostertagia and other bovine gastrointestinal nematodes, it is clear that eradication of these parasitoses is not a simple task. The persistence of L3s in grass and the relatively rapid use of favourable climate conditions by the parasites means that gastrointestinal nematodoses are still considered to be significant processes in cattle breeding worldwide.

Despite the existence of numerous control strategies related to the various cattle production and management systems almost all of them are based on one or two basic tactics: the administration of anthelmintics and grazing systems.

Since the development and registration of the first benzimidazole carbamates in the early 1960s, the control of gastrointestinal nematodoses in grazing cattle has been based on the routine application of broad-spectrum anthelmintics despite the existence of other practices that form part of the so-called comprehensive control for these parasitoses.

The validity of strategic parasite control programs involving the administration of anthelmintics became clear once the epidemiological aspects, which provided an understanding of the contamination models of grass with L3s and allowed the risk of severe infections to be prevented, were

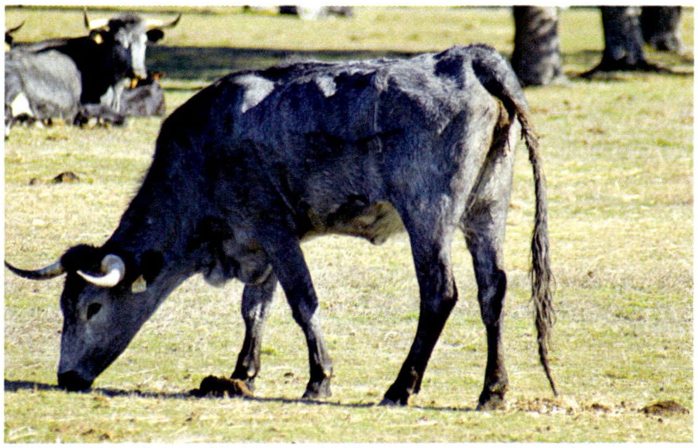

Diarrhoea, which is not always constant in parasitic gastroenteritis, appears to be mainly linked to *Trichostrongylus* and *Nematodirus* infection. Atrophy of the villi results in functional disorders, with a decreased surface area available for absorption, decreased enzymatic activity in the intestinal mucosa and malabsorption syndrome. The diarrhoeal symptoms in ostertagiosis coincide with exit of the larvae from the mucosa and are preceded by motility changes, with marked reticuloruminal and gastric inhibition which, together with biochemical alterations, can lead to an increased bacterial population that contributes to the onset of diarrhoea.

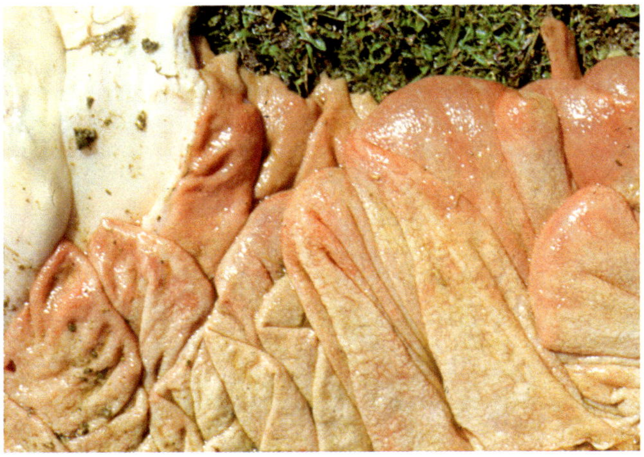

Infection of the abomasum by ostertagia initially results in dilation of the affected gland and marked protrusion of that gland above the mucosal surface. The cells in its epithelium (mucosal, parietal and principal) are replaced by mucous secretion cells. Exit of the larvae from the glands leads to epithelial cells lysis in the upper edge of the glands, thus resulting in marked hyperplasia with mucosal thickening, submucosal oedema and increased plasma cell levels. *Image courtesy of Dr. P. García Palencia.*

determined. Clearly, as environmental contamination with infective forms is closely related to climate, strategic control programs vary as regards time of year and number of treatments required, and may also differ widely between regions, even though the final goal is to reduce grass contamination.

In practical terms, prevention by the administration of anthelmintics has become synonymous with "safe pastures", and the administration of effective drugs and subsequent transfer of treated animals to clean/safe pastures with very low or non-existent levels of contamination, forms an important part of such control programs.

"Clean pastures" are not easily available, and, according to some authors, this may not even be necessary if anthelmintics are used tactically. Despite some contraindications, repeated antiparasitic treatments at different times of year reduce the numbers of L3s in grass to very low levels. The number and times of anthelmintic administration vary by region and animal production method.

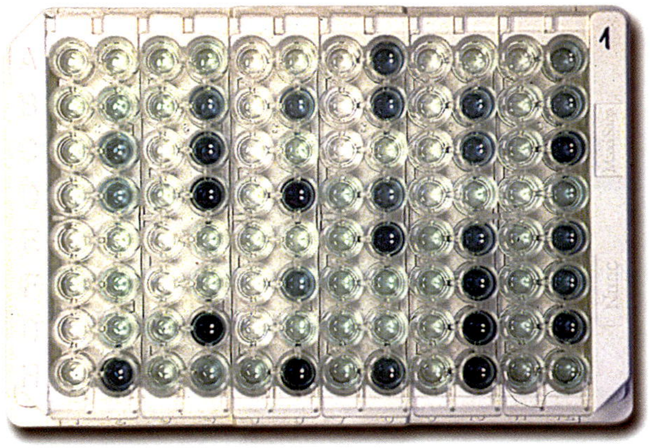

Lesions and functional alterations to the abomasal mucosa reduce hydrochloric acid secretion, thus meaning that pepsinogen is not correctly transformed into pepsin, allowing the passage of macromolecules, such as untransformed pepsinogen, into the blood stream via the binding complexes between damaged endothelial and epithelial cells. In addition to the larva-related lesions, the simple presence of larvae stimulates the production of pepsinogen, which passes directly into the blood stream.

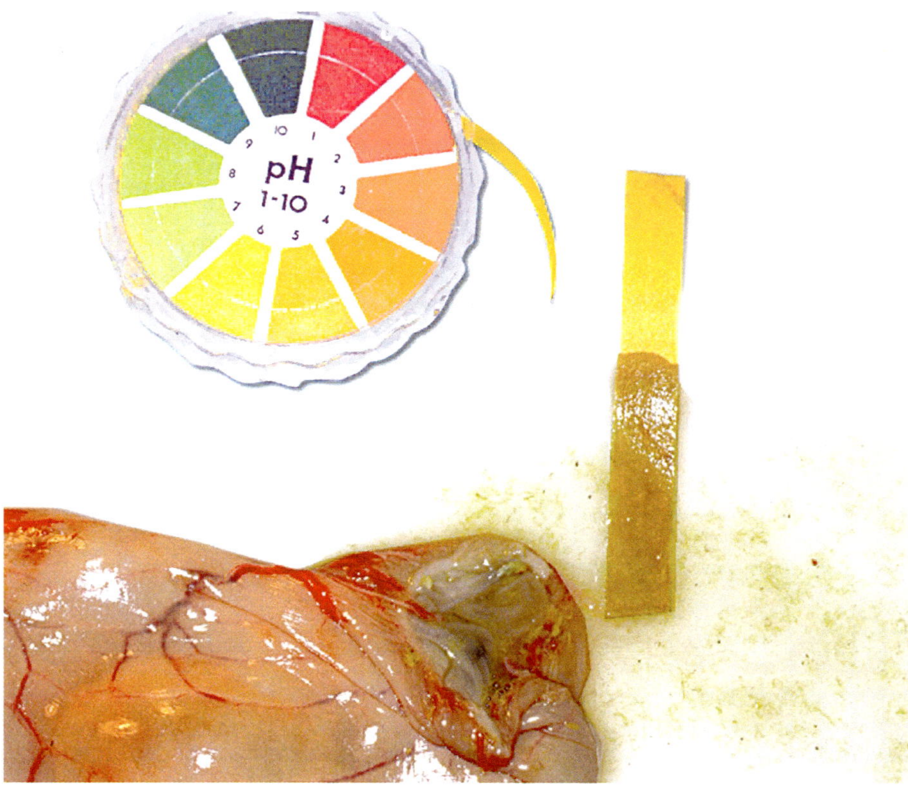

The abomasal pH in infected animals increases to more than 7, particularly when the larvae exit the gastric mucosa. An inhibition of acid secretion induced by the presence of the parasite and related parietal cell loss also occurs. The increased pH has a negative effect on protein digestion as pepsinogen is not transformed into pepsin. As is the case with other gastritic processes, this pepsinogen can be detected in the animals' serum and acts as an indicator of this disease.

8 Are all small worms in cows trichostrongylidae?

Clinical signs characterised by postration, anorexia, ruminal atony, lateral decubitus position and the death of 12 animals in 5 days were observed in a herd of 30 Limousin yearlings in November. Over half the remaining animals presented similar, although less severe, signs. Necropsy showed macroscopic lesions, in the form of nodules, consistent with the presence of nematodes in the abomasum and small intestine. The parasite burden was high and numerous white worms around 2 cm in length were collected from the small and large intestine using forceps. Smaller worms were also collected upon filtering the digestive contents. Some of these were dark red in colour, thus highlighting their blood-feeding habits.

1. Which nematodes can parasitize the bovine digestive tract?
2. Can all bovine digestive parasites produce specific clinical signs?
3. How is acute cooperiosis diagnosed?
4. What causes intestinal nodules in oesophagostomosis?

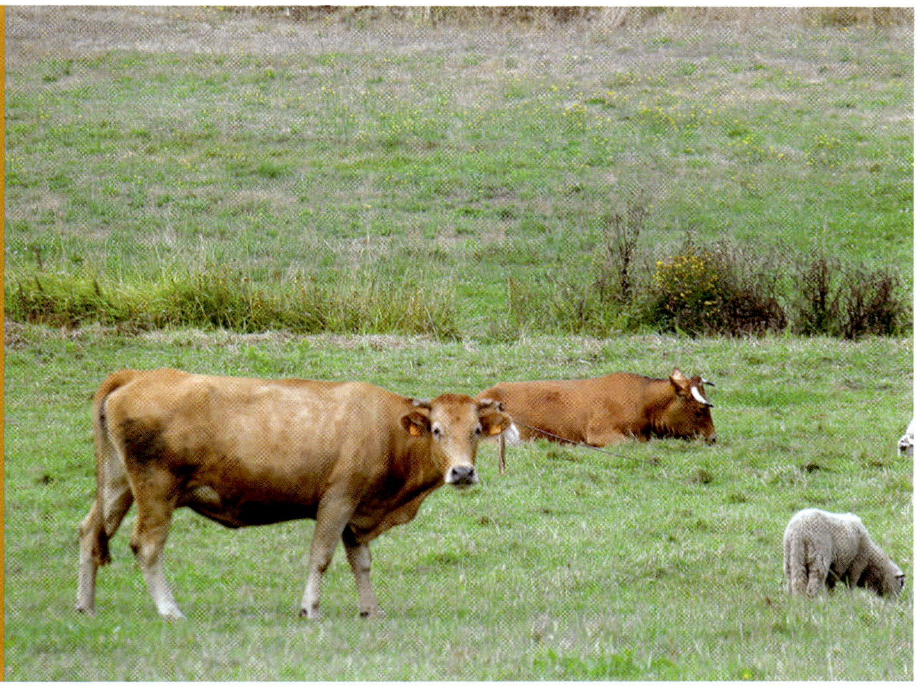

1 Which nematodes can parasitize the bovine digestive tract?

Gastrointestinal nematodoses have varying aetiologies. The parasites concerned belong to several families and genera, although the *Trichostrongylidae*, *Molineidae*, *Strongylidae* and *Ancylostomatidae* families tend to be the most important.

Trichostrongylidae are of greatest interest. In some Spanish regions their incidence can reach 51-96 %. The most important genera are *Ostertagia, Haemonchus, Trichostrongylus, Cooperia* and *Nematodirus* (the latter belongs to the Molineidae family).

Strongylidae and *Ancylostomatidae* are represented by *Oesophagostomum* and *Bunostomum* spp., respectively, although they are much less prevalent.

However, these are not the only nematodes involved and, from a clinical point of view, it is very difficult to identify gastrointestinal disorders caused by nematodes of less significance and prevalence. Some examples are *Trichuris*, which is found in the caecum, or *Strongyloides papillosus,* although the latter can be found in highly localised enzootic foci, especially in poorly maintained rural cowsheds.

Infections caused by trichostrongylidae species that live in the abomasum and small intestine (*Haemonchus, Cooperia, Nematodirus, Ostertagia* and *Trichostrongylus* spp.) almost always appear concomitantly with others such as those caused by *Oesophagostomum* or *Bunostomum*, which are located in the final stages of the small intestine and early stages of the large intestine (colon).

In practical terms, together they cause what has traditionally become known as parasitic gastroenteritis.

Depending on the region, some species can be more prevalent than others in countries with temperate climates such as Spain. However, the majority are present and infect young cattle, causing important infections, especially in the first grazing season. It should be noted that *Ostertagia* species are particularly important in bovines due to the repercussions of their infections.

2 Can all bovine digestive parasites produce specific clinical signs?

Under natural conditions, infections are mixed and involve various genera and species, although the proportion of each depends, above all, on the time of year, and therefore on environmental factors, as well as other aspects such as the animal's age. However, certain signs are related to the majority presence of one species or another.

For example, when *Haemonchus* predominates, the disease is characterised by intense anaemia and its effects such as tiredness, metabolic alterations, intermitent lack of appetite and weight loss. Younger animals tend to be more intensely infected. Generally speaking, such animals eliminate stools with a normal consistency containing large quantities of parasite eggs.

Infections in which *Trichostrongylus* species predominate tend to be chronic in nature and progress more slowly. More intense infections may result in anaemia and diarrhoea with dark grey, sticky or liquid stools, which dirty the rear third of infected animals. Digestive alterations result in weight loss, weakness and, in the absence of appropriate feeding, cachectic states.

Nematodirus infections can also have undesirable effects, such as diarrhoea, weight loss and growth disorders, especially in young animals.

The clinical signs of both type I and type II ostertagiosis appear as the larvae begin to exit the gastric glands. This occurs at around 16-18 days post-infection in type I and after a period that can reach as long as 6 months in type II. Irrespective of the time at which they present, symptoms include lower weight gain accompanied by diarrhoea and, occasionally, thirst due to dehydration.

In type I ostertagiosis the stools are dark green in colour due to the high content of chlorophyll that remains undegraded due to the altered gastric pH. There is no anaemia or pyrexia but in advanced stages the animals present dull and bristly hair and sunken eyes. Mortality is usually low.

The clinical signs of type II ostertagiosis include a marked weight loss that leads to emaciation and profuse watery brown or light-brown diarrhoea. Together with dull hair, the rear third of the infected animals is completely covered with stools. Many animals remain prostrate, especially towards the end of the process. Oedemas may be present on the lower parts of the body, especially in the submandibular region. Normocytic and normochromic anaemia is not accompanied by fever. As this form typically presents in stabled animals,

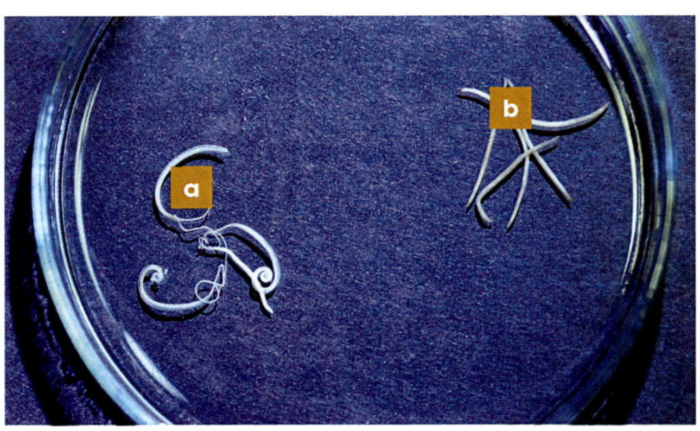

Trichuris (a) and *Oesophagostomum* (b). The parasites in the large intestine are larger and can readily be seen with the naked eye. They measure more than 1 cm and can be recognised from their cylindrical or rectangular developed buccal capsule, with or without cervical fins (*Oesophagostomum*) or a characteristic morphology of a whip-like worm with a thicker posterior end (*Trichuris*).

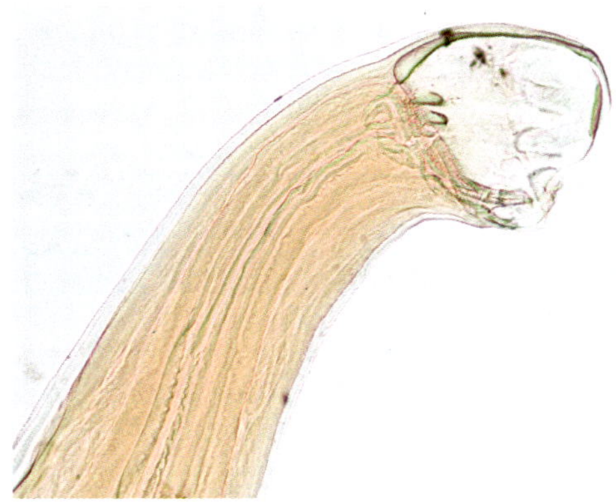

Image showing the anterior end of *Bunostomum*. The intestinal alterations caused by adults are due to their feeding habits, which result in ulcerative enteritis. The emigration of some *Bunostomum* larvae via the lungs may cause bronchopneumonic foci and lymphadenitis in ganglia in that region. Adults are characterised by possessing a well-developed buccal capsule lacking teeth but with a pair of lancets at its base.

inappropriate feeding may have an additive effect on the pathogenesis. In some regions, ostertagiosis is complicated by fasciolosis, which worsens the anaemic symptoms. In contrast to type I ostertagiosis, mortality can be high, with death occurring as soon as one or two weeks after the appearance of symptoms.

3 How is acute cooperiosis diagnosed?

Cooperia infections affect younger animals and are normally mild. Their presence in animals older than 4 months rarely has pathogenic effects.

The symptoms of cooperiosis can only be considered to be useful for the diagnostic process in endemic regions in which seasonal outbreaks occur from time to time in calves. In such cases loss of appetite and weight, emaciation and submaxillary oedema, together with profuse intermittent diarrhoea, are of clinical utility.

A *post mortem* study of an animal is useful to confirm an outbreak, although the elimination of around 1000 EPG (eggs per gram faeces) in young calves and endemic regions can also be used to confirm infection.

4 What causes intestinal nodules in oesophagostomosis?

Oesophagostomum radiatum infection is generally well tolerated by adult bovines. Disease is only observed in young animals, although it generally progresses subacutely ending with death of the infected animals at two or three months post-infection.

Although adult worms are located in the large intestine, the nodules in which the *Oesophagostomum* larvae are found are present throughout the intestine, with the pathogenic action being especially related to infection of the small intestine. This is particularly evident when a large number (thousands) of nodules are present, although alterations may also be observed in "normal" infections with a burden of a few hundred (around 400) nodules.

The nodules are around 1-5 mm in diameter and their contents are often yellowish or grayish red in colour and serosanguineous, creamy or caseous. They also contain fourth stage (L4) larvae. The caseous material can calcify in the final stages.

In severe cases, thickening of the stomach wall, swelling of the regional lymph nodes and oedematous infiltration of the colonic mesentery may also occur.

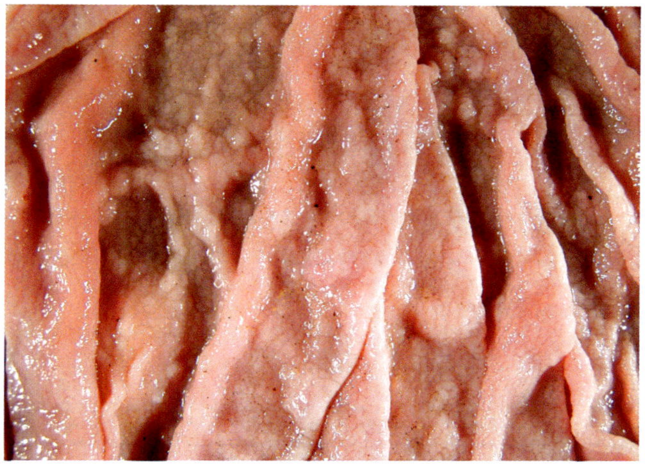

Ostertagia spp. infections result in an intense hyperplastic gastric reaction, with the presence of visible nodules 2-3 mm in size that possess a central orifice if the larva has already exited into the gastric lumen. In severe infections, this nodular reaction means that the mucosa acquire a characteristic "embossed leather) appearance.

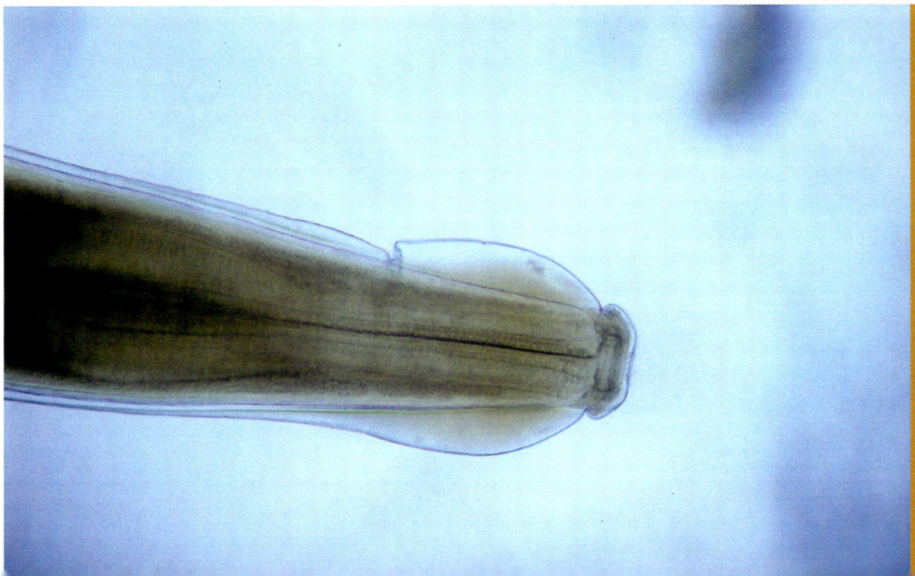

Image showing the anterior end of *Oesophagostomum*. *Oesophagostomum* species have cuticular extensions in the cephalic region that characterise them. The cuticle that surrounds the buccal orifice leads to a cervical from which structures such as highly developed cervical vesicle protrudes.

9 Is it the same finding eggs in faeces as diagnosing trichostrongylidae-related gastroenteritis?

During professional activities in a diagnostic laboratory, it is common to receive samples lacking the information required for parasitological analysis. Correct stool sample collection and submission is almost as important as providing the lab with the clinical and zootechnical information that allows the analyst to select the most appropriate methods for detecting the possible agents involved.

1. How are samples submitted to a laboratory?
2. What is the method of choice for detecting nematode eggs in bovines?
3. What clinical and zootechnical information should be taken into account when submitting a sample?
4. What other tests can help diagnose an outbreak of trichostrongylidosis?

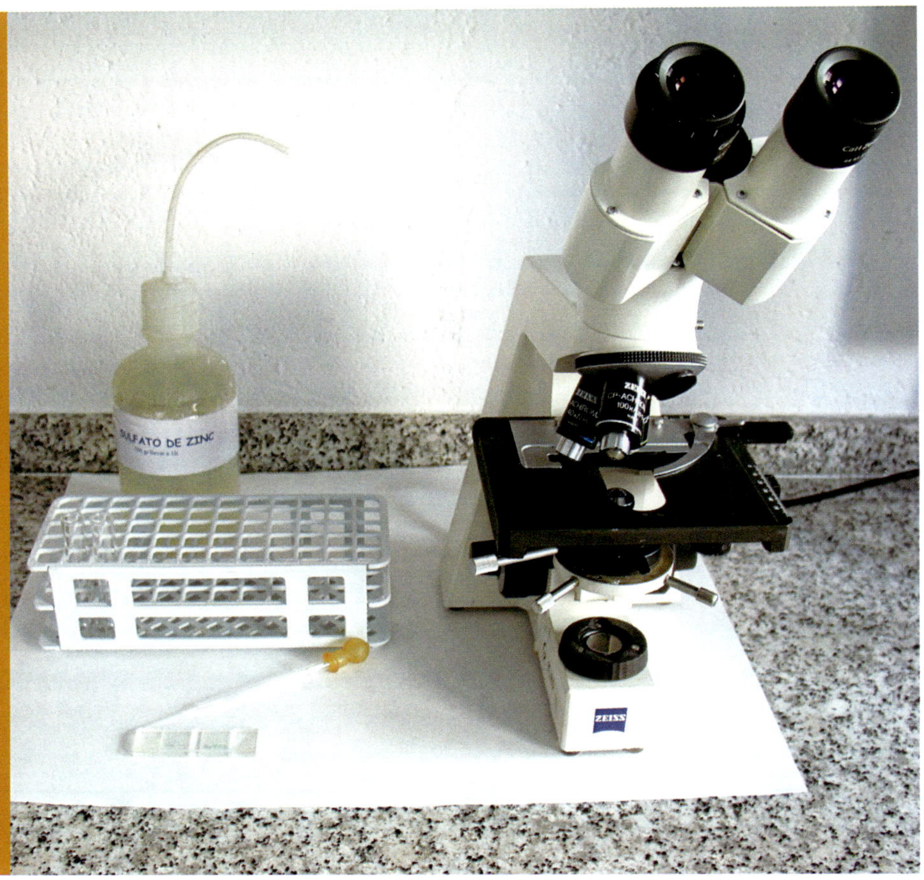

1 How are samples submitted to a laboratory?

If the results obtained by a laboratory are to have any meaning, samples must be correctly collected and stored under the best possible conditions to prevent them from deteriorating prior to their arrival at the laboratory. Results obtained using incorrectly stored samples are of little use. To avoid this, some laboratories destroy such samples prior to analysis.

If vets do not want to waste their own time, or that of others, they must be aware of exactly what the laboratory requires prior to collecting samples.

Irrespective of the type of analysis to be requested and the type of sample to be submitted, certain important aspects must be taken into account. For example:

- The sample(s) must be fresh and must be correctly collected and stored.
- Each sample must be correctly labelled and identified.
- The following information must be submitted together with the samples: owner's name, clinical signs of the animals, number of animals affected or at risk of being affected, *post mortem* alterations, proposed diagnosis and type of sample submitted.

Generally speaking, stool samples can be collected and submitted in the extraction gloves themselves or placed in clean glass or, even better, plastic recipients. They should be correctly packaged to prevent breakage. A knot should be tied close to the faecal matter and the air removed in order to prevent further development of the parasitic forms. Due to the high humidity of the gloves when extracting the faeces, they should be identified using a specific marker pen or by inserting a paper containing the note and tying another knot. If necessary (especially when sampling early in the day in hotter months and with no access to a fridge), samples must be stored cold using ice or any cold accumulator for 8-24 hours. They must obviously be submitted using a fast or express courier service.

2 What is the method of choice for detecting nematode eggs in bovines?

The first diagnostic step is analysis of the stools of suspect animals. Macroscopic analysis is important as it provides interesting information as regards interpretation of the results. Faecal consistency and visible particles that appear in the depositions, as well as the colour, presence or absence of blood, smell, etc. should also be taken into consideration. Mature rings of cestodes or eliminated worms may also be observed.

A microscopic examination, which allows a qualitative analysis that may offer a very interesting overview of the status of the problem animal(s), is then undertaken. Even the simplest methods provide important information, although concentration or special methods for each particular case are recommended.

Direct methods involve emulsifying a small amount of faeces, with the help of a glass rod or similar instrument, directly on a microscope slide, together with one or more drops of water if the sample is very dry. If the stools are diarrhoeal they can be spread directly on the microscope slide. It should be noted, however, that this is a fairly unreliable method if the infection is mild or when the faecal mass is large, as is the case with bovines.

Whenever possible, indirect methods, which basically comprise concentrating the parasitic forms by emulsifying the stools in a solution with a higher density than water, thereby concentrating the eggs, larvae, oocysts, cysts, etc. by flotation, should be used.

Flotation methods involve emulsifying the faeces in 20-30 times their volume of a saturated salt solution (1.15) or any

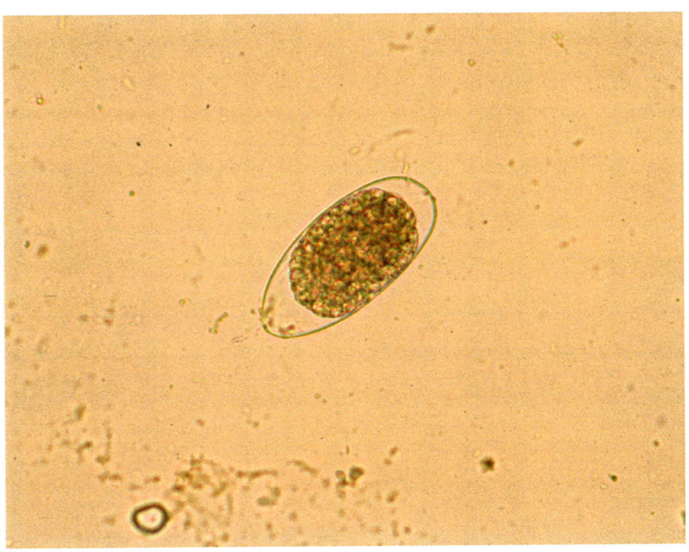

Strongyle eggs are ovoid, colourless and thin-shelled. They range between 70-90 µm in length and 40-60 µm in width, except for those of *Nematodirus* and *Marshallagia*, which are more than 150 µm in length. Generic identification on the basis of their morphology is very difficult. As such, they are identified on the basis of the infective third stage larvae obtained after incubation of the eggs in coproculture, which involves maintaining the faeces in a humid environment at a temperature of around 25 °C for 7-10 days.

other solution of sufficient density (1.280-1.440). After removing the faeces by filtration, the solution is allowed to stand for 25-30 minutes and various samples are taken from the surface of the liquid using a bent platinum loop or inverted haemolysis tube. The samples obtained are placed on a microscope slide and examined under the microscope without a cover-glass.

Egg elimination must always be quantified. Although there are various techniques available for this, the most widely used is the McMaster technique, or any of the modifications thereof, which requires the use of a McMaster slide. This slide has two transversally opened chambers, with a cover-glass on their upper part etched with two 1 cm^2 squares, one for each chamber. Each of these cells is 1.5 mm in depth. The steps to be followed and variations on the original method can be consulted in any book on parasitology techniques. The number of eggs in the stool sample is calculated by a simple rule of three that takes into account the volume of the chamber, the amount of sample analysed and the mean number of eggs counted in each of the McMaster device chambers.

3 What clinical and zootechnical information should be taken into account when submitting a sample?

Trichostrongylidosis is associated with a series of clinical signs, the most important being diarrhoea. The clinical presentation is usually accompanied by lower weight gain, poor general health status and lack of appetite, together with other more or less characteristic alterations to blood composition, such as hypoalbuminaemia with diminished total protein concentration, and anaemia, which is a characteristic sign of infection by haematophage species such as *H. placei*, although it may also present in animals with a chronic condition caused by non-haematophage species.

Infection is often clinically non-obvious, tends to be chronic and it is difficult to identify signs compatible with gastrointestinal nematodosis (mainly trichostrongylidosis).

Animal production yields usually decrease, therefore zootechnical parameters are often of great interest. The nutritional deficiencies associated with anorexia and the excessive loss of plasma proteins via the digestive mucosa enhance the deterioration presented by some infected animals.

4 What other tests can help diagnose an outbreak of trichostrongylidosis?

Apart from the clinical and production data for the herd, other analyses and tests can be used to establish a definitive diagnosis.

As trichostrongylidae eggs are very similar and their size for the various genera and species overlaps, and considering that the pathogenicity of these species also differs, the most important species in terms of pathogenic potential and presence in the faeces to be tested must be identified whenever possible. This requires the faeces to be cultured in the laboratory to obtain L3s, which can be readily identified by an experienced technician following certain guidelines.

To this end, the faeces are placed in suitable recipients at the temperature (approximately 25 °C), humidity (water and/or charcoal should be added every two days, if required, to maintain the correct humidity) and oxygen level (the sample is mixed regularly to ensure it is correctly aerated) required for post-embryonic development to the L3 stage. This stage is reached after some 7-10 days. After this time, the sample is wrapped in a double gauze and placed in water in a device (Baermann-Wetzel apparatus) containing a few

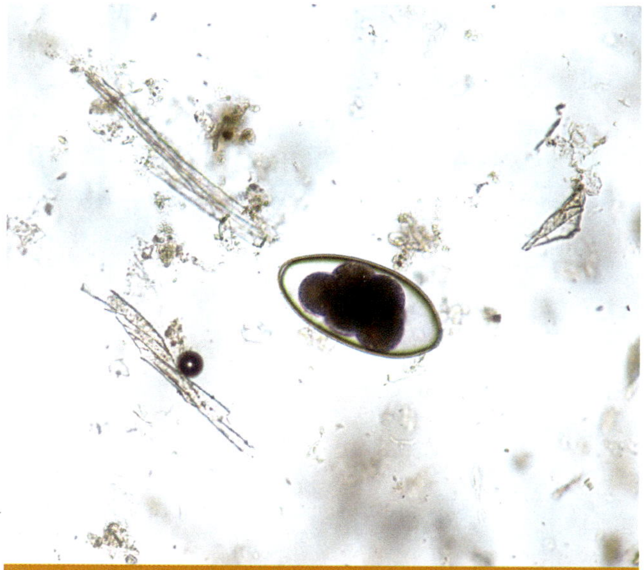

Nematodirus eggs are large and contain eight blastomeres. The first two moults occur inside the egg, with the infective larva breaking the shell and emigrating to the grass. This biological characteristic is of interest from an epidemiological viewpoint.

drops of dispersant to prevent the larvae remaining attached to the surface due to surface tension. Finally (after a further 5-8 hours), the first 10 mL of water, which contains the L3 that have been concentrated by sedimentation, is collected and placed in a test tube.

A single drop of this sediment, together with a drop of Lugol's solution, is placed between a microscope slide and cover-glass and observed under the microscope to identify the larvae.

A simple technique has been recently described that facilitates the identification of the eggs of the species *H. contortus*, which is characterised by a marked degree of haematophagy. This method is based on the affinity shown by the shell of eggs from the ovine species *H. contortus* for a lectin, namely PNA (*peanut agglutinin*), that is not seen in other species of gastrointestinal nematodes. The use of PNA with fluoresceine isothiocyanate allows *Haemonchus* eggs to be visualised when observed under fluorescence due to their bright yellow colour, which distinguishes them from the eggs of other parasite species.

For various reasons, many of which depend on the worm and host concerned or are environmental in nature, faecal egg and larvae counts do not always provide a clear picture of the infection severity. As a result, and whenever possible, attempts should be made to count and identify the worms from either an animal from the herd that has died or by performing a necropsy on a slaughtered animal.

The alterations present in the carcass such as anaemia, gastritis, enteritis, emaciation, etc., also provide important information, which can often prove definitive. One of the most characteristic alterations caused by trichostrongyliases is hypoproteinaemia, with a marked decrease in albumin levels.

The use of complementary techniques that demonstrate blood and enzymatic alterations, such as haemoglobin and haematocrit levels, etc., may also be of great use. Determination of the immunoglobulin levels may also be helpful, although more from an epidemiological viewpoint.

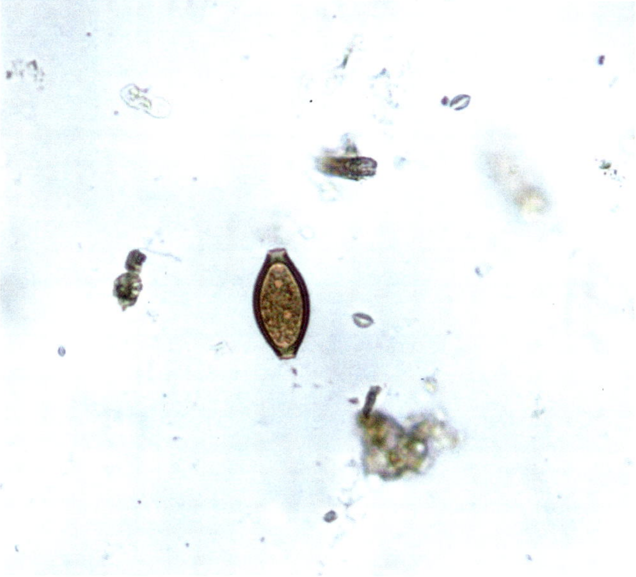

Trichuris eggs are lemon-shaped, with very curved sides and a very thick shell, and are yellowish-brown in colour. The mucous layer surrounding the egg can easily be seen on both sides, extending beyond the outline of the egg itself. They are not segmented when eliminated to the exterior. They measure 70-80 × 30-42 µm.

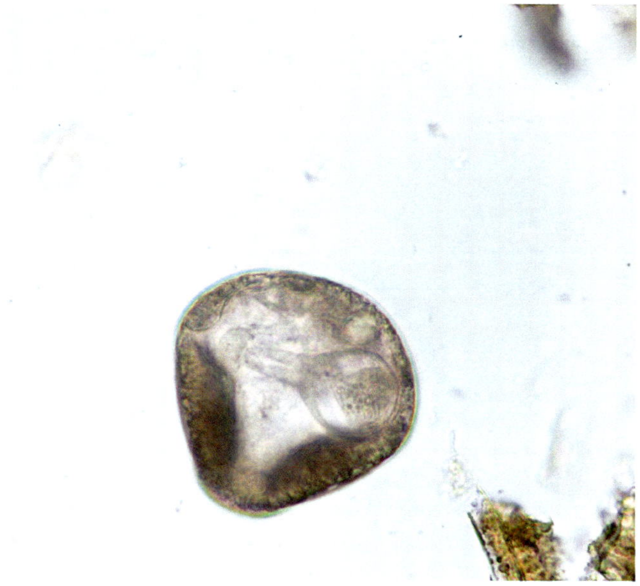

Moniezia eggs have a thick covering, or embryophore, with a quadrangular (*M. benedeni*) or triangular morphology (*M. expansa*). The hexacanth embryo or oncosphere in their interior is surrounded by a structure typical of the pyriform group or apparatus. Eggs from *M. benedeni* (>75 µm), the most common species in bovines, are larger than those from *M. expansa* (56-67 µm), which is more common in smaller ruminants.

10 Which trichostrongylidae do bovines share with other animal species?

The vet is notified of a case of diarrhoea in a Friesian heifer aged 11 months, from the north of Spain, belonging to a farmer with 20 cows stabled over the winter months. In February, the animals had already been almost three months without grazing. The family lives in the upper floor, which can be accessed by a stairway from the cowshed itself. The shed has a traditional distribution, with a manger along one wall and a large door that the cows use in spring and summer to access the common pasture, which is also grazed by horses from neighbouring areas. Various flocks of sheep pass through these pastures early in the morning and late in the evening. The coprological analysis for the heifer showed a large quantity of strongyle eggs.

1. Do all strongyle eggs in cows come from trichostrongylidae?
2. Which species are shared by bovines and other herbivores?
3. How was winter ostertagiosis discovered in stabled animals?

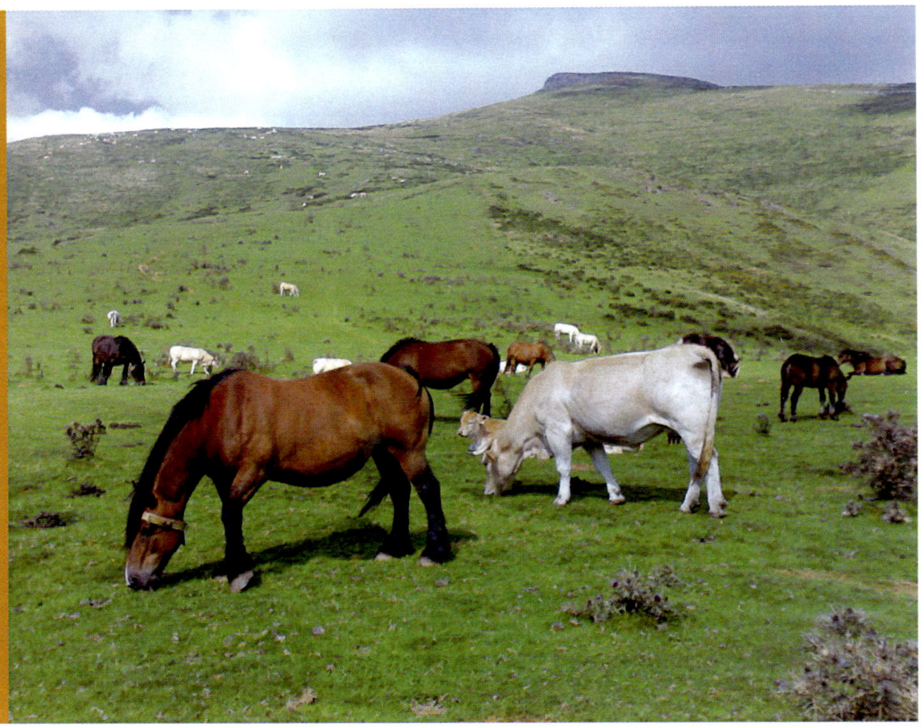

1 Do all strongyle eggs in cows come from trichostrongylidae?

Obviously not. Other nematode species can also be found alongside trichostrongylidae in the bovine digestive system, although the latter tend to be the most abundant. Irrespective of their relative importance, the following parasite species have been found in cattle from the Iberian peninsula: *Bunostomum phlebotomum, Capillaria bovis, Toxocara vitulorum, Oesophagostomum columbianum* and *Oesophagostomum radiatum*. However, trichostrongylidae are the most important for various reasons. Infections are normally mixed, although some tend to predominate under certain circumstances or in certain geographic regions.

As the clinical diagnosis of trichostrongylosis is very often imprecise, a coprological analysis is of considerable use. However, the fact that infections are mixed under natural conditions, with the involvement of various representatives from the most prevalent genera, means that it is by no means easy to determine which species is of greatest pathogenic importance on the basis of the morphological characteristics of the eggs excreted in faeces.

It must also be taken into account that, despite the morphological differences between trichostrongylidae species, it is very difficult to identify them, even for a person with some experience in the field. The eggs have a thin shell, contain more than 16 blastomeres when eliminated in faeces and differ slightly in terms of shape and size (70-90 µm on average). Some characteristics are, however, of use. For example, *Haemonchus* eggs are barrel-shaped, with curved sides and identical poles, whereas those of *Trichostrongylus* are thinner and have one pole more pointed than the other. *Ostertagia* eggs are also thin, have a somewhat oblique longitudinal axis and one of the poles is more pointed, whereas those of *Cooperia* are thin, with parallel sides and rounded poles. Eggs from *Nematodirus* species are around 2-3 times larger and always present fewer than 16 blastomeres, thus making them easy to identify.

As such, except for *Nematodirus*, the differences between the eggs of the other genera do not allow their identification in order to establish a diagnosis. Consequently, coprocultures must be performed to obtain larvae whose morphological characteristics allow a specific or generic diagnosis.

The best medium for growing eggs and larvae (L1, L2 and L3) is unaltered faeces eliminated by the animals. This medium contains sufficient oxygen, humidity and temperature to guarantee suitable growth conditions. If possible, the culture should be maintained at 25 °C and should be regularly aerated. L3s develop after 7-10 days and, once recovered, can be identified under a microscope following the corresponding guidelines. These guidelines take into account the length of the larva, including the cuticle surrounding it, the length from the tip of the tail to the posterior end of the sheath, the number and shape of intestinal cells, and other characteristics.

2 Which species are shared by bovines and other herbivores?

The following table shows that some of the gastrointestinal nematode species of greatest pathogenic importance in bovines (which we can term "primary pathogens") are also able to infect other domestic ruminants (sheep and goats).

This is particularly true for the most important species from the genera *Haemonchus, Oesophagostomum* and *Ostertagia.*

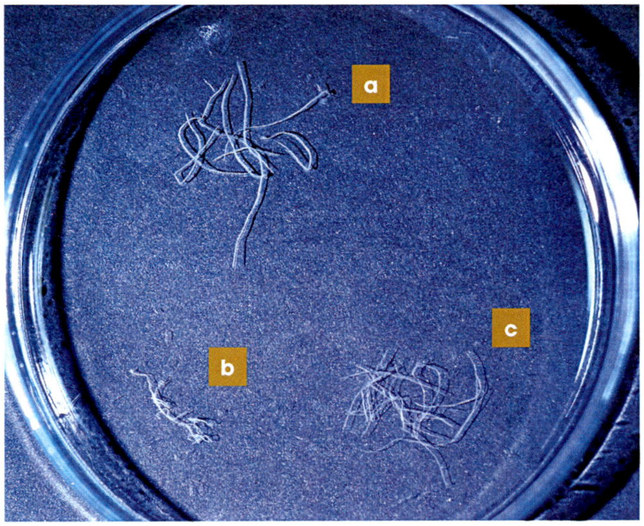

Haemonchus (a), *Trichostrongylus* (b) and *Ostertagia* (c). *Haemonchus* is the largest of the abomasal parasites: the female measures more than 2 cm and the male is slightly smaller. Male *Teladorsagia* tend to measure less than 1 cm, with the females being slightly larger. *Trichostrongylus* is the smallest: females measure less than 8 mm and males around 6 mm. Males can easily be differentiated from females as they are smaller, thinner and present an extension at their posterior end that resembles the head of a pin.

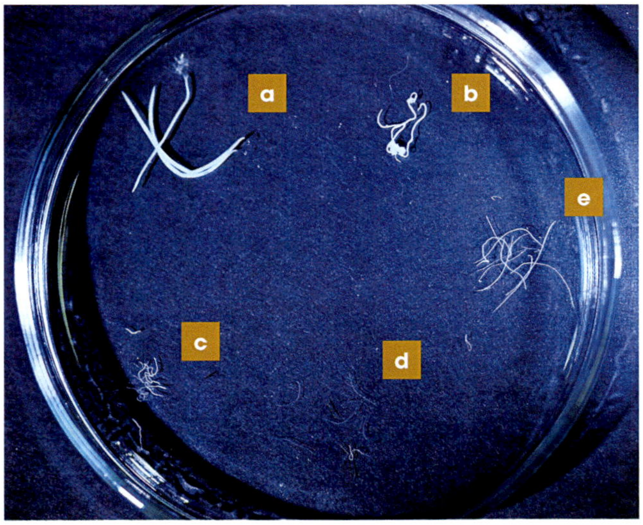

Bunostomum (a), *Nematodirus* (b), *Trichostrongylus* (c), *Strongyloides* (d), *Cooperia* (e). Small reddish worms with a slightly swollen anterior end (*Cooperia*) can often be found in the small intestine along with other, very small (around 5 mm) whitish worms from the genus *Trichostrongylus*. The various species of *Nematodirus* are large and generally coiled. The largest nematodes, which are easily recognisable from their buccal capsule, are from the genus *Bunostomum*.

Some species from the genera *Trichostrongylus* (*T. axei*, which is also an equine parasite), *Cooperia* (*C. oncophora*, *C. punctata* and *C. macmasteri*) and *Haemonchus contortus* are also shared. The species *Nematodirus helvetianus*, which predominates in bovines, has also been found in sheep.

The significance of this lack of host specificity is that, in order to be fully effective, prophylactic and control measures must take this fact into account. As the establishment of measures targeting only one of several herbivore species that share a pasture may prove ineffective and fail to control the problem.

3 How was winter ostertagiosis discovered in stabled animals?

The importance of *Ostertagia ostertagi* infection increased markedly in 1957 when Martin, Thomas and Urquhart discovered 10 outbreaks of chronic severe diarrhoea and emaciation in heifers aged 12 to 18 months from milk herds in the west and south of Scotland. In eight of these 10 outbreaks the affected animals had grazed for the first time between October and January prior to winter stabling. In most herds the heifers had grazed alongside adult cows sharing the same areas, whereas in others they had grazed alone, although the same pastures had been used by adult animals the previous year.

None of the animals presented diarrhoea prior to stabling, although the physical condition of the majority of them was somewhat poor.

After stabling for a period of between 3 and 10 weeks, most animals presented profuse and persistent diarrhoea, except for short remission periods, accompanied by weight loss, lack of appetite and thirst. These symptoms continued for several weeks, and the majority of animals subsequently died, with antiparasitic and antibiotic therapy having no effect.

An individual clinical examination of some animals confirmed their poor physical status and extreme weakness, and found that their hind third, limbs and tail were completely covered with faeces. These faeces were very liquid, with a normal colour and free from blood. Defecation was not

Major gastrointestinal nematodes in bovines that also infect other domestic herbivores

	Cow	Sheep	Goat	Horse
Bunostomum phlebotomum	X	X		
Cooperia macmasteri	X	X		
Cooperia oncophora	X	X		
Cooperia punctata	X	X		
Haemonchus contortus	X	X	X	
Haemonchus placei	X			
Nematodirus helvetianus	X	X		
Oesophagostomum columbianum	X	X	X	
Oesophagostomum radiatum	X		X	
Teladorsagia circumcincta	X	X	X	
Ostertagia crimensis	X	X		
Ostertagia lyrata	X			
Ostertagia ostertagi	X	X	X	
Trichostrongylus axei	X	X	X	X
Trichostrongylus colubriformis	X	X	X	
Trichostrongylus vitrinus	X	X	X	

accompanied by tenesmus in any case. The faeces occasionally recovered their normal consistency for short periods of time, although the diarrhoea subsequently reappeared.

Weight loss was very marked and subcutaneous and submandibular oedema was observed in a few animals.

Some animals presented mild anaemia and decreased plasma protein levels and eliminated faeces containing varying quantities of gastrointestinal nematode eggs, although the count exceeded 1000 EPG in most cases (the highest value was 3500 EPG). In a few cases parasite elimination by the heifers was sufficiently low to allow the presence of a parasitic gastroenteritis to be ruled out; the animals that recovered eliminated very low quantities of eggs.

Paratuberculosis was ruled out in all cases using various methods. The only change observed in all autopsies performed was found in the abomasum and concerned a thickening of the fundal mucosa, intense hyperplasia and the presence of nodules 2-3 mm in diameter, with a central orifice and pink or dull red edges, and small ulcers. This nodular hyperplastic reaction led to a characteristic "embossed leather" appearance. The gastric contents of autopsied animals showed a high but variable number of adult nematodes and immature forms (between 11,000 and 250,000), approximately 25 % of which belonged to the genus *Ostertagia*. These findings confirmed that the symptoms (severe diarrhoea) were compatible with ostertagiosis, as traditionally described in bovine pathology textbooks.

Assuming that the heifers had not become infected whilst stabled, the authors were surprised that, in all outbreaks, the clinical signs presented between 3 and 10 weeks after the animals had been stabled. In some animals, the clinical signs only presented 5 months later, thus suggesting an aetiological process that was not parasitic in nature.

In the absence of more information and experimental studies, Martin *et al.* suggested that the clinical signs were due to inhibition of some of the larvae, with this delayed development being responsible for extending the prepatency period and the "late" onset of the clinical signs.

This particular presentation, which appeared in other countries as well as Scotland, was soon resolved and termed type II ostertagiosis. This disease is characterised by the appearance of clinical signs weeks or months after stabling and coincides with the de-inhibition and sexual maturity of fourth stage larvae shortly after moulting from L3 (*Early* L4 or EL4) ingested during previous grazing.

The epidemiological, pathological and therapeutic consequences of type II ostertagiosis are of major importance and deserve special attention in both dairy and beef herds.

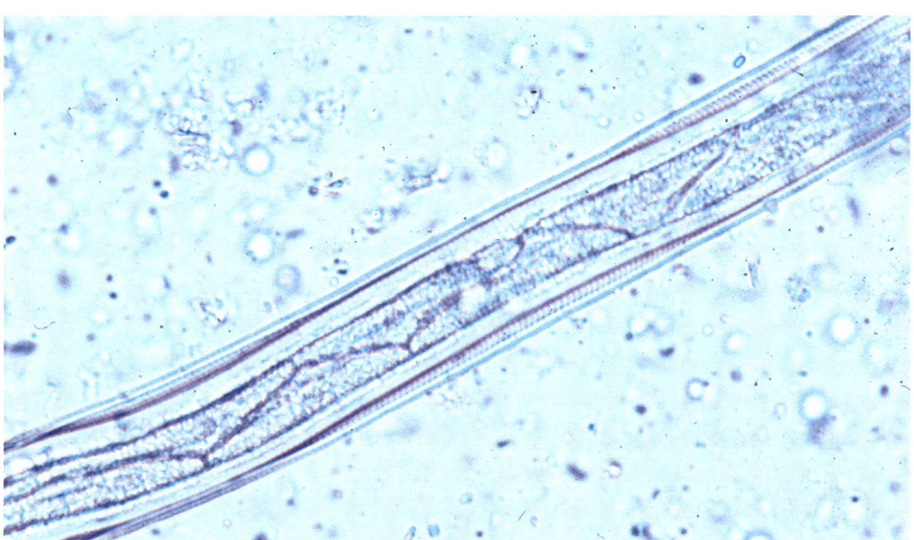

Third stage larvae are vermiform, measure between 600 and 1500 µm in length by 20-30 µm wide and possess a strongyliform-type oesophagus. They are characterised by being surrounded by the cuticle from the previous stage. The space between the distal end of the larva and the end region of the cuticle constitutes the "tail", which is used to classify larvae as short-tailed (20-40 µm), medium-tailed (40-80 µm) or long-tailed (>80 µm). In some genera the cells in their interior are imperceptible (*Bunostomum*), whereas other contain 8 cells (*Nematodirus*) and yet others 16 (*Haemonchus, Teladorsagia, Cooperia* and *Trichostrongylus*). Finally, some contain 32 cells (*Chabertia* and *Oesophagostomum*).

Biological cycle of *Trichostrongylidae*

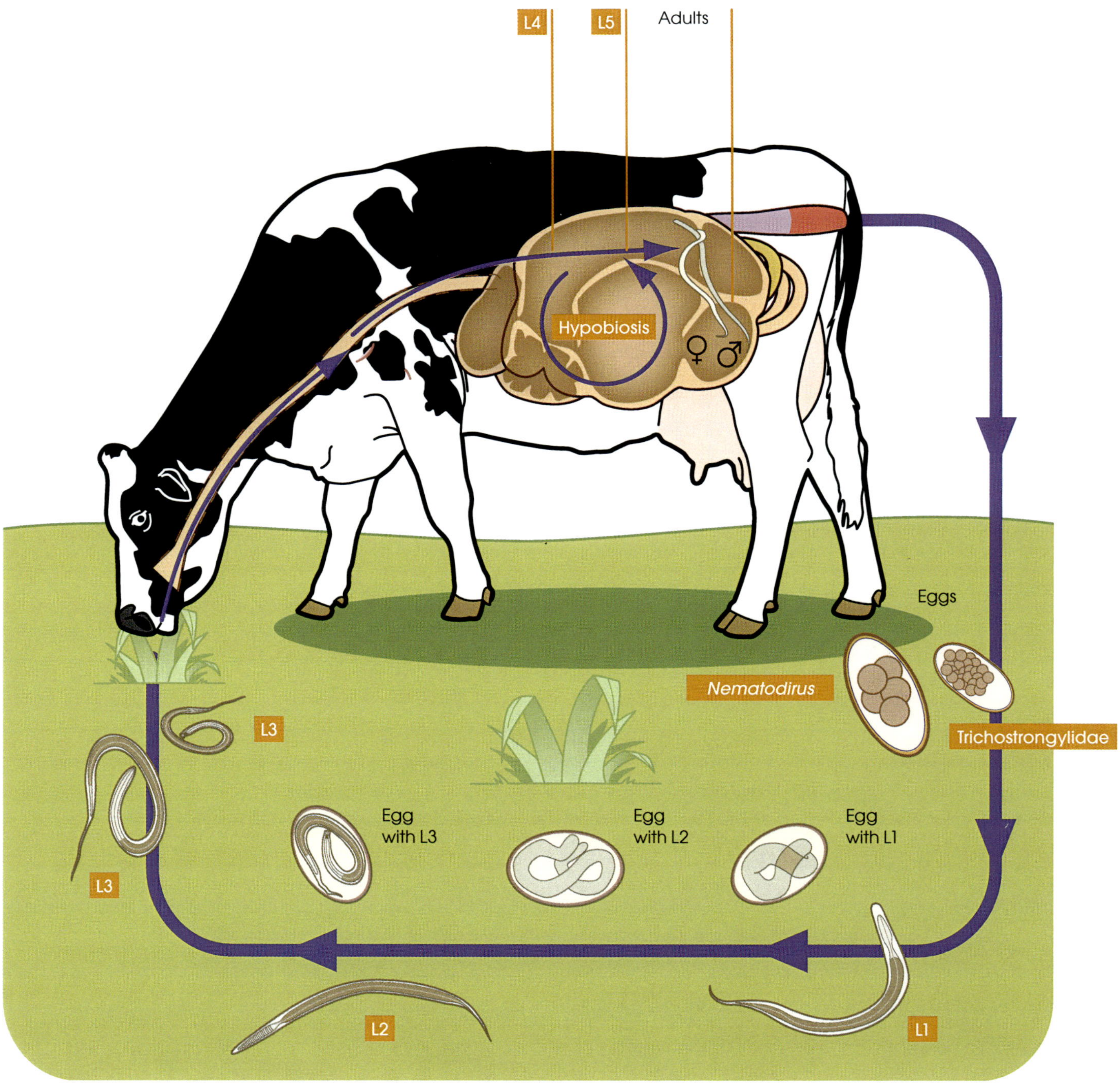

11 Have populations of antiparasitic-resistant helminths been detected?

There is a farm on the outskirts of Calahorra (La Rioja, Spain) on which two herds of cattle are each managed by a brother from the same family. The younger brother has 23 nursing cows and a bull enclosed in a shed with a small neighbouring corral. The other brother has 73 cows and a bull, which are housed in larger corrals, a small portion of which is roofed, equipped with feeders with tethers. Adult animals are accompanied by younger ones, which feed from their mothers, and adjacent corrals containing heifers and calves. All corrals are adjacent to a large, shared family estate. The animals are derived from French Limousin stock purchased 8 years previously. Both brothers had a falling out several years ago and different health control systems The former owns a veterinary products store and deworms his animals monthly, whereas the other only administers macrocyclic lactones to dry cows. The first-season animals from both herds have diarrhoea and, as they share pasturage, the elder thinks this could be due to resistant nematodes selected as a result of incorrect use of the products applied by his brother.

1. What evidence is available regarding the presence of resistant nematode populations in cattle?
2. What type of products exist to control trichostrongylosis?
3. Is it appropriate to treat animals and move them to clean pastures?

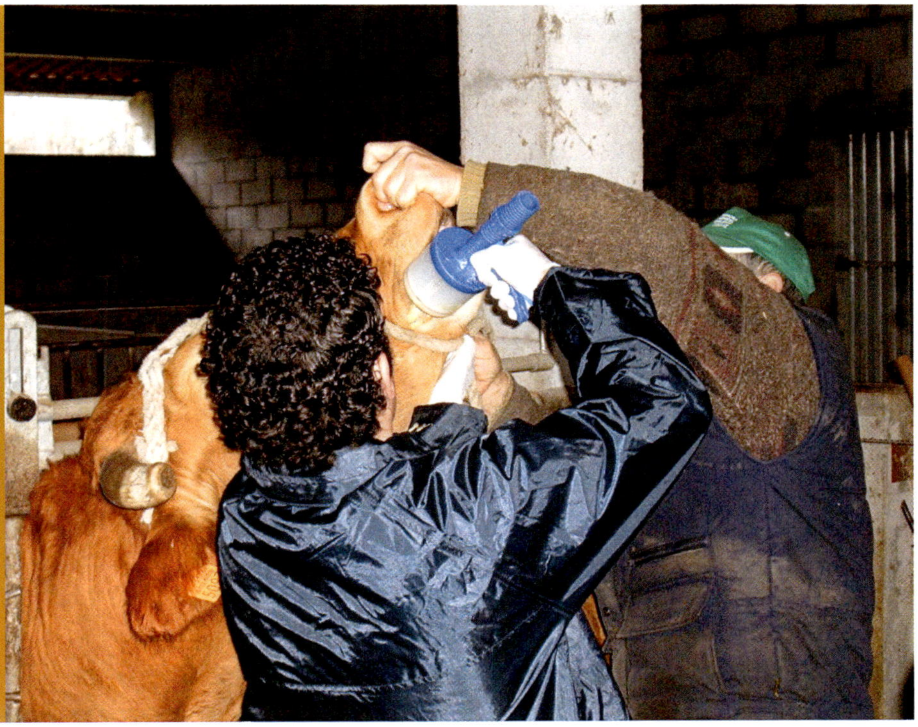

Image courtesy of Dr. A. Paz.

1 What evidence is available regarding the presence of resistant nematode populations in cattle?

Three years after the launch of thiabendazole in 1961, studies noting the varying efficacy of this anthelmintic against *Haemonchus contortus* in mixed infections in sheep began to appear. Reports concerning the resistance of some trichostrongylidae species from different regions to benzimidazoles were published in the 1970s and 1980s. These initial reports were followed by others concerning resistance to other chemical groups, such as imidazothiazoles and macrocyclic lactones, although almost of all of them referred to trichostrongylidae parasites in sheep and goats. However, some reports regarding bovine parasites, such as the resistance of *Cooperia* spp. to moxidectin in Australia, were also published.

It is curious that, irrespective of the chemical group concerned, anthelmintic resistance tends to appear earlier in countries in the southern hemisphere.

Indeed, the situation in sheep has reached such a high level that breeding and farming is now almost impossible on farms in some countries. However, for reasons that remain unclear, the incidence of anthelmintic resistance in bovines is much lower than that found in sheep.

Although some European *Ostertagia ostertagi* "strains" are known to be resistant to morantel tartrate and fenbendazole, the situation in other countries is much more worrying due to their spread, with reports of severe situations in South America and New Zealand, where resistance, mainly of *Cooperia* spp. to ivermectin, was detected on more than 90 % of farms surveyed. However, it appears that anthelmintic resistance has been observed more frequently in sheep than in cattle worldwide, although there is nothing to prevent the development of resistance by bovine parasites. It is possible that one of the reasons for this inequality between sheep and cattle is the fact that the sheep and goats share parasite species and that the difference in pharmacokinetic profile for anthelmintics in goats means that the effective dose of these drugs is significantly higher than in sheep. Or it may simply be that the administration frequency is higher in small ruminants for production reasons and lower in cattle due to the production type and the need to avoid residues.

2 What type of products exist to control trichostrongylosis?

Although the majority of anthelmintics are able to cure parasite infections, or at least reduce their effects, very few reduce the parasite burden to levels at which the risk of reinfection is insignificant.

Although it is becoming increasingly clear that control of animal parasitoses in general, and trichostrongylosis in particular, must involve comprehensive control comprising the use of various different methods (chemical, biological, genetic, immunological, management, feeding, etc.) depending on the biology and epidemiology of the parasites concerned, and assuming that 100 % efficacy is never achieved if these methods are applied separately, current practice places greater emphasis on chemical control. This is based on molecules with a highly effective anthelmintic action that are able to eliminate the parasite populations hosted by an animal or to prevent the infective forms ingested by the animal with grass from becoming established and developing.

Despite the importance of helminth infections in veterinary medicine, very few broad-spectrum anthelmintics for the control of parasitoses in farm animals have been developed and marketed over the past half century.

First of all, it should be remembered how the efficacy of an anthelmintic is defined. According to the recommendations of the World Association for the Advancement of Veterinary Parasitology (WAAVP), the efficacy for each genus/species concerned should be expressed as a percentage as follows:

- Very high efficacy anthelmintic: >98 %.
- Effective anthelmintic: 90-98 %.
- Moderately effective anthelmintic: 80-89 %.
- Insufficiently active or inactive anthelmintic: <80 %.

In practical terms, any new anthelmintic must have an efficacy of at least 95 % against all, or the majority of, gastrointestinal nematode species.

The chemical groups contained in the most effective anthelmintics in veterinary medicine are described below.

Benzimidazole carbamates

Thiabendazole and albendazole belong to this group. The discovery of the first of these, thiabendazole (which was initially used as a fungicide), followed, shortly afterwards, by other benzimidazoles and pro-benzimidazoles, launched the era of broad-spectrum anthelmintics for the control of gastrointestinal nematodes in production animals. These anthelmintics are highly effective against various genera, including trichostrongylidae and other gastrointestinal nematodes, and their action is not restricted to adult worms: some are ovicides and many are also effective against the inhibited larvae of some species. The registration of thiabendazole was followed by that of other drugs from the same family, such as mebendazole, fenbenzadole and albendazole. Pro-benzimidazoles such as thiophanate and netobimin also showed high efficacy.

The limited solubility of these products means that their absorption is slow, with peak concentrations in circulation being reached at 24-36 hours post-administration. They act by interfering with β-tubulin polymerisation in parasites.

Imidazothiazoles and tetrahydropyrimidines

These groups, which are included in the same section as they share the same mode of action, include drugs such as levamisole and morantel tartrate. The first imidazothiazole was tetramisole, which is a 50 % racemic mixture of L and D isomers in which the L isomer is more active.

These compounds are also highly effective against adults and inhibited larvae from the majority of gastrointestinal nematodes. Depending on the route of administration, peak plasma levels are reached between 1 and 6 hours post-application. They act as nicotinic agonists, producing spastic paralysis in the parasites, which are expelled from the host.

Macrocyclic lactones

Avermectins and milbemycins belong to the group of macrocyclic lactones. The marketing of ivermectin as an oral anthelmintic for antiparasitic control in farm animals was revolutionary as, alongside its efficacy against a long list of helminths, it also proved to be effective against arthropods, and all at much lower doses than other anthelmintics. Avermectins are produced by fermentation of an actinomycete (*Streptomyces avermitilis*), with ivermectin and its natural precursor (abamectin), doramectin and eprinomectin being the most common. The milbemycins include moxidectin, which is obtained by fermentation of *Streptomyces cyanogriseus* subsp. *noncyanogenus*.

Lactones are also highly effective against the adults and inhibited larvae of numerous parasite species. Although moxidectin is the most effective against gastrointestinal nematodes, its efficacy against some arthropods is somewhat inferior to that of ivermectin.

The kinetics of ivermectin depends on the route of administration, with peak plasma levels being achieved within one day when administered orally but longer times being required when administered subcutaneously or as a bolus, etc. Moxidectin reaches its peak plasma level rapidly but its half-life is longer. These drugs bind to chlorine channel receptors and membrane transporters such as glycoprotein P and produce flaccid paralysis in the parasites.

Organophosphates

Main organophosphates include naphthalophos and trichlorfon. Although initially used as insecticides, their anthelmintic efficacy against gastrointestinal nematodes in ruminants was soon demonstrated. Naphthalophos was used until the 1980s, and occasionally in the 1990s, to combat anthelmintic resistance. However, their use in ruminants has been limited due to their low efficacy against some parasite species and their toxicity, although they are effective against inhibited forms of *Haemonchus*. They act by inhibiting cholinesterase activity in worms, thereby interfering with neurotransmission and inducing paralysis.

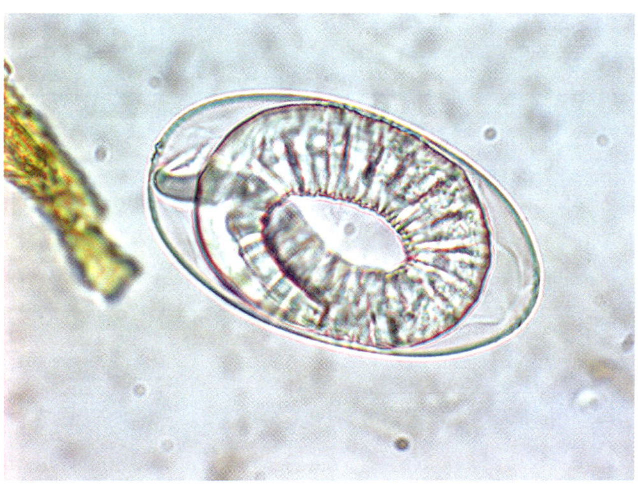

Resistance to benzimidazoles is easily detected due to the absence of an ovicide effect for these anthelmintics during both egg hatching (egg hatching test) and embryonic development (embryonic development inhibition test). Although the first analysis is easier to perform, and therefore more widespread, the correlation with respect to the resistant population detected *in vivo* is not always good and is strongly influenced by the age of the worms.

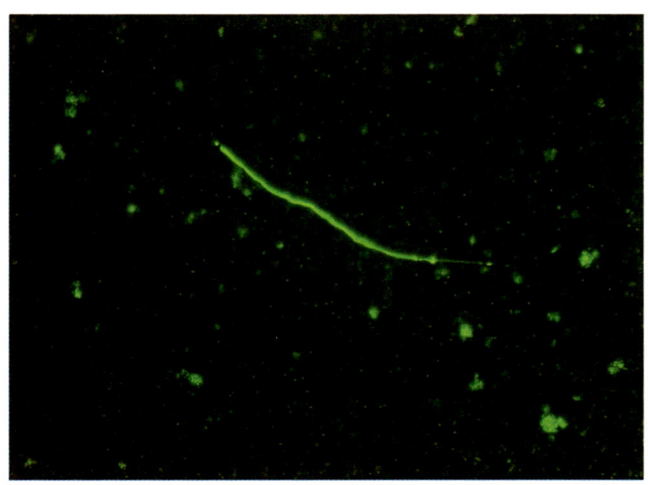

Worm populations resistant to macrocyclic lactones can be detected *in vivo* by feeding cultured larvae 1. The technique involves administering various concentrations of the drug to a culture medium containing *E. coli* bearing a fluorescent substance. The action of the drug is confirmed by the absence of this fluorescent substance in the digestive tract of the larvae as, if they are sensitive to the drug, they will present muscle atony.

Salicylanilides

Closantel is a substituted salicylanilide with narrow anthelmintic spectrum although it is highly effective against trematodes. Its activity against nematodes is more limited, except for *Haemonchus* and other species that live in bile ducts or neighbouring regions, possibly due to its albumin-binding affinity. The peak plasma concentration is achieved at between 8 and 48 hours post-administration, with a half-life of 2-3 weeks, thus implying good protection against infections that occur several weeks after initial administration of the drug.

Amino acetonitrile derivatives (AADs)

Although currently only marketed in a few countries, monepantel is the latest generation of anthelmintics to demonstrate a very high efficacy against many gastrointestinal nematodes in ruminants (cattle and sheep) at a dose of 2.5-5 mg/kg. It is rapidly absorbed after oral administration, with plasma levels decreasing after around 2 days. It acts as a nicotinic agonist but mediated by a single nicotinic acetylcholinesterase receptor.

It is sometimes necessary to broaden the spectrum of an anthelmintic or to increase its efficacy. Thus, in regions in which cestode or trematode infections have a similar importance to those produced by gastrointestinal nematodes, the need often arises to broaden the action to these parasite groups. The combination of two or more anthelmintics is often a good solution, and increased efficacy is often also required in the event of anthelmintic resistance.

3 Is it appropriate to treat animals and move them to clean pastures?

Generally speaking, for many years the main gastrointestinal nematode control strategies in ruminants worldwide have tended to involve one or both of the following methods: application of an anthelmintic and grazing management.

The foundations on which strategic treatments are based is a reduction in the number of infective larvae (L3) contaminating the grass. Obviously, the model and intensity of contamination with different parasite species varies widely according to various factors, such as climate and animal management.

Irrespective of this, attempts must be made to both reduce the risk of exposure of the animals to high L3 doses and to remove the parasite burden affecting the productivity. However, it must be noted that although sustained treatments tend to be advantageous, various key factors must be taken into account when designing control programs.

First of all, when the proportion of resistant worms in the population is low, any measure that is able to reduce the size of the parasite population favours resistance genes. Likewise, any practices that reduce contamination of the grass, whether by anthelmintics or management, also favour the selection of resistant worms.

A good example of how deworming and grazing programs promote the development of resistance is the practice of "deworming" and changing the animals to "clean" pastures. Under these conditions, all the parasites present in the host are exposed to the anthelmintic action. Subsequently, upon transferring the dewormed animals to a free (uncontaminated) areas, only resistant worms will contaminate the "clean pastures", which have very low contamination levels or, even worse, have not been grazed since at least the previous season. As there is no population of sensitive L3s in the grass to dilute or replace those that have survived the anthelmintic treatment, the resulting population will be resistant and parasite control programs will be affected and prove ineffective to some extent.

In the absence of the selection pressure exerted by the anthelmintics used to eliminate the parasite burden from the hosts, the practice of rotating grazing provided something similar. This was based on the fact that allowing a plot to rest for a certain period of time was considered to reduce or eliminate contamination of the grass, and therefore the risks to the animals, when that plot was grazed again.

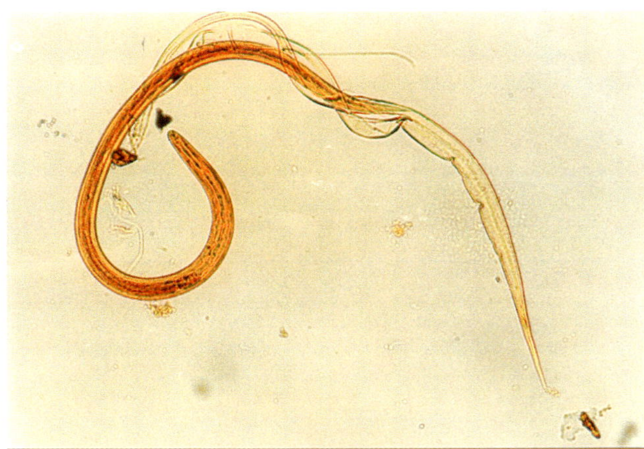

Various tests that detect benzimidazole resistance in third-stage larvae have been developed as an alternative to the ovicide effect of drugs. The effect of various types of anthelmintics (benzimidazoles, levamisole and ivermectin) can be measured using the larval development inhibition test with good correlations. In this technique, eggs are incubated in the presence of a food source (usually heat-treated *E. coli* bacteria) and the anthelmintic concerned up to the third stage. Developmental inhibition is readily identified.

12 What losses arise due to *Fasciola hepatica* on a dairy farm?

At an organic farm with 350 cows where the animals are maintained under living conditions as similar as possible to those that would be encountered in nature, the highest profits are obtained from those products derived from the very high quality milk produced. The farmer's computer system, which allows him to determine the quantity of milk produced by each animal and the steps each animal takes on the large expanse of land available for grazing fresh grass, has detected possible health problems. The animals do not receive any chemicals, including antiparasitic agents, and last year the farmer purchased 20 animals from a nearby farm. In the faeces from 80 % of the cows, the vet did not see Fasciola eggs in faecal samples from the animals during the prior year's examinations. Fasciola eggs are present now.

1. How has *Fasciola* appeared on this farm?
2. How many litres of milk are lost in a subclinical infection?
3. What methods exist to detect this infection in dairy cattle?

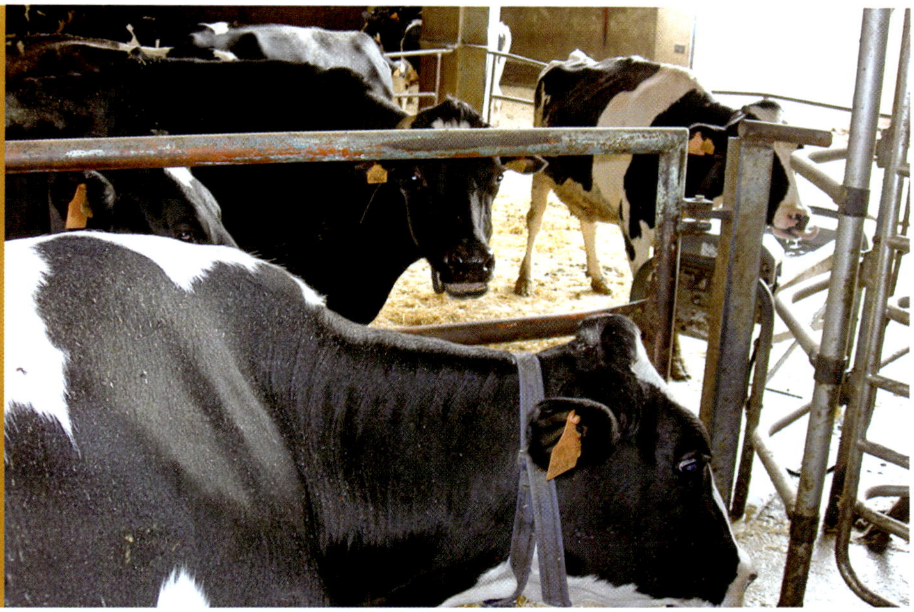

1 How has *Fasciola* appeared on this farm?

The key to establish fasciolosis control measures lies in understanding the factors involved in its transmission. The epidemiology depends on exposure of the animals to the risk of ingesting metacercariae present in the environment. Likewise, the ingestion of metacercariae depends on pasture management and the animal farming system used, as well as climate factors, pasture availability, humidity, etc.

The presence of *F. hepatica* depends on the existence of habitats suitable for lymnaeid snails, which have a very high biotic potential (a single snail can produce 25,000 infective stages in only three months), and appropriate temperature and humidity (>10 °C) for the reproduction of intermediate hosts, which can remain active essentially throughout the year. These factors are also essential for miracidia development and cercaria formation in molluscs.

Pastures become contaminated by animals with chronic infections, as liver flukes can live in the host for long periods of time (8-10 years). The continual elimination of liver fluke eggs by infected animals has been observed throughout the year. Wild animals may also be reservoirs.

In Spain, the most favourable period for cercariae emergence is between September and December, in other words autumn is the period of highest risk for animals. Moreover, the existence of metacercariae in autumn coincides with pasture depletion and the use of irrigated areas, which are generally highly contaminated.

The resistance of metacercariae to unfavourable environmental conditions means that some may remain in the grass if there is a mild winter.

As such, the incorporation of animals that could potentially be parasite reservoirs, climate conditions that favour parasite development both in the external environment and in intermediate hosts, and the ecological nature of the farm, especially an absence of anthelmintic use, can contribute to the presentation of clinical cases of fasciolosis in any given region.

2 How many litres of milk are lost in a subclinical infection?

Subclinical endemic parasitisms often go unnoticed in the event of decreased production yields. Helminth infections of the digestive system and annexes leads to a marked loss of appetite, which in fasciolosis may be as high as 15 %, thus affecting feed conversion indices, etc. After 6 months, subclinical bovine fasciolosis can lead to an 8-9 % variation in calf weight and up to a 5 % decrease in milk production. It should also be noted that the effects on animals in their growth period are much clearer, because their high feed conversion ability is wasted, sexual maturity is delayed and compensatory growth is often not achieved in animals freed from parasites using the appropriate treatment.

A significant relationship between anti-*F. hepatica* antibody levels in milk, as determined by an ELISA assay, and milk production has been demonstrated. The mean reduction in daily milk production in positive animals compared to their negative counterparts was 2 kg, whereas the difference between the latter and mildly positive animals was not statistically significant. Other reports have noted a decrease in milk production of up to 8 %.

However, such calculations are by no means easy and, in the best of cases, are of only limited value, even when estimates are obtained using experimental animals. Moreover, their value is minimal and they really only serve to support something that is already widely known, namely the economic and health repercussions of many parasitoses, and to confirm the importance of parasitic diseases in animal farming.

3 What methods exist to detect this infection in dairy cattle?

As well as more traditional methods, which attempt to demonstrate directly the presence of reproductive forms of liver flukes (eggs) there are other methods that aim to provide an understanding of the infection dynamics in herds without the need for individual analyses, the value of which is often limited.

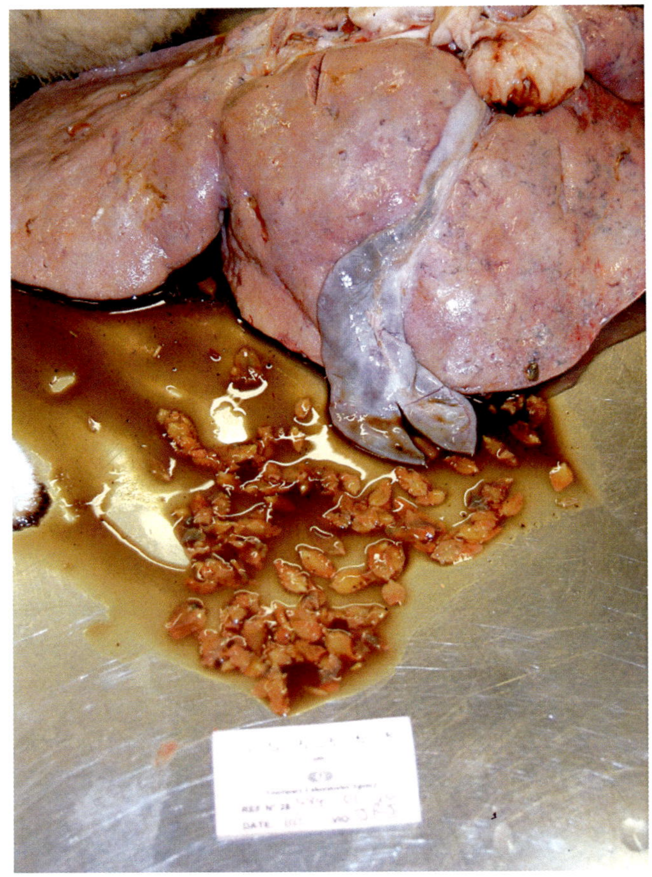

Although adult *F. hepatica* worms are found in the bile ducts of numerous mammals, in contrast to other species, bovines have a moderate receptivity to the presence of this helminth. Proline, which is synthesised and excreted in large quantities by *F. hepatica*, could mediate the hyperplastic response that occurs in the bile ducts.
Image courtesy of Dr. S. Mitchel.

The diagnosis of an infection has traditionally been performed by faecal analysis of a pool of faeces from groups of animals or randomly selected animals. Such analyses are of limited use given the poor sensitivity of techniques that use faecal samples (flotation and sedimentation), thus meaning that numerous false negatives may be obtained. Moreover, the prolonged endogenous development of the parasite means that the results are always negative in the early stages of a primary infection.

The cost and difficulty of this type of analysis also means that attempts have been made to develop other techniques for detecting such infections.

An assessment of the impact of fasciolosis on dairy herds requires appropriate methods and techniques that provide correct information which can be used to identify those animals that really need to be dewormed.

In this context, various studies have been undertaken over the past few years in an attempt to determine the utility of immune techniques for detecting the antibodies present in milk so that the milk tank samples taken for other tests can also be analysed for this purpose.

A test has been developed the sensitivity and specificity of which have been confirmed using the serum of suspect animals, that appears to be able to determine *F. hepatica* infection levels in herds by detecting antibodies in milk.

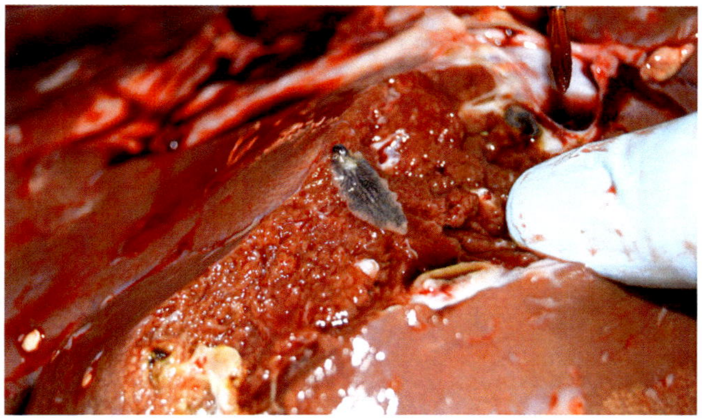

The organic reaction in cattle is more energetic than in sheep and leads to an intense tissue reaction, fibrosis and calcification of the bile ducts, which act as a mechanical barrier and confer significant resistance to future reinfections.

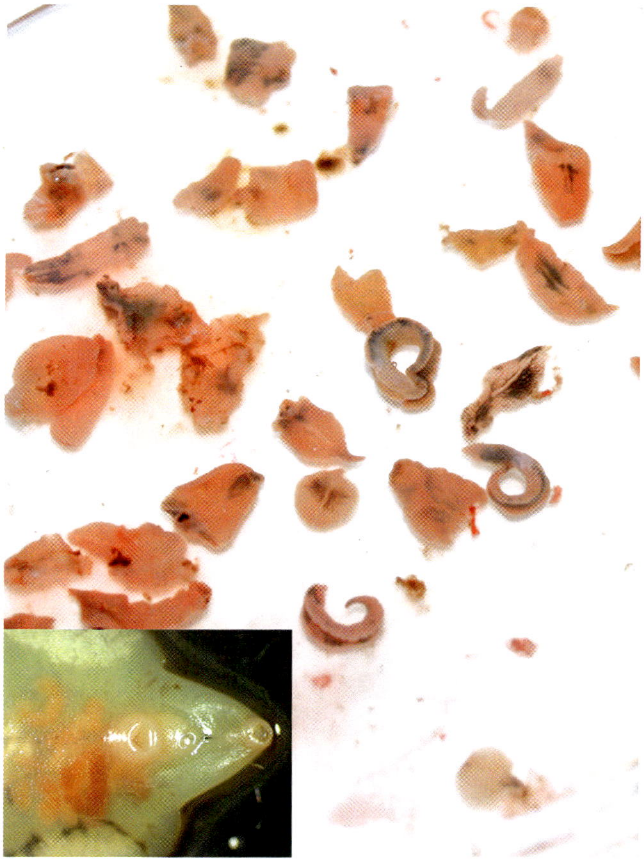

This wide-bodied, dorsoventrally flattened hermaphrodite helminth measures between 20 and 50 mm. Its most distinguishing features include the presence of two very closely located suckers, with the ventral sucker being larger than the oral, and a conical projection at its anterior end in which the oral opening is located. The main internal organs (digestive and reproductive apparatus) are highly branched.

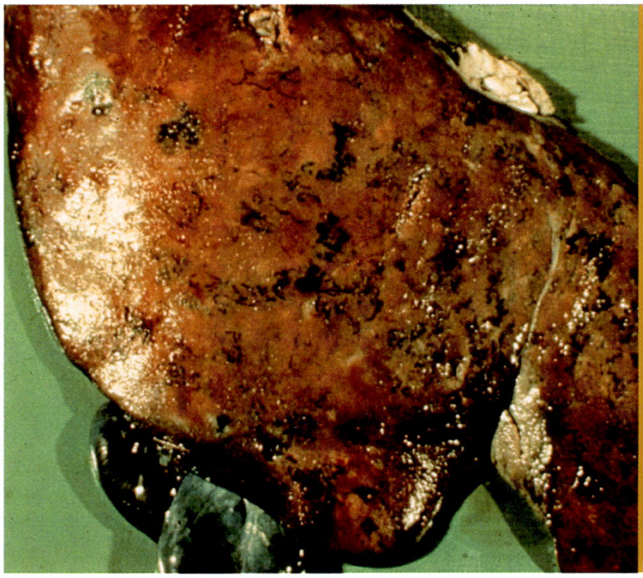

Acute fasciolosis is caused by the almost simultaneous ingestion of large quantities of metacercariae over a short period of time and normally affects animals exposed to the parasite for the first time. In contrast to sheep, it is an uncommon disease in cattle. Death occurs due to the extensive tissue trauma caused by the intrahepatic migration of immature liver flukes. *Image courtesy of Dr. C. Novoa.*

Biological cycle of *Fasciola*

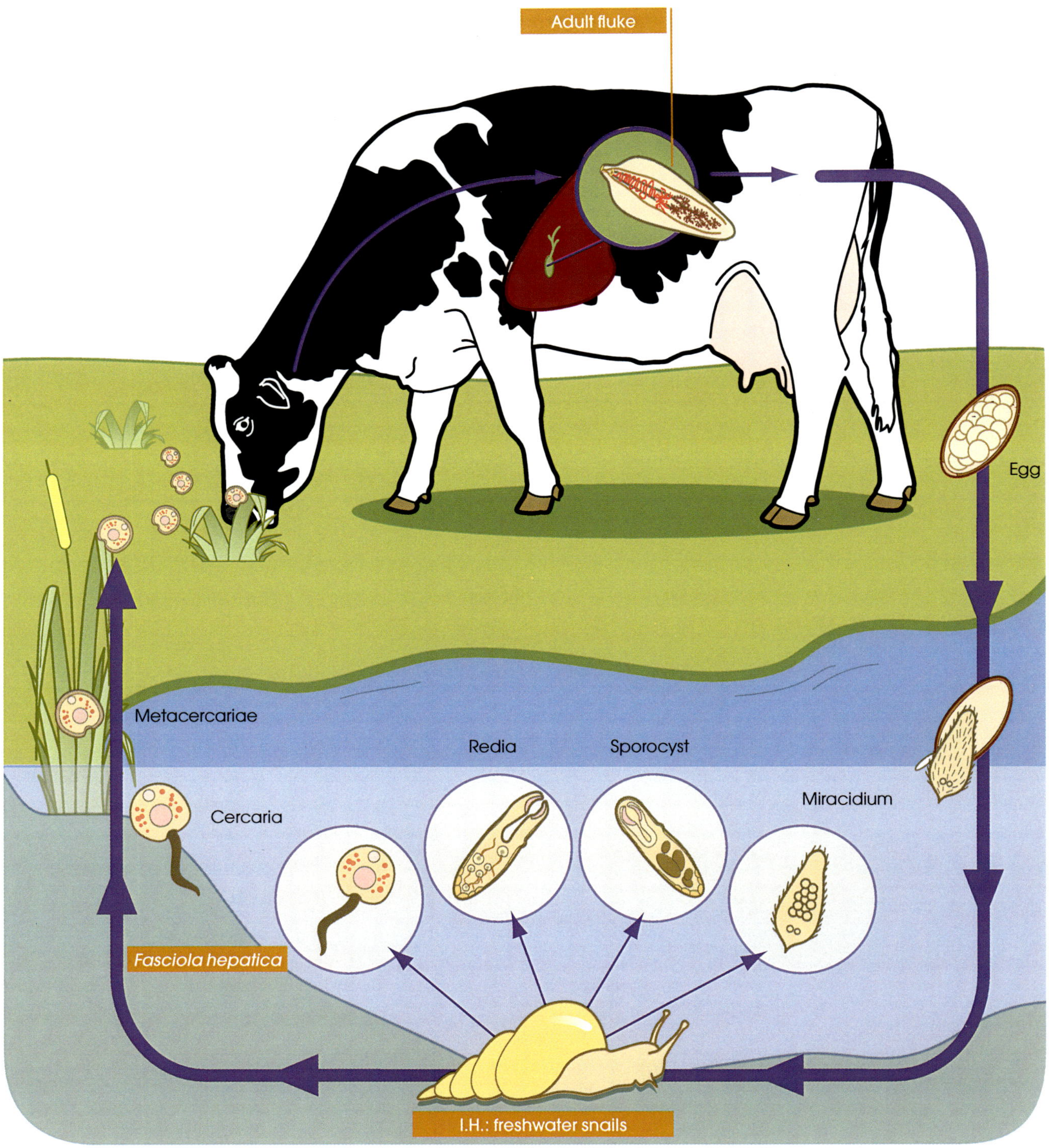

13 Is climate change affecting the biological cycle of *Fasciola hepatica*?

Several calves from the same farm present signs consistent with traumatic peritonitis, such as fever (41 °C), anaemia and extreme tiredness that causes them to become separated from the group. After the sudden death of two calves aged 8 and 14 weeks, routine necropsy confirms the presence of hepatic lesions consistent with acute fasciolosis. This parasitic infection had already been detected in adult animals on the farm by the presence of both eggs in faeces and antibodies in the milk tank samples, and fasciolicides were used as part of the parasite-control program, although the affected animals had not been treated due to their age.

1. Is acute fasciolosis common in very young calves?
2. Could this be due to climate change?
3. What measures can be taken in such cases?

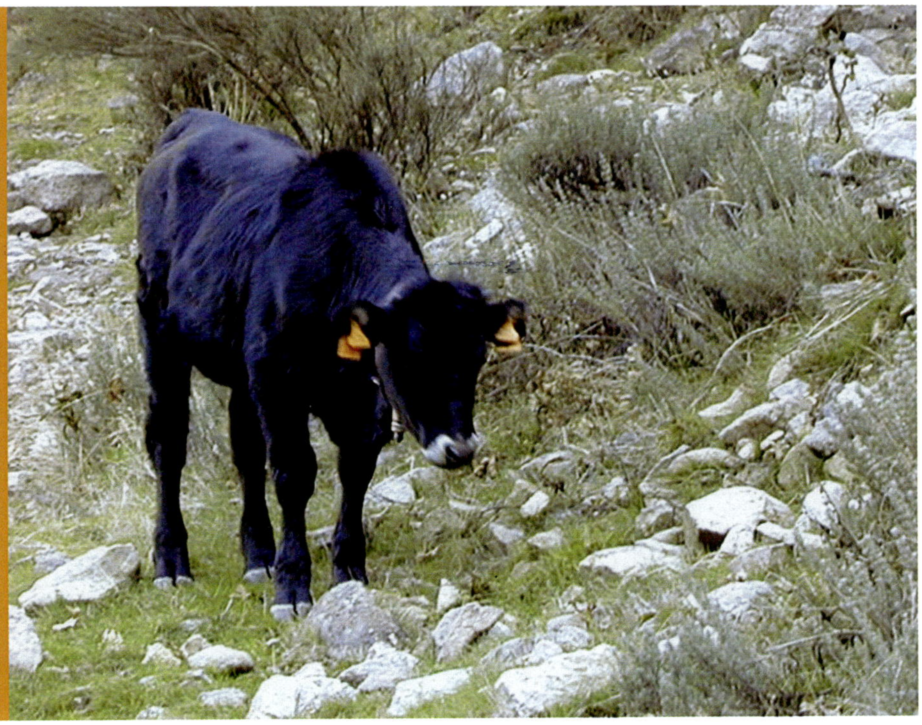

1 Is acute fasciolosis common in very young calves?

The appearance of acute or hyperacute fasciolosis in bovines is not common. Clinical signs related to the presence of this parasite vary widely, ranging from digestive alterations such as diarrhoea or lack of appetite to more general signs such as poor physical state, anaemia or oedema in the flanks. The organic lesions caused by a primary *Fasciola hepatica* infection are considered to be intense and serious due to the traumatic action of the parasite. Outbreaks in this species tend to be chronic.

After the ingestion of metacercariae when grazing, the immature flukes, are released in the duodenum and, after around 24 hours, the majority are found in the abdominal cavity. After a further 15 hours they cross Glisson's capsule and begin to migrate through the hepatic parenchyma. This process normally passes unnoticed except when a large quantity of metacercariae have been ingested. Only around 30 % are thought to reach the bile ducts, with the remainder being retained in other regions of the body or in the hepatic parenchyma. During the migratory phase they cause tissue destruction with the onset of haemorrhagic paths; the parasites can be found at the end of these paths. As they move randomly, the paths are serpentine, around 2-3 mm in diameter, and are caused both by feeding of the fluke and the trauma

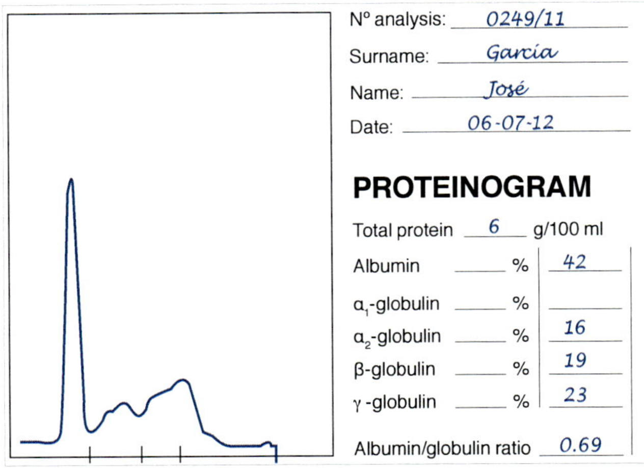

The onset of infection is marked by an increase in total plasma proteins due to an increase in immunoglobulin levels, mainly the gamma fraction, which subsequently decrease due to the loss of albumin at 10-11 weeks post-infection, coinciding with a loss of red blood cells and the onset of anaemia. A very marked peripheral eosinophilia also presents.

arising due to their spiny external coating. The secretion of toxic substances plays a key role in the onset of anaemia and hepatic tissue necrosis. The haemorrhagic paths are gradually replaced by cellular infiltrates over time, becoming grey or white in colour.

Once in the bile ducts, especially those of the left lobule, the appearance of an intense fibrous reaction and, after around four months, calcification of the duct walls, is common in bovines. This reaction usually prevents infections from being long-term as the flukes die and, if there is no reinfection, the connective tissue epithelialises and can be fully restored under experimental conditions.

A higher incidence of fasciolosis in bovines has been reported recently in young animals in northern regions in which winters were traditionally colder and this disease was considered to be a relatively well controlled endemic infection.

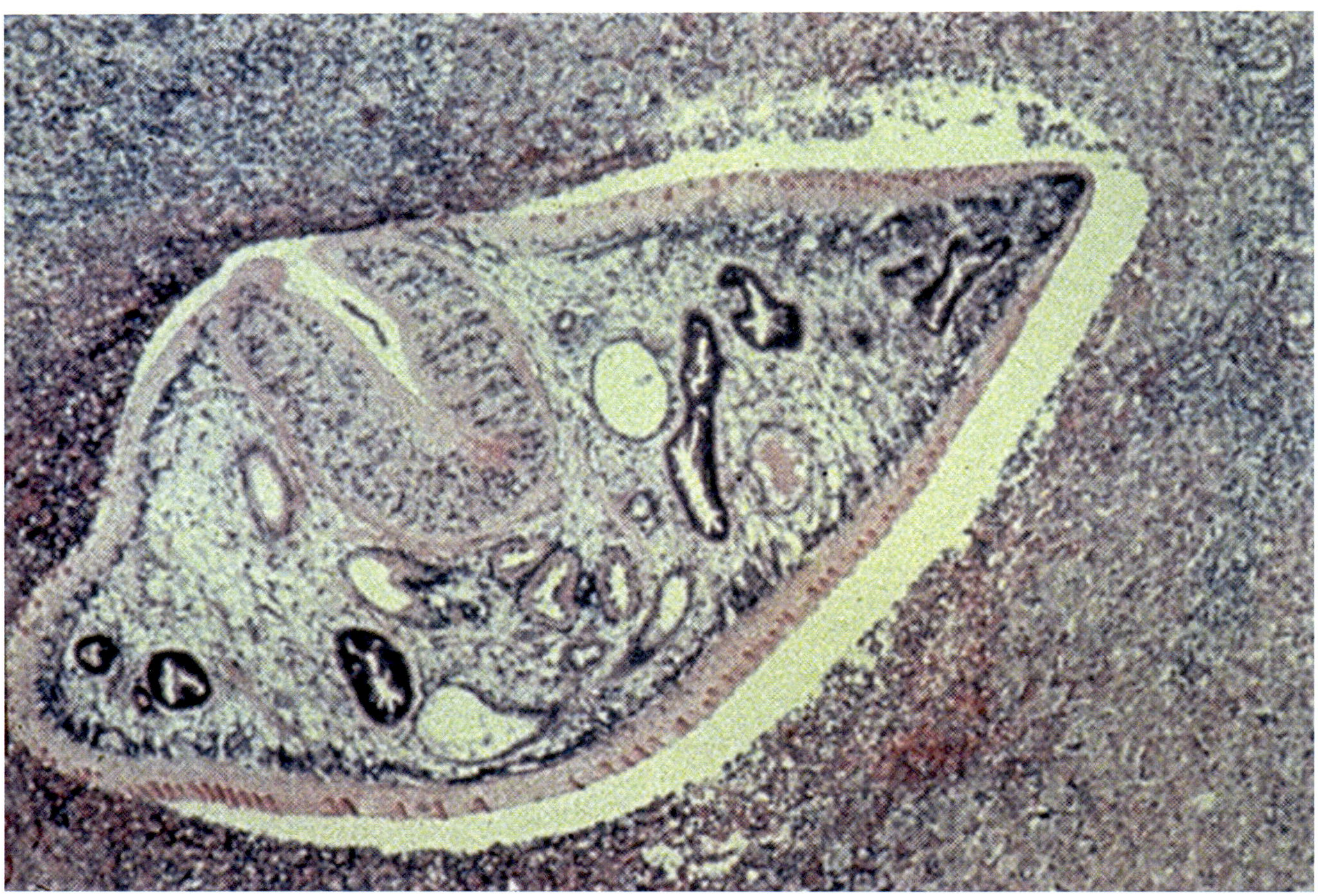

The worms reach the liver, where they cause a pathological condition characterised by necrosis and haemorrhage, one week after ingestion of the metacercariae. Acute processes often result in death due to the extensive trauma caused by the intrahepatic migration of immature flukes.

Fasciola hepatica is a flat, leaf-shaped trematode whose surface is covered with microscopic spines that, together with the action of the suckers, produce intense irritation of the epithelial cells, which modify their structure as a defensive reaction.
As a result of the extensive erosion and necrosis of the biliary mucosa, a marked inflammatory reaction that affects the neighbouring lamina propria develops in bovines.

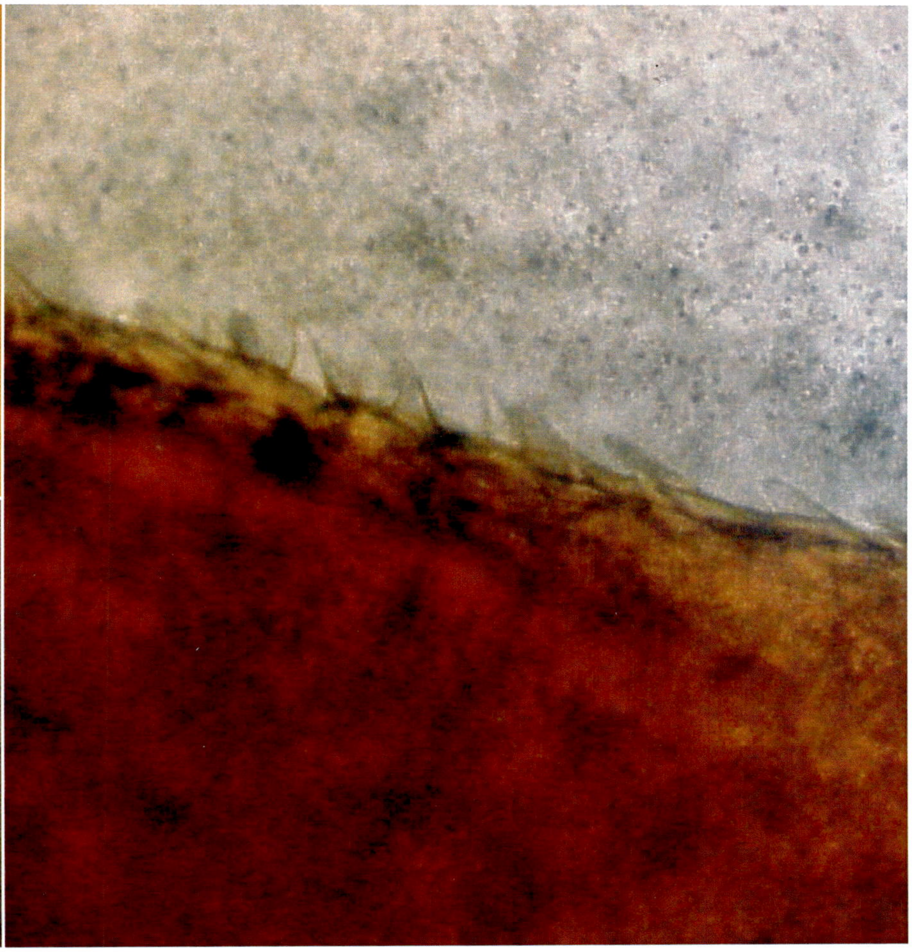

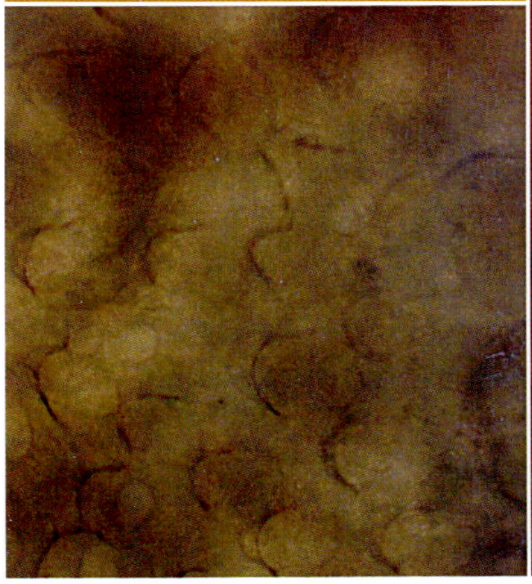

2 Could this be due to climate change?

Various reports over the past few years have indicated a change in the epidemiological model for fasciolosis, with a higher incidence of acute clinical disease and deaths in endemic regions of northern European countries. Recent findings suggest that metacercariae can survive the winter if the temperatures are not extreme, thus meaning that the animals are more exposed to infection under those conditions.

This situation is not new to countries in the south of Europe, such as Spain, where it has been common for many years. For example, in Spain the parasite is known to evolve in snails throughout the year, although at higher rates in the warmer months from the end of winter until the end of autumn. As very few snails survive below 0 °C, mild winters may result in greater pasture contamination in spring, which is when young animals begin to graze and are more sensitive to infection.

Despite this, other factors may also be involved in this increase in the appearance of clinical cases of fasciolosis. Disease control has tended to be based on the use of a product that is highly effective against all parasitic forms, including immature migratory forms, namely triclabendazole. However, the incorrect and excessive use of this drug appears to have led to the development of resistant populations.

There is general agreement regarding the relationship between climate change and higher temperatures and rainfall, with the winter period being most strongly affected due to a reduction in the number of cold days and increased humidity. In Scotland, for example, some models suggest an increase in the average temperature of around 4 °C by the end of this century taking into account the 1 °C increase observed between 1961 and 2004. Similarly, the grazing period has been extended by almost 30 days over the same period and the number of days with frost has decreased by around 20.

These epidemiological changes have been related to increased, or more localised, rainfall flooding the affected region and the maintenance of suitable microhabitats. All the above, together with the appearance of populations resistant to triclabendazole, are currently causing great concern.

3 What measures can be taken in such cases?

Although very little can be done as regards the seasonal changes in fasciolosis due to the influence of temperature and humidity, the fact that the intermediate snail host tends to be found in flooded or very wet zones may be an advantage when it comes to infection control. Indeed, the latest acute clinical cases in calves have been linked to the release of young animals to pasture immediately after the grass had been cut for silage and before it had begun to grow again, thus forcing the animals to graze on the edges of the pastures where more grass was present. The conditions in these zones are ideal for snails and, as a result, contamination with metacercariae can be very high. One measure that can be taken involves fencing off these potentially hazardous zones.

Other factors that should be taken into account include the current trend in agricultural and farm production towards more ecological methods (organic agriculture), greater extensification and the current higher likelihood of being able to graze year round in some regions, which may also explain the changes being detected in the free-living phases of the parasite and, consequently, the epidemiology of infection.

The presence of *Galba truncatula* in wet zones such as that seen in the picture is essential for the spread of *F. hepatica*. The biotic potential of these molluscs is very high, with a single individual being able to produce 25,000 new examples in only 12 weeks under favourable environmental conditions. The snails live in wet and clayey zones and "expel) the cercariae, which lose their tail and encyst in grass and water, transforming into the infective forms for animals: metacercariae.

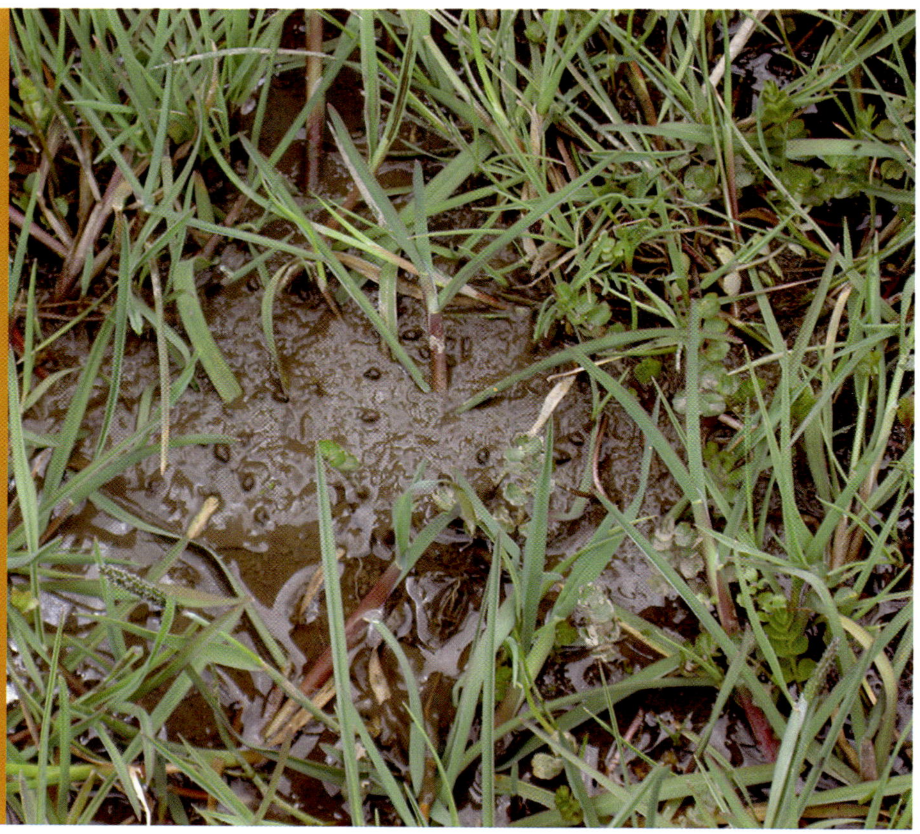

14 How is fasciolosis diagnosed in cows?

Our services are requested to optimise the antiparasitic program for bovines in their first grazing season. These animals are grazed for around 10 months (from February to November) on a traditional farm and receive anthelmintic treatment as an intraruminal bolus. For the past two years, the calves have suffered clinical fasciolosis. The farm has also experienced fertility problems and reduced milk yields for the past three years. Since then all animals have received treatment with oxyclozanide once a year (in February). In light of current legislation, which prohibits the use of anthelmintics in lactating animals, the intention is to reduce the load in young animals and to control the need to administer drugs by determining the antibody levels in the milk tank.

1. What is the method of choice for detecting liver flukes in young animals and adults?
2. Does the resistance of bovines increase with age?
3. Why do clinical signs of anaemia and oedema appear in fasciolosis?
4. What other blood parameters may be affected?

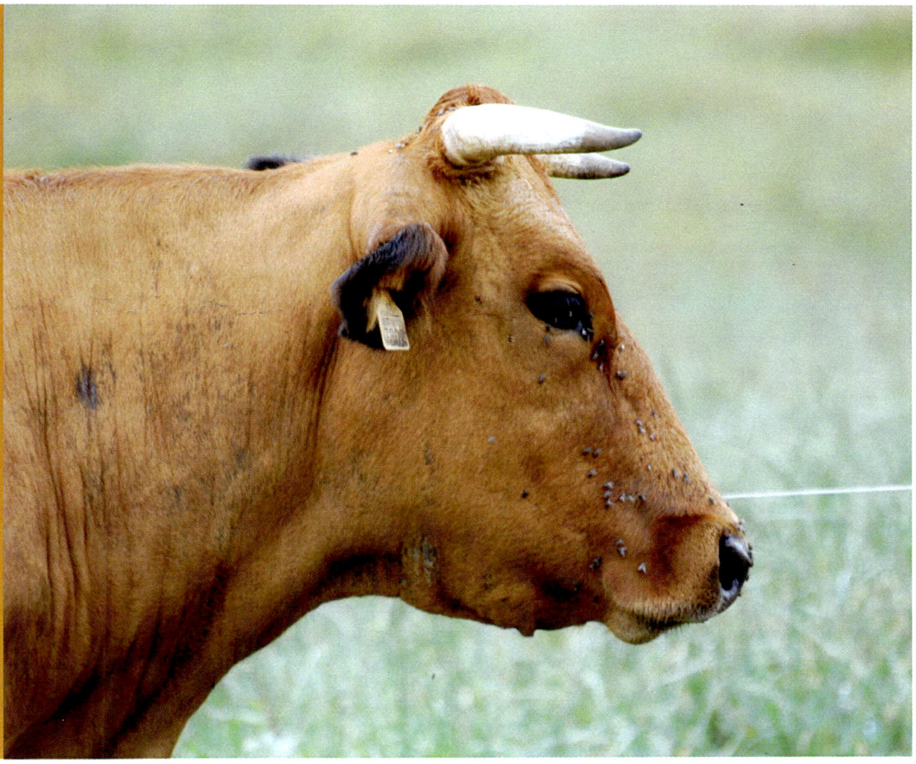

1 What is the method of choice for detecting liver flukes in young animals and adults?

As is the case for any parasitic disease, the diagnosis of fasciolosis is based on the incidence of the disease, clinical signs, parasitological and biopathological analyses and necropsy.

As far as the incidence is concerned, fasciolosis mainly affects young animals, although they do not tend to present highly specific signs. Although acute and subacute fasciolosis may also present in bovines, the chronic form, which can be observed in winter and early spring (December to March), is clinically the most common. The most characteristic symptoms are weight loss, anorexia and anaemia-related mucosal pallor, submandibular oedema and ascites, although this is not constant.

The parasitology techniques used include direct techniques, which detect the presence of the parasite (faecal analysis, antigen detection) and indirect techniques, which indicate current or incipient infection using immune reactions.

Faecal analysis is highly specific but poorly sensitive and, in primary infections, only serves as a "late" diagnosis of the disease as liver fluke eggs appear in faeces at around 10 weeks post-infection. Moreover, it should be considered that the diagnostic value is affected by large variations in the faecal excretion of parasite eggs, especially when results are negative.

Methods for determining the plasma activity of some liver enzymes are of great diagnostic utility.

Immunodiagnosis is also of great use. Several serological, agglutination, immunofluorescence, immunoenzyme assays (ELISA) and complement fixation techniques have been described. The most widely used is an ELISA, or one of its many modifications, using somatic or excretion/secretion antigens from the parasite.

One of the techniques used to detect active infections is the double ELISA, which detects circulating antigens in the serum or faeces of suspect animals well before prepatency finishes. However, this technique is more suitable for diagnosing fasciolosis in naturally infected herds and its use in individual cases is not recommended. Although some ELISA tests for detecting infections using milk or serum samples have been registered, they are not widely used in Spain.

Very recently, the ability to diagnose an infection shortly after contagion by PCR using a specific fragment of mitochondrial DNA has been demonstrated. This test allows positive results to be obtained at three weeks post-infection (standard PCR) or even earlier (two weeks post-infection) if nested PCR is used.

Fibrotic tracks in the liver, which result from reorganisation of the lesions caused by the worms during intraparenchymal migration and hyperplastic cholangitis, which occurs once the flukes reach the bile ducts and gall bladder, are observed upon necropsy. The organic reaction in cattle is highly energetic and leads to an intense tissue reaction with calcification of the bile ducts, which act as a mechanical barrier to reinfection. Moreover, marked emaciation of the carcass and a variable number of fasciolae in the bile ducts (average: 300) are also observed. Lesions can also be seen in the periportal and mesenteric ganglia, which are enlarged and a have greenish brown colour, and in the peritoneum.

2 Does the resistance of bovines increase with age?

For many years it was thought that beef cattle acquired immunity to *Fasciola hepatica*, although "field" observations do not appear to confirm this.

Animals naturally exposed to *Fasciola* infections are readily reinfected and studies of the intensity of infections with age have shown that adult bovines do not exhibit lower parasite burdens than their younger counterparts. Thus, there is no evidence that age confers resistance to fasciolosis.

It appears that *Fasciola hepatica* is able to "divert" the hosts immune response towards a strong Th2 response, which favours its survival in the animal.

3 Why do clinical signs of anaemia and oedema appear in fasciolosis?

The pathogenesis of fasciolosis is related to the number of parasites that invade the liver and is associated with the migration of immature fasciolae via the hepatic parenchyma and, subsequently, the haematophagous activity of the adult fluke already present in the bile ducts.

Fasciolosis proceeds with anaemia, hypoalbuminaemia and hyperglobulinaemia and, depending on the intensity and duration of the infection, hyper- or hypoproteinaemia. Anorexia and weight loss or growth retardation are also characteristic.

The anorexia that accompanies fasciolosis is partially responsible for the hypoalbuminaemia and weight loss, although it apparently has no effect on the anaemia.

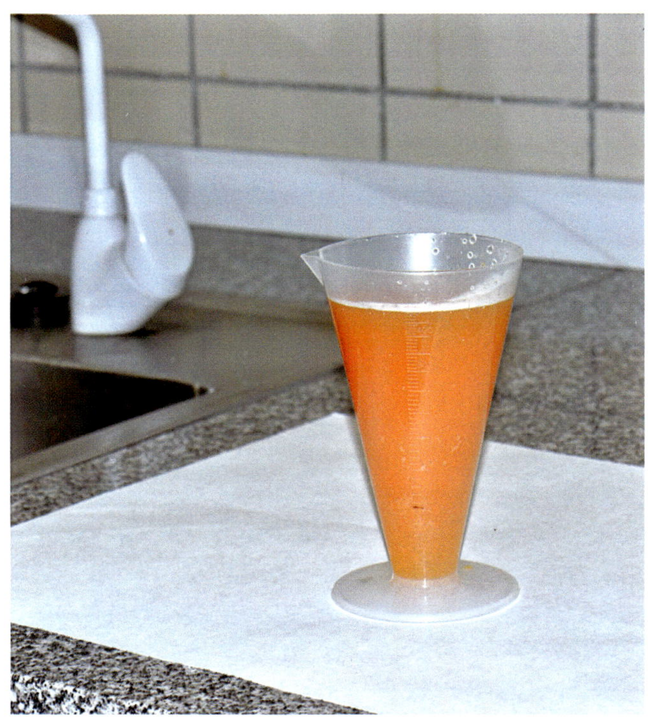

The sedimentation cup is used to concentrate those trematode eggs with a higher density than the detritus found in faeces, thus allowing them to be obtained in the sediment after repeated washing. Addition of a contrast dye to the sediment makes their identification easier by allowing the golden yellow colour of the eggs to stand out.

Voluntary food intake progressively decreases post-infection and reaches its low point at the end of the prepatency phase, at which stage the hepatopathy caused by immature fasciolae is highest. There is some degree of correlation between the appearance and intensity of the lack of appetite with decreased hepatic metabolic capacity and the onset of anaemia and loss of plasma proteins associated with adult fasciolae. In light of this, the anaemia, hypoalbuminaemia and loss of extravascular protein stores may somehow affect ingestion.

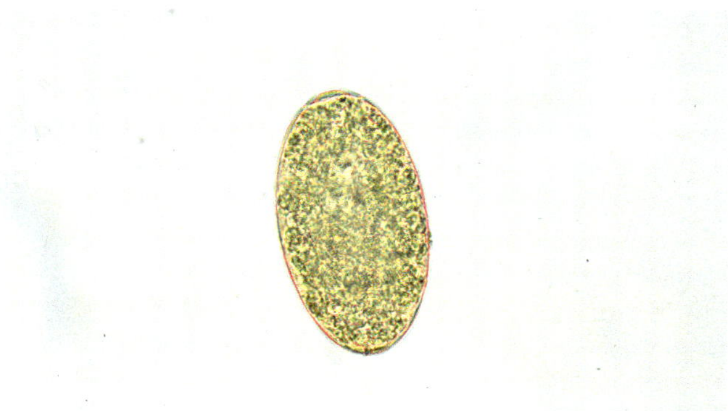

An adult liver fluke lays between 2000 and 5000 eggs, which pass into the intestine mixed with bile and exit to the exterior in faeces, per day. These eggs are highly characteristic due to their large size and colour, they are ellipsoidal, operculated, yellow coloured and measure 130-150 μm. The finding of 100-200 eggs per gramme of faeces in cattle indicated a probably pathogenic infection that requires the application of a fasciolicide. Coprological analyses in primary infections are usually negative.

Some animals may exhibit submandibular oedema ("bottle jaw") and ascites. Normochromic and macrocytic anaemia gradually develops. A marked reticulocytosis (8-30 %), which is only observed in animals with a haematocrit value of less than 25 %, may also be present. Alterations to blood values are accompanied by alterations to serum protein levels. This initially leads to hyperproteinaemia, mainly due to an increase in formed elements (mainly immunoglobulins) in response to parasitic antigens, followed by hypoproteinaemia, especially due to the marked decrease in albumin plasma levels.

4 What other blood parameters may be affected?

Blood analyses highlight the presence of anaemia at around 12 weeks post-infection, with a haematocrit that may reach values of 20-24 %. The anaemia is haemorrhagic, macrocytic and normochromic.

Other parameters are also of great diagnostic utility. For example, increased glutamate dehydrogenase activity is indicative of a recent acute process. Levels of other enzymes, such as aspartate aminotransferase and sorbitol dehydrogenase, also increase during migration of the worms through the hepatic parenchyma, although they are less specific. Likewise, γ-glutamyltransferase levels peak once the parasites have reached the bile ducts. These enzymes can also be used to check the treatment efficacy.

Other hepatic function tests, such as sulfobromophthalein and antipyrine, have also been used.

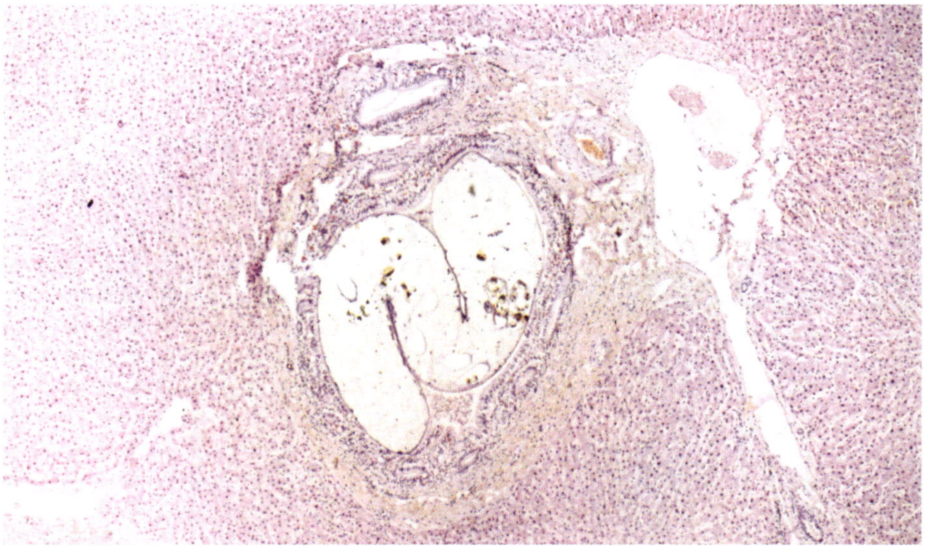

Post-necrotic fibrosis occurs as a result of reorganisation of the migratory paths caused by liver flukes. This can be seen throughout the liver, although it is more common in the ventral lobe as this is the preferred entry site for the flukes. The response to the presence and activity of parasites in the bile ducts results in hyperplastic cholangitis.

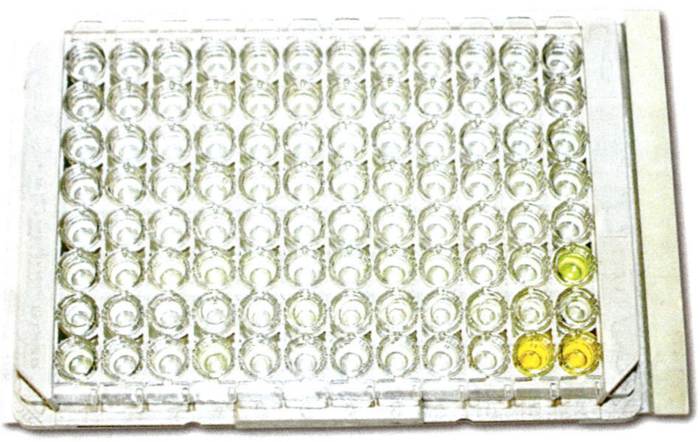

The most widely used immunological technique is ELISA, or one of its many modifications, using somatic or excretion/secretion antigens from the parasite. Recent improvements in antigen purification methods have markedly improved the sensitivity and specificity of this test, which is available on the market. However, maximum efficacy as regards results interpretation is obtained for the diagnosis of fasciolosis in naturally infected herds, and its use for individual cases is not recommended.

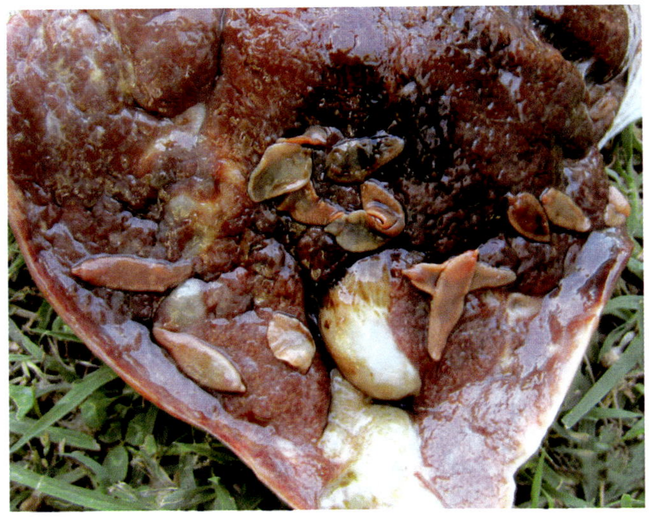

The diagnosis of chronic fasciolosis in a dead animal involves the observation of hepatic fibrosis and hyperplastic cholangitis and the presence of adult worms in the bile ducts and gallbladder. An intense tissue reaction, fibrosis and, finally, calcification of the bile ducts, occurs.
Image courtesy of Dr. J. Villalba.

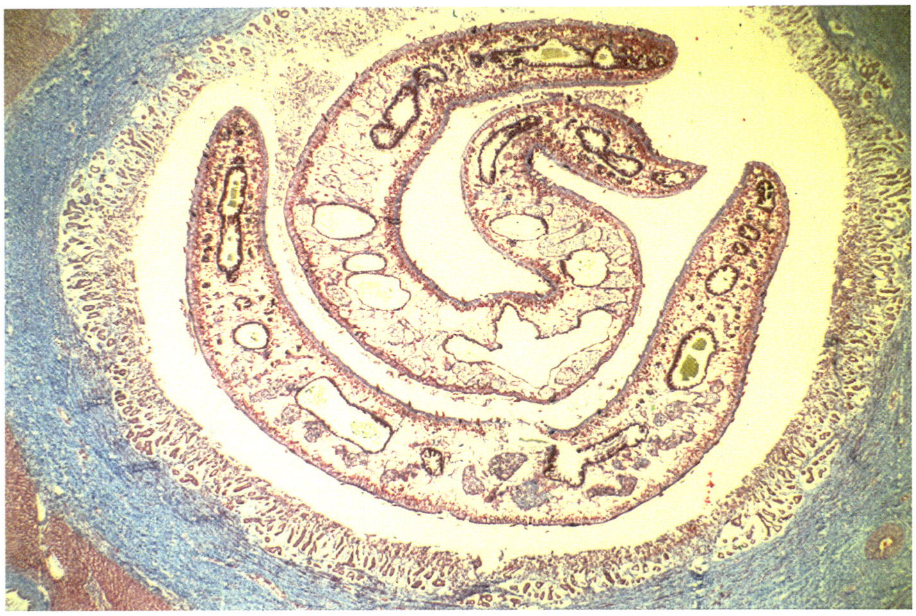

Fasciolosis. A histological section showing the presence of liver flukes in a bile duct, cellular inflammation and infiltration and other alterations (hyperplasia and periductal fibrosis).

15 Are parasites found in the rumen?

During preparations for the Noreña food festival in the north of Spain, the butchers detected the presence of parasites in many of the entrails purchased to prepare the typical tripe (*callos*). They complain of the time required to remove these fat, pear-shaped one-cm-long pinkish white worms with a rosy end, from the surface of the rumen. The worms were only rarely seen in the reticulum or abomasum, but in some cases the wall of the reticulum was so damaged that it has to be discharged. The older villagers claim that this is because it has rained a lot and hasn't been very cold, which was more common in the past than currently.

1. What are paramphistomes?
2. Are they pathogenic in adult animals?
3. What is the relationship between climate and their prevalence?
4. Why do they appear in dewormed animals?

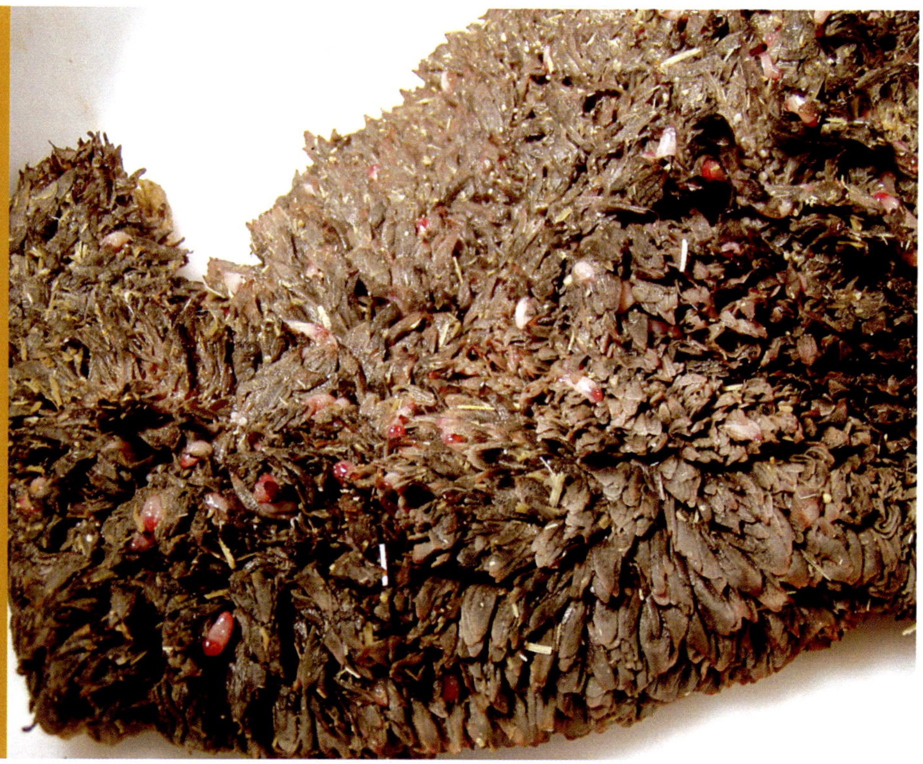

1 What are paramphistomes?

Paramphistomes live in the reticulum and rumen and are also known as "gastric trematodes". These fleshy pinkish or pale-red trematodes are conical or pyriform and are dorsally convex and slightly ventrally concave, measuring 5-12 mm × 2-4 mm. Immature worms are smaller (1-2 mm in length). As is the case for all digenean trematodes possesses two suckers: a large and powerful posterior ventral sucker, known as the acetabulum, and a smaller, pyriform oral sucker.

They are found embedded between the rumenal papillae in varying numbers. It is fairly common to find several hundred paramphistomes in a single animal with no clinically detectable alterations, although if they coexist with other helminths, such as *Fasciola hepatica*, they may contribute to the alterations produced by fasciolae, the effects of which are very noticeable.

Many parasitic amphistomes are found in domestic animals. However, as their biology and pathogenic action are very similar, they can be considered jointly. The most important are those located in the rumen and reticulum, including the genera *Paramphistomum*, *Calicophoron*, *Cotylophoron* and others.

2 Are they pathogenic in adult animals?

Infection is more common in young animals in which small successive infections lead to a strong immunity, the result of which is both a marked reduction in the number of worms and a less intense pathogenic action.

The most important pathogenic action arises due to the activity exerted by immature forms of the parasite in the duodenum. Once excysted in the small intestine, they penetrate the mucosa producing disorders such as erosions, petechiae and necrosis, all of which lead to loss of appetite. Plasma albumin levels also decrease, thus resulting in hypoalbuminaemia with generalised oedema. Hydropericardium, hydrothorax, pulmonary oedema, ascites and submandibular oedema, amongst others, may also be observed.

The disorders caused by adult parasites in the intestinal mucosa are less important than those caused by immature paramphistomes, which can lead to gastroenteritis and blood-stained diarrhoea, especially in young animals.

In most cases adult parasites tend not to produce clinically detectable disorders, although they are known to cause chronic ulcerative rumenitis with atrophy of the rumenal papillae if large numbers of worms are present. Paramphistomosis is diagnosed in animals aged 4-18 months and is associated with the presence of a large number of parasites (up to 30,000) in the duodenum and jejunum. The clinical signs include the onset of diarrhoea at approximately two months of commencing grazing.

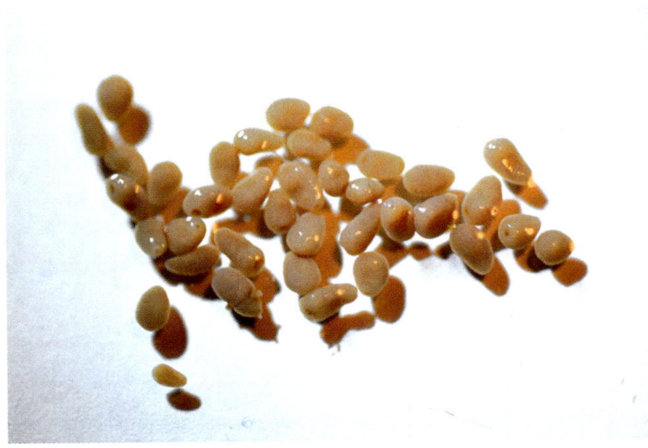

Paramphistomes are slightly flattened, moderately small, conical, oval, pyriform or elliptical parasites with a larger and more powerful ventroterminal sucker than its oral counterpart. The average lifespan in their definitive hosts can be as long as 4 years.

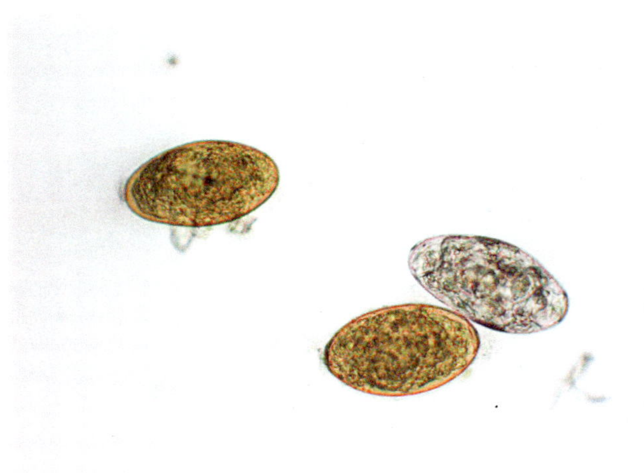

The parasites present in the rumen deposit incompletely embryonated eggs which are excreted in the faeces. These eggs are morphologically very similar to those of liver flukes but are grey coloured, and each worm produces 75 eggs per day on average.

The clinical disorders produced by adult worms attached to the ruminal mucosa are less important than those caused by the migrant juvenile forms. The immature forms exit the cyst in the first part of the small intestine and penetrate the mucosa, causing erosions, petechiae and necrosis, which themselves produce gastroenteritis together with blood-stained diarrhoea, especially in young cattle. *Image courtesy of Dr. S. Mitchel*

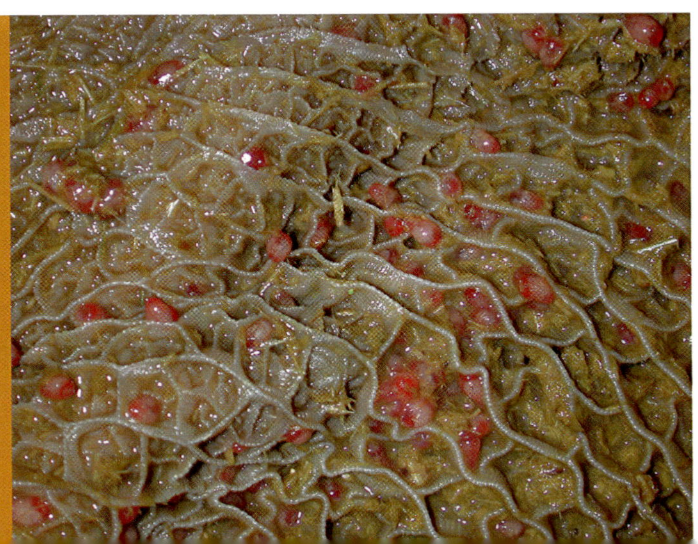

3 What is the relationship between climate and their prevalence?

The exogenous cycle of *Paramphistomum* spp. is indirect and very similar to that of *Fasciola hepatica*. Some phases are fully exposed to environmental factors (eggs and metacercaria), whereas others —those which develop in the intermediate host mollusc— are only indirectly affected by climate.

The eggs eliminated in the faeces of infected animals need water to continue developing, a process that also requires temperatures of at least 28 °C. Under these conditions, the miracidia, which must invade a snail to continue the cycle, hatch after around two weeks. However, if the environmental conditions are unfavourable, the time required for embryo formation in the eggs and subsequent hatching of the miracidia can be much longer.

Gastropod molluscs from the Planorbidae, Bullinidae and Lymnaeidae families act as intermediate hosts. In these hosts, the recently hatched larvae (miracidia) transform into sporocysts, rediae and, finally, cercariae, which leave the snail and encyst in the grass or in water, where they can survive for up to three months. As such, it is normal that climate conditions affect the life cycle of paramphistomes, speeding up or delaying their development. Likewise, the number of cercaria finally produced also varies a great deal, thus determining whether there is a risk of a severe infection or, as is usually the case, the animals only suffer mild infections.

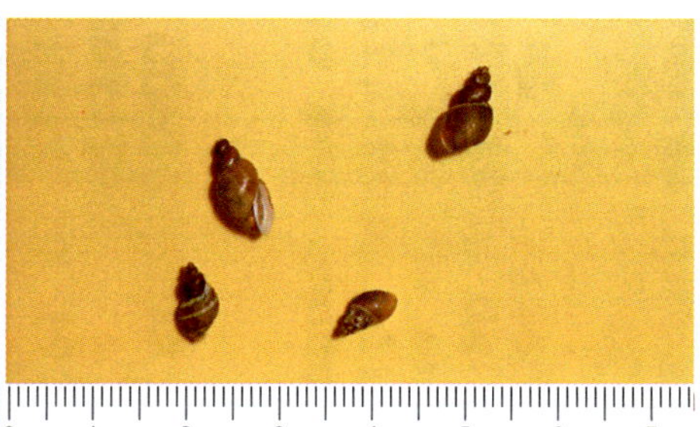

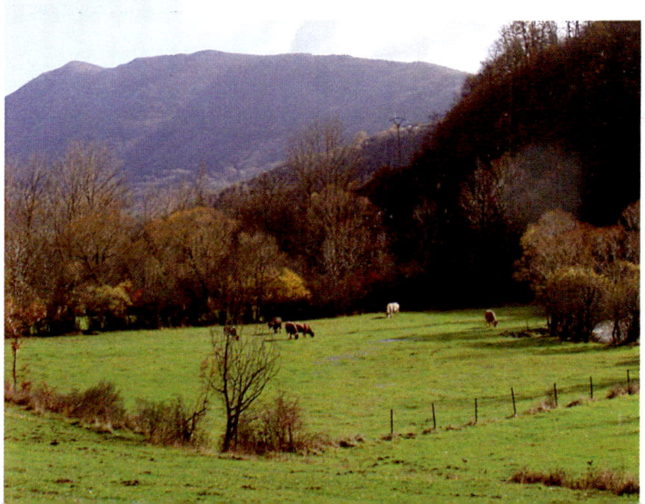

4 Why do they appear in dewormed animals?

The antiparasitic treatments most widely used for chemoprophylaxis in cattle include macrocyclic lactones and benzimidazole carbamates.

Of these, macrocyclic lactones are ineffective against paramphistomes and the activity of the majority of benzimidazoles is limited to the adult forms of the parasite, although in any case their efficacy is not particularly high.

For various reasons, in current practice parasitological analyses are not usually undertaken prior to administering an anthelmintic; one of the most widely used such drugs, which as noted above have limited efficacy against this parasite group, is applied instead. As a result, "routine deworming" is ineffective at eliminating paramphistome infections. Although it would be advisable to administer a "narrow spectrum" anthelmintic, this requires a prior analysis to confirm the need for treatment and the drug of choice in each specific case.

Oxyclozanide is the most effective anthelmintic for the treatment of both acute (due to juvenile forms) and subacute and chronic presentations (caused by adults). Two treatments separated by two days should be administered and other measures, such as fencing off hazardous areas and targeting the intermediate hosts that play a role in the biological cycle, should also be put into place. In this sense, the use of molluscicides to restrict the population of intermediate host snails and the removal of vegetation from some areas of pasture may help to decrease the infection risk for the animals.

Access to the definitive host occurs by ingestion of grass contaminated with metacercariae. They develop in a similar manner to *Fasciola hepatica*, requiring an intermediate host that may be a freshwater mollusc such as *Galba truncatula*. Prior infections in adult animals provoke a sufficient degree of immunity to protect against subsequent reinfections, which is why paramphistomosis is a disease of young animals.

16 What are bovine cestodes like?

A fattening farm in Zaragoza province, in Spain, has purchased a group of calves with a slightly lower weight than on previous occasions (around 60-70 kg each). Following the *Good hygiene practice* guidelines for fattening cattle published by the Spanish Ministry of Agriculture, Food and Environment, they are provided with water and a vitamin/mineral complex. A deworming treatment was also applied. The following day, the floor where they are kept is covered in white strands several metres in length, thus forcing the keepers to remove the bedding prepared the previous day.

1. Which cestodes can be found in bovines?
2. What are oribatid mites?
3. Which products are cestocides?

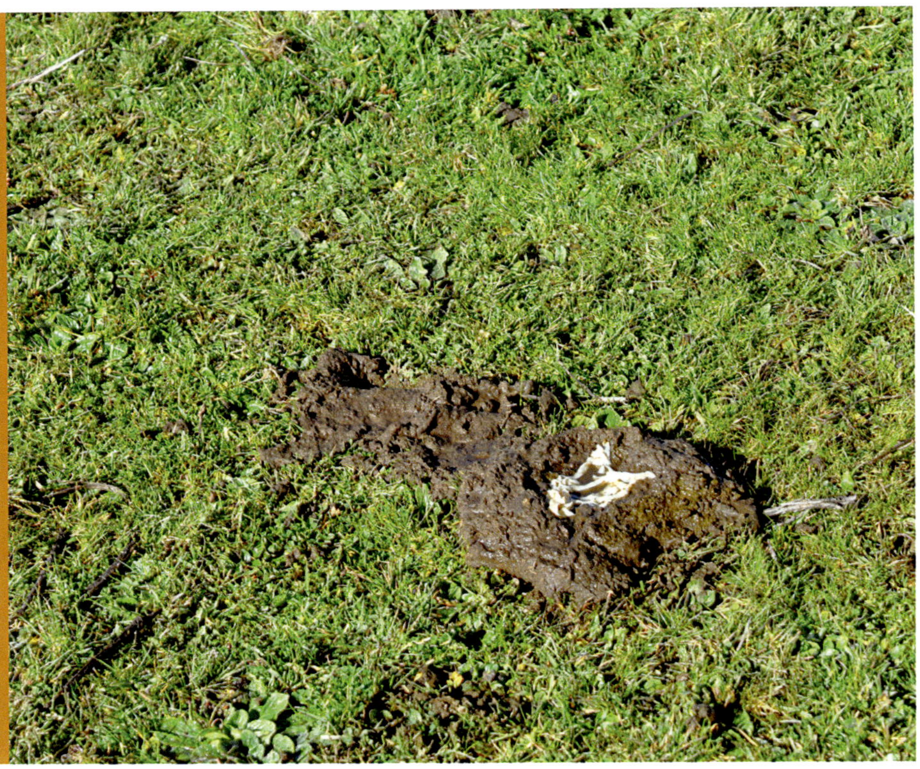

1 Which cestodes can be found in bovines?

Although bovines host a wide variety of parasites, cestodes are not the most numerous. However, a distinction must be made between those species that live in the digestive tract of these animals in an adult state and those which use bovines as intermediate hosts but which live in other animal species as adults. This is the case of larval cyst forms, especially echinococcal cysts, cysticerci and coenuri, which are less common in bovines than in small ruminants.

The most important adult cestodes hosted by bovines include infections by species from the genus *Moniezia* and to a lesser degree, the genera *Avitellina, Stilesia* and *Thysaniezia*, which infect both domestic animals and some species of wild ruminants such as deer, mountain goat, etc.

The species *Moniezia benedeni* is by far the most important from the *Moniezia* genus. This large cestode possesses two pairs of genital organs and cuticular glands arranged dorsally and ventrally between two proglottids, in multiple groups, known as interproglottidal glands. The eggs are triangular or polygonal, with a well-developed pyriform apparatus, and measure 80-85 µm. Adult worms live in the intestine, are almost half a metre long (around 40 cm) and 1.6 cm wide. They possess a cuboid scolex with four forward-facing suckers with circular openings.

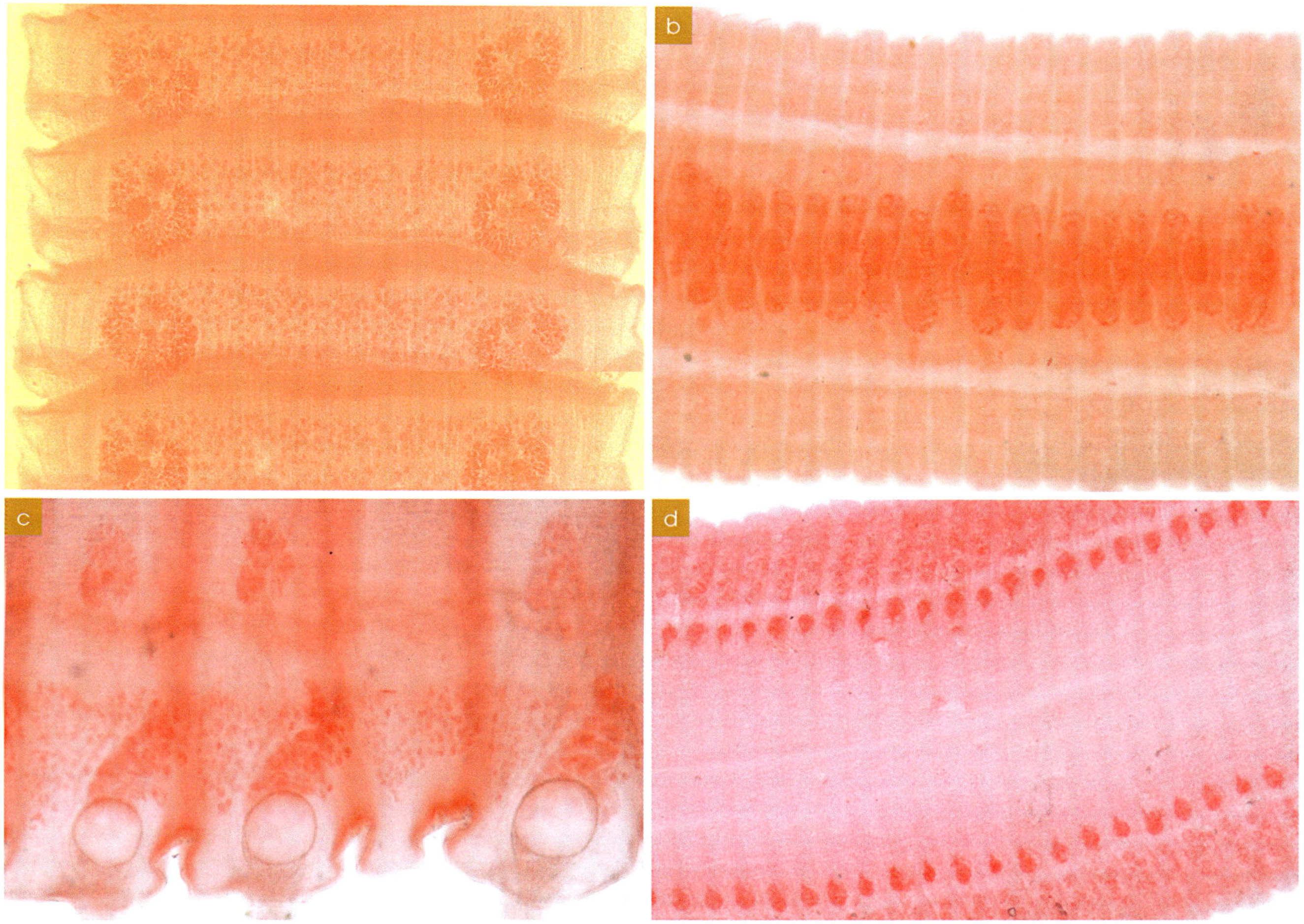

(a) *Moniezia benedeni*, (b) *Avitellina centripunctata*, (c) *Thysaniezia giardi*, (d) *Stilesia globipunctata*. Long cestodes possess several layers of muscle fibre beneath their surface that allows them to perform truly acrobatic movements in order to copulate with other individuals or with different sections of themselves. To fulfil this reproductive function they possess very well developed male and female genital organs, which can be singe or double in each ring and open laterally into the atrium via the genital pore either continuously, on one side or the other, or alternating regularly or irregularly.

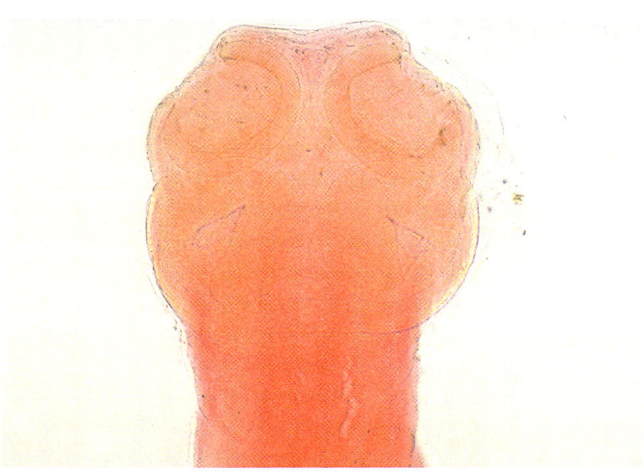

Moniezia species are normally large tapeworms (0.2-1 m) with a strong scolex and four suckers but lacking a rostellum and hooks. They possess numerous proglottids with full and independent morphofunctional provisions.

2 What are oribatid mites?

The last segments (proglottid) of the adult worm, which are replete with eggs, detach from the strobilus in the host's intestine. Once expelled with the contents of the intestine, the eggs exhibit an ability to move that persists even in the external medium. In other cases, the proglottids fracture in the intestinal sinus, where they release their eggs, which reach the exterior mixed in with the host's faeces.

The involvement of an intermediate host is required for the cycle to continue in the external medium. Grass mites from the order Oribatida act as intermediate hosts. There are numerous species able to participate in the life cycle of these cestodes. Furthermore, oribatid mites are very abundant, which means that it is almost certain that the cycle will continue.

The families of greatest epidemiological significance are Scheloribatidae, Oribatulidae, Galumnidae and Ceratozetidae, with the genera *Scheloribates, Galumna, Adoristes, Oribatula, Oppia,* etc. being the most important. Of these, the species *Scheloribates laevigatus* is the most commonly infected worldwide. As far as Spain is concerned, it appears that, due to both its presence and abundance, *Scheloribates laevigatus* is the main culprit responsible for contamination in the majority of pastures grazed by cows and sheep.

When an egg is ingested by a mite that acts as an intermediate host, the oncosphere remains free and perforates the intestine to the abdominal cavity, where it forms a larval cyst around 0.2 mm in size known as a cysticercoid.

3 Which products are cestocides?

The limited efficacy and high toxicity of some older formulas of taeniafuge preparations based on copper sulfate, with or without nicotine, tin arsenate, dichlorophen, etc. have passed into the annals of pharmacopoeia.

Some conventional cestocides, such as bunamidine (25-50 mg/kg b.w.), niclosamide (100-150 mg/kg b.w.) and resorantel (70 mg/kg b.w.), continue to provide good results. These compounds are both safe and effective

However, the most effective cestodicide is praziquantel, administered in doses of 25-100 mg/kg b.w. The efficacy of this compound against species found in the bile ducts is also good. It acts rapidly, safely and effectively, causing rupture and vacuolation of the integument, especially in mature proglottids.

Benzimidazole carbamates, which block the energy metabolism of cestodes, are highly recommended as they also act against other flat or round helminths that parasite ruminants and often, coexist with anoplocephalidae. In this sense, fenbenzadole (5-25 mg/kg b.w.), oxfendazole (5 mg/kg b.w.), luxabendazole (7.5-10 mg/kg b.w.) and, particularly, albendazole (7.5 mg/kg b.w.) can be used with excellent results.

Oral or injectable doses of 7.5-20 mg/kg b.w. of some guanidine-derived probenzimidazoles, such as netobomin, are also useful against cestodes. trematodes and nematodes in cows and sheep.

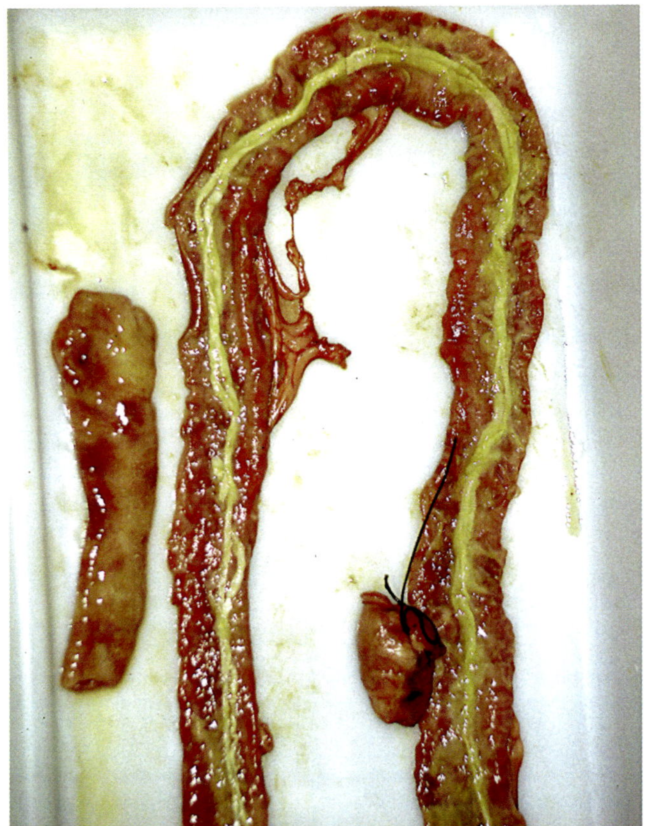

The irritating and inflammatory effects caused by these cestodes are mainly felt at the sites to which they attach to the intestinal mucosa. Their traumatic and mechanical action may cause acute or chronic blockages of the lumen and, rarely, fatal perforations of the intestinal wall. The intestine may present symptoms ranging from a simple cold to severe enteritis and mucosal congestion, local oedema and abundant cellular infiltrate.

Biological cycle of *Moniezia*

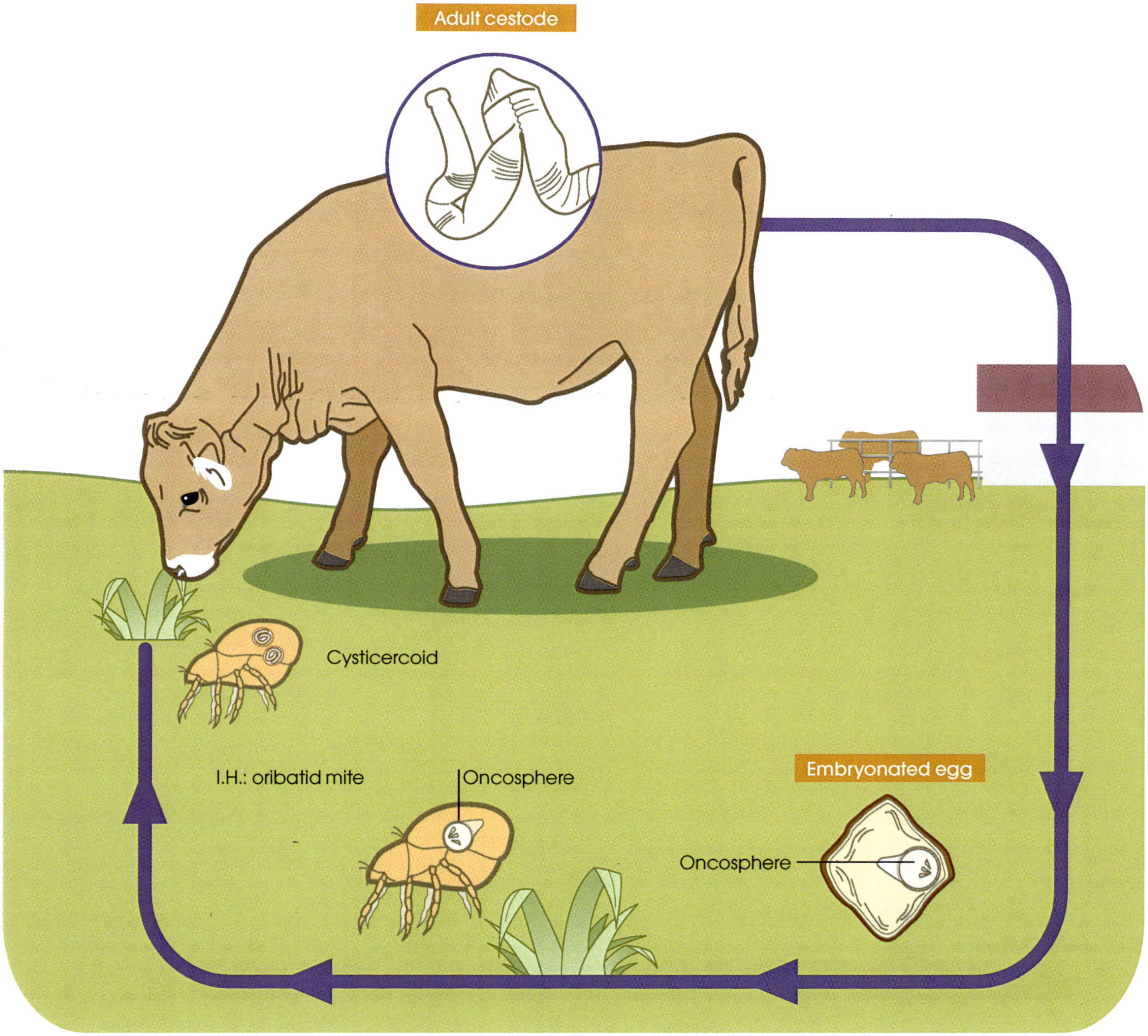

17 Does age influence cestode infections?

Fifty extensively raised calves from Palencia province (Spain) were selected to conduct an efficacy test on an antiparasitic treatment. The presence of cestodes from the genus *Moniezia* was confirmed in all of them, with egg morphology allowing these parasites to be identified as *Moniezia benedeni*. Seven days later they were transported to facilities in Madrid province, close to the Veterinary School where the assay was being performed. Transfer was performed by day by staff specifically hired for that purpose but with no experience in handling this type of animal, therefore loading was especially problematic. Once installed, and after resting for 24 hours, stool samples were taken in order to distribute the animals into groups according to the test protocol. To the investigators' surprise, none of the stool samples contained cestode eggs. After repeating the analysis, with identical results, five animals were slaughtered and found to be completely free from endoparasites.

1. How can what happened be explained?
2. Are cestodiases common in adults?
3. What repercussions do they have?

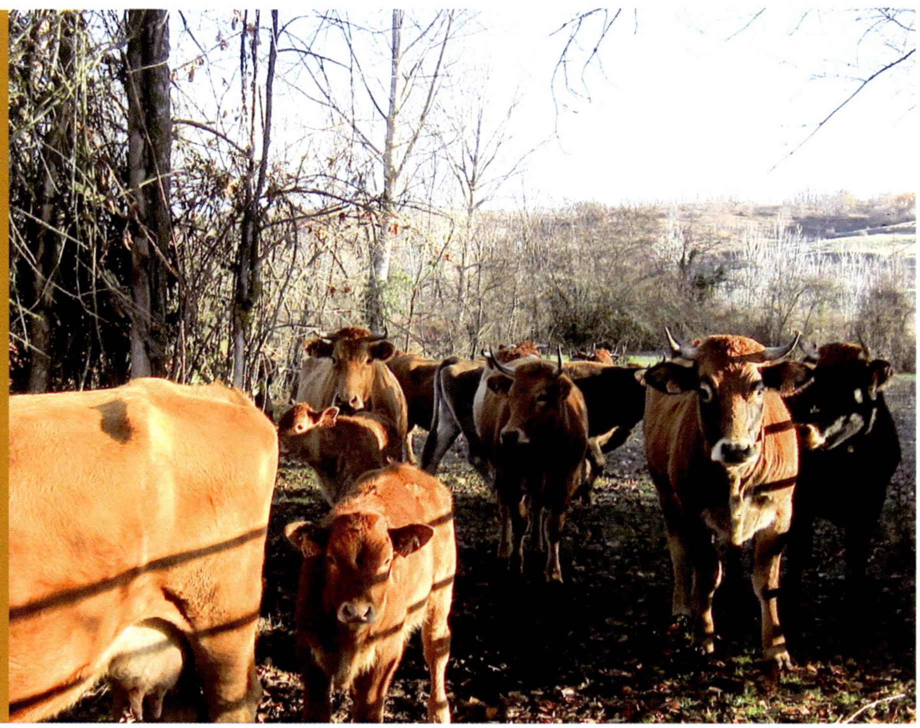

1 How can what happened be explained?

As the half-life of tapeworms, which disappear from the host in just a few months, is short, the reservoir and persistence of contamination in grazing areas depends very strongly on the quantity of eggs released onto the land and the specific biology of the intermediate oribatid hosts.

Larger animals tend to be resistant to reinfection and adult worms appear to cause antibody production when in contact with tissues in the intestinal lumen. This, and epidemiological factors arising from the farming models used and the biology of the intermediate hosts, means that this disease tends to be linked to young animals (lambs and calves), with locally well-defined seasonal presentation patterns.

Animals infected by *Moniezia* spp. acquire some degree of immunity as the majority of parasites are eliminated within 2-4 months post-infection. Moreover, it appears that stress may contribute to this "self-healing" phenomenon.

Symptoms go unnoticed when few cestodes are present. High burdens with digestive symptoms accompanied by anaemia, progressive weight loss and growth retardation may be found in young animals.

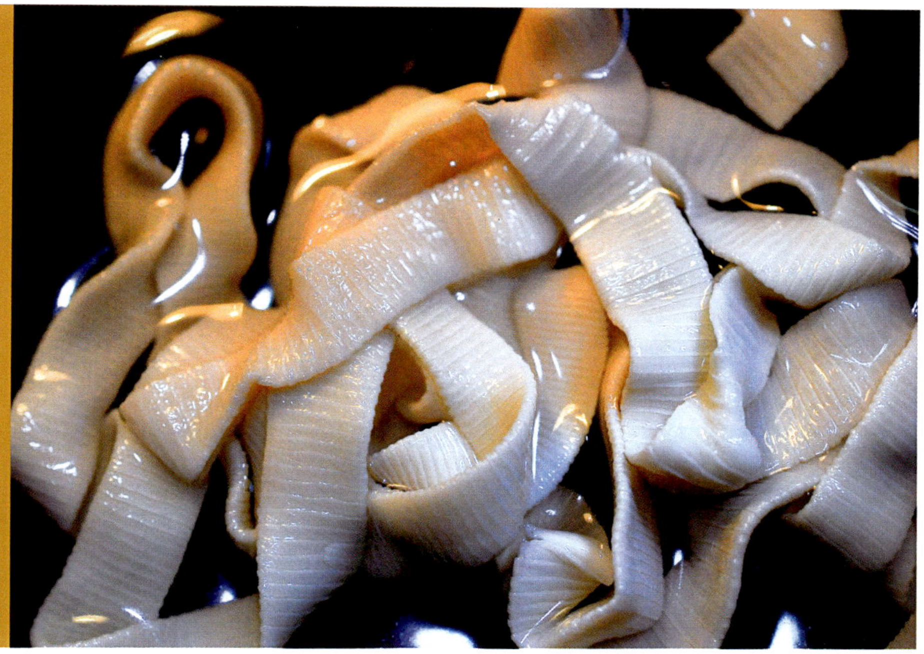

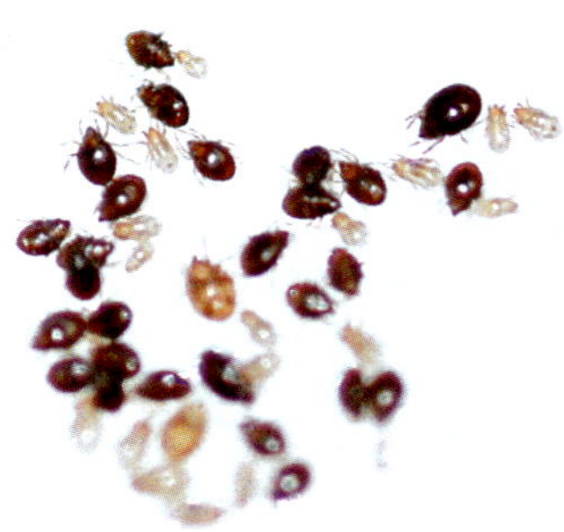

The intermediate hosts are pasture mites from the order Oribatida. More than 100 mite species can host cysticercoid larvae in their interior. Animals are infected upon accidental ingestion when grazing.

2 Are cestodiases common in adults?

The main bovine cestodiases are widely distributed, occurring endemically in many regions and causing harmful effects in young animals that, on occasion, have very negative repercussions for the growth of these animals and the economic health of their farms.

On the Iberian peninsula, high prevalences have been reported in breeding cows and sheep as well as in wild ruminants (deer, mountain goat, etc.). Processes caused by various species from the genera *Moniezia* and, to a lesser extent, *Avitellina, Stilesia* and *Thysaniezia* predominate.

The species found in Iberian bovines are *Avitellina centripunctata, Moniezia benedeni, M. expansa, M. trigonophora, Stilesia globipunctata, Thysaniezia giardi* and *T. ovilla*.

3 What repercussions do they have?

The pathogenic picture is governed by a series of actions that harm the host. These actions are strenghthend when combined. These depend particularly on the size of the worms and the intensity of the infection.

Attachment of the worms to the intestinal mucosa induces an irritating and inflammatory action. It normally results in mild intestinal catarrh, which may develop into severe enteritis and mucosal blockage, local oedema and an abundant cellular infiltrate.

Some species, such as *Stilesia hepatica* and *Thysanosoma actinioides*, which are found in the bile ducts, provoke a chronic inflammatory reaction, with hyperplasia and sclerosis of these ducts.

The presence of adult cestodes in the intestine leads to a traumatic/mechanical action that results in intestinal obstruction and erosion or perforation of the intestinal wall, which may have serious consequences. Other pathogenic actions, such as a pyogenic reaction, are infrequent, abdominal oedema and erosions or perforation trigger abscess formation and peritonitis, respectively.

However, morbid symptoms are rarely observed in cattle and then only when infection is intense. On such occasions, digestive disorders, chronic tympanites or recurrent diarrhoea are observed. The animal's hair becomes bristly and it loses weight and develops mild anaemia.

Despite the limited pathogenic role played by these parasites, farmers commonly demand that their animals be treated when proglottids are observed in faeces.

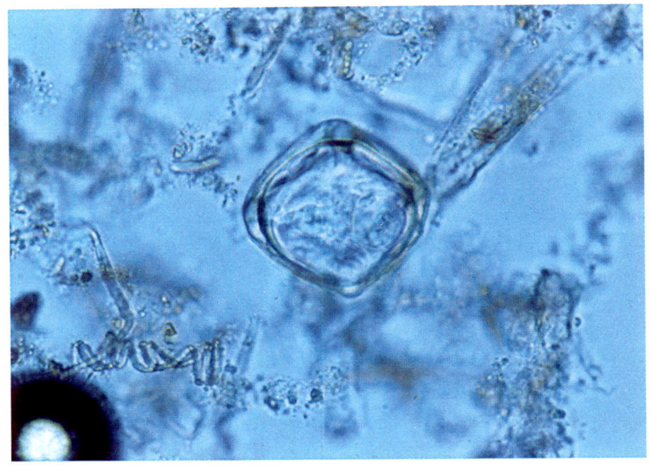

The observation of eggs in faeces, and the identification of proglottids, allows the presence of cestodes to be confirmed. The morphology, size, involucrum thickness and, above all, typical pyriform apparatus are characteristic of this parasite group. The most common species in bovines, namely *Moniezia benedeni*, has a clearly quadrangular morphology, in contrast to the ovine species *M. expansa*, which is triangular.

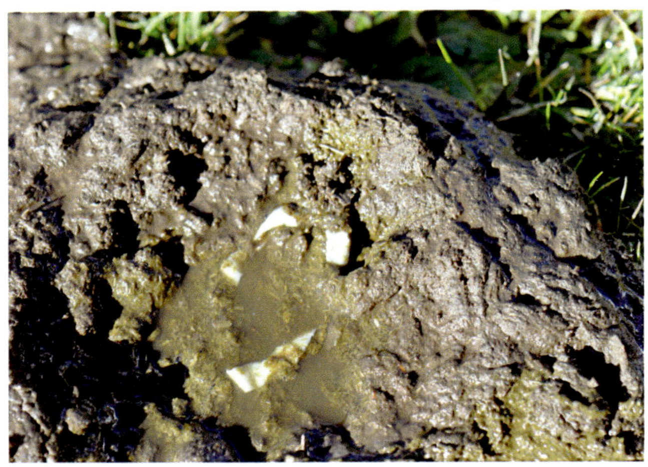

Mature proglottids, isolated or in groups, are eliminated through faeces and break open in the environment, releasing the eggs. In other cases, they dissolve in the intestinal tract and the eggs are released in the faeces.

18 Are adult animals resistant to *Cryptosporidium*?

During a school visit to a high yielding dairy farm, the students find small white huts on the floor in the neighbouring field turned over on their sides, with the interior exposed to sunlight. The farm managers explain that this is the best method for preventing diarrhoea caused by a small parasite, bacteria or viruses in the calves. Since the huts have been "sunbathing) there have been no major cases of diarrhoea in newborn and weaned animals. In the last outbreak some 5 years ago all the calves, but no adult cows, died.

1. Why does it affect newborn animals?
2. Can the bovine variety infect humans?
3. What characterises the biological cycle of *Cryptosporidium*?

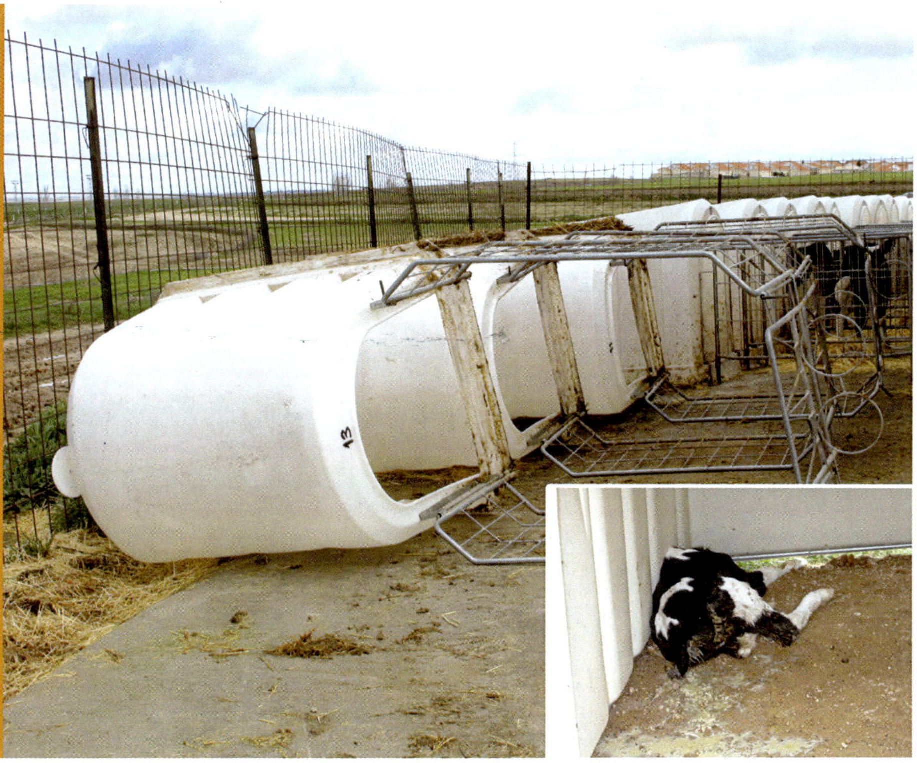

Image courtesy of Dr. J. V. González.

1 Why does it affect newborn animals?

From a contagion, severity of infection and host age point of view, various studies of cryptosporidium isolates from domestic ruminants have highlighted a significant aetiological complexity. The four species currently known in bovines (*Cryptosporidium parvum, C. andersoni, C. bovis* and *C. ryanae*) are found at different times throughout the animals' life. Thus, the former (*C. parvum*) predominates in suckling calves, participating in the aetiology of the diarrhoeal syndrome found in newborn animals, whereas the other three are more common in weaned calves and in adults. This means that newborn calves are a public health risk, with infection prevalences of 85 % that drop to only 6 % in calves aged more than two months.

2 Can the bovine variety infect humans?

The genus *Cryptosporidium* includes a multitude of intracellular and extracytoplasmic parasite species that affect around 150 host species, including numerous mammalian species such as humans and various domestic animals. Their morphological and biological characteristics are unique: they form a special group amongst the apicomplexan protozoa.

The application of biochemical and, more recently molecular techniques has highlighted the enormous genetic diversity of this genus and has allowed the existence of numerous species in different host vertebrates to be confirmed. As regards this genetic diversity, the genotypes of some parasite species have been described. Without going into great detail concerning the accepted species and those which are currently only considered to be genotypes, 24 species from the genus *Cryptosporidium* are currently considered to be valid, with around 60 genotypes in different animal species that have also been found to be parasitic in humans.

Out of the ones found in cattle, the species that commonly is associated with zoonotic infection is *Cryptosporidium parvum*. Others such as *C. andersoni* or *C. ubiquitum* rarely infect humans and *C. bovis* does not infect people. In short, the genus contains species that are initially parasitic in animals, especially bovines, but which can reach humans via various pathways, thus constituting a zoonotic problem of varying importance that is closely related to various epidemiological and socioeconomic factors (immunodeficiency, immunosuppressant treatments or infections) of the huma population in various regions.

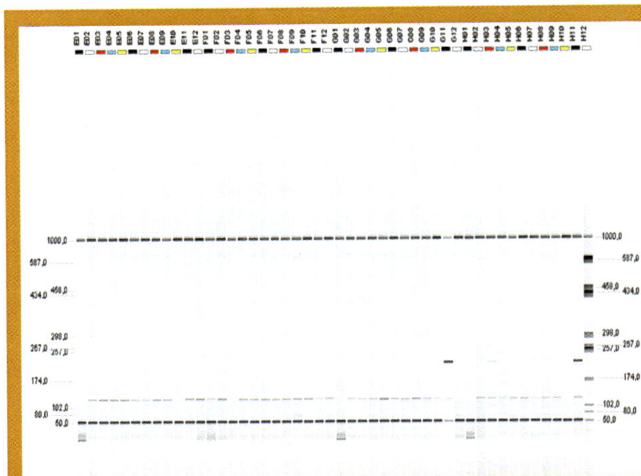

The broad genetic diversity of the genus and the fact that many species can be transmitted to humans means that molecular techniques are essential for their correct identification. Moreover, *C. parvum* infection in calves is commonly associated with other enteropathogens, such as enterotoxigenic *E. coli* and other pathogenic *E. coli* strains, rotavirus, *Clostridium* perfringens and *Salmonella*.

3 What characterises the biological cycle of *Cryptosporidium*?

The biological cycle is monoxenous and all its phases, both sexual and asexual, occur in the same host. In domestic ruminants, the cycle commences upon ingestion of the oocyst, which is followed by excystation in the host's gastrointestinal tract, where the four sporozoites are released. The mammalian body temperature (around 37 °C), bile salts and, possibly, trypsin all markedly affect this phase.

Once released, the sporozoites reach the luminal border of enterocytes by contraction/extension and gliding movements. There they invaginate, similar to a finger in a glove, and are enclosed by the host cell membrane, which encapsulates the parasite inside a parasitophorous vacuole.

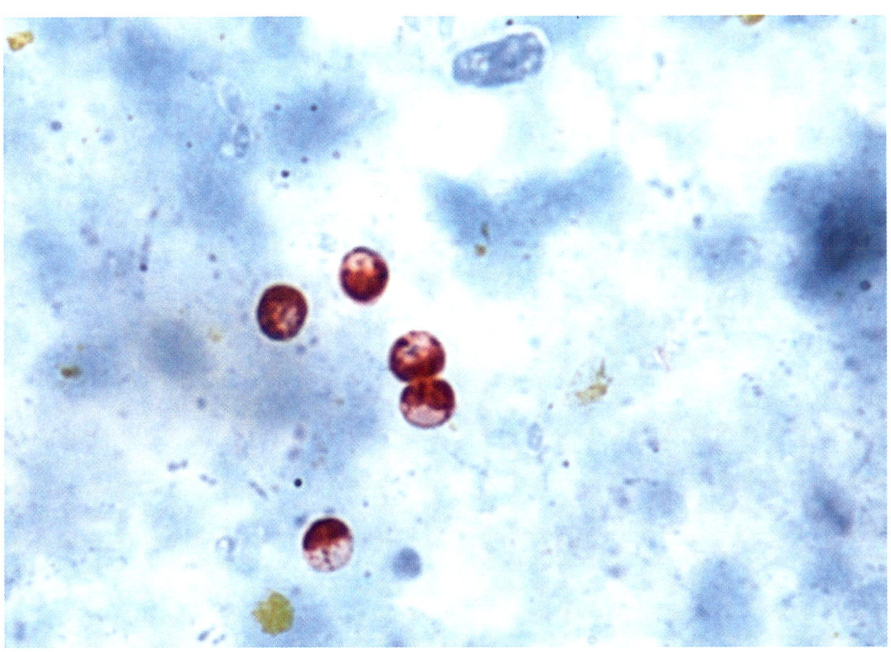

As a large quantity of oocysts are excreted in the faeces during the course of the infection, their study thereof can be considered to represent a sampling of the intestine as a whole. The oocysts excreted can be detected using a large number of techniques, including classical techniques such as staining for acid-fast microorganisms (modified Ziehl-Neelsen staining technique), which allows them to be visualised with an intense pink colour.

Four or eight merozoites are formed during merogony (ectomerogony) depending on whether a first- or second-generation schizogony is underway. Two types of schizonts are known to exist, namely type I, which is the first to appear during the biological cycle and has eight merozoites, and type II, which has four merozoites. Type I merozoites can generate new first-generation schizogonies or form type II schizonts, which go on to form macro- and microgametes. Most type II merozoites that enter the host cell are destined to form macrogametes, with just a few forming microgametocytes containing 16 microgametes in their interior.

The macrogametes contain polysaccharide (amylopectin) granules in their basal part and wall-forming bodies around their edges. The microgametes lack a flagellum and move towards the macrogametes following the intestinal flow or by contraction and extension of the intracytoplasmic microtubules. Fertilisation is accompanied by penetration of the microgamete via the parasitophorous vacuole and membrane of the macrogamete. Sporogony occurs inside the host cell.

Formation of the oocyst wall occurs prior to spore formation, which results in the formation of four sporozoites. The 80 % of oocysts, known as thick-walled oocysts, that present a double oocyst wall are the resistant forms found in the environment and are responsible for inter-host transmission. Thin-walled oocysts (20 %) are surrounded by a single membrane unit and are responsible for autoinfection. Their relatively weak wall breaks shortly after their release from the host cell and the sporozoites penetrate neighbouring epithelial cells, thereby restarting the endogenous cycle.

The prepatency period in domestic ruminants is 3-4 days, although this can be extended up to 6-7 days depending on age and infective dose.

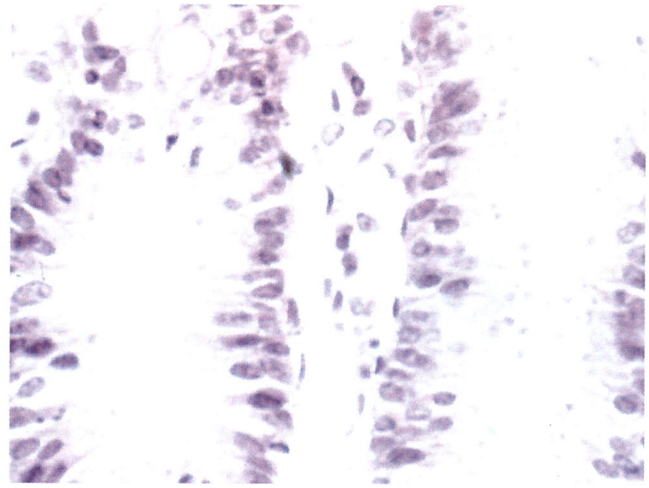

The majority of the endogenous stages of the parasite are found in the jejunum and ileum, with some also being found in the duodenum, caecum and colon. The apical part of the villi presents zones with aggregates in various stages of degeneration and often includes endogenous forms of the parasite. The lamina propria is normally infiltrated with macrophages and lymphocytes.

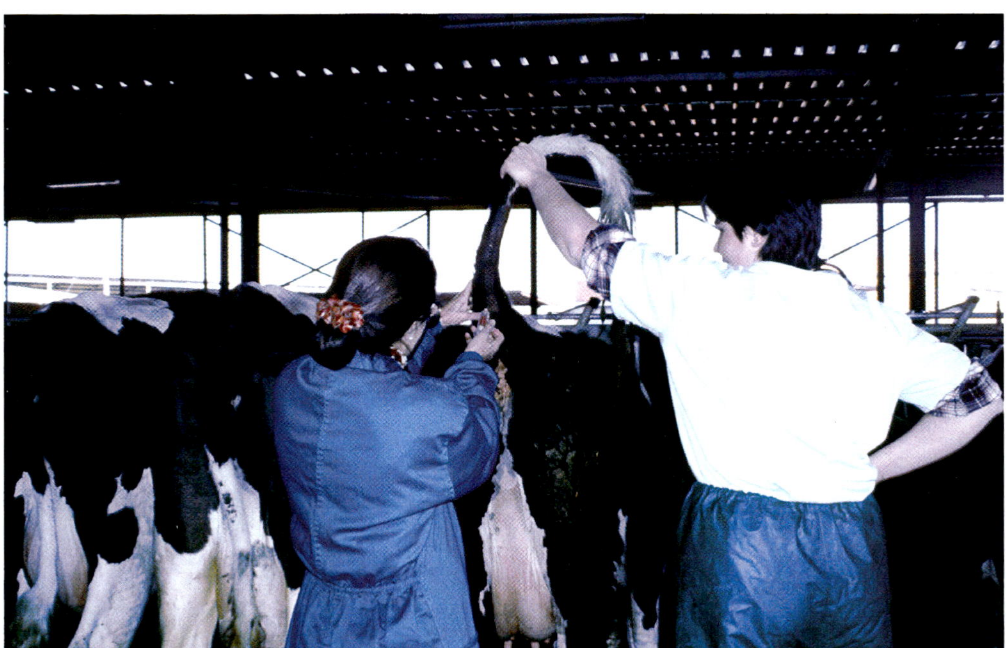

Methods for detecting blood antibodies are not widely used in domestic ruminants and present some specificity problems, such as the reaction of colostral antibodies or the cross-reaction with other Apicomplexa in older animals.

19 What measures can we take to prevent cryptosporidiosis outbreaks?

Like most years, outbreaks of diarrhoea occur in calves on a dairy farm in Somosierra, Madrid. Initially, the farmer only detects staining of the hindquarters and the tail in two almost newborn animals. As instructed by the vet, he separates the animals from their mothers and houses them in a clean quarantine station to observe their evolution. He confirms an increased number of bowel movements, which are increasingly liquid, and calls the vet at night. By the time the vet arrives a further three animals have diarrhoea and the first animals affected have worsened considerably —their faeces are aqueous, smell very badly, are very light (yellow or white) in colour, they show clear signs of dehydration, their limbs are cold, they have stopped eating and have great difficulties in standing and remaining standing.

1. How are cryptosporidia maintained from one calving season to another?
2. How can calf deaths be avoided?
3. How is cryptosporidiosis diagnosed?

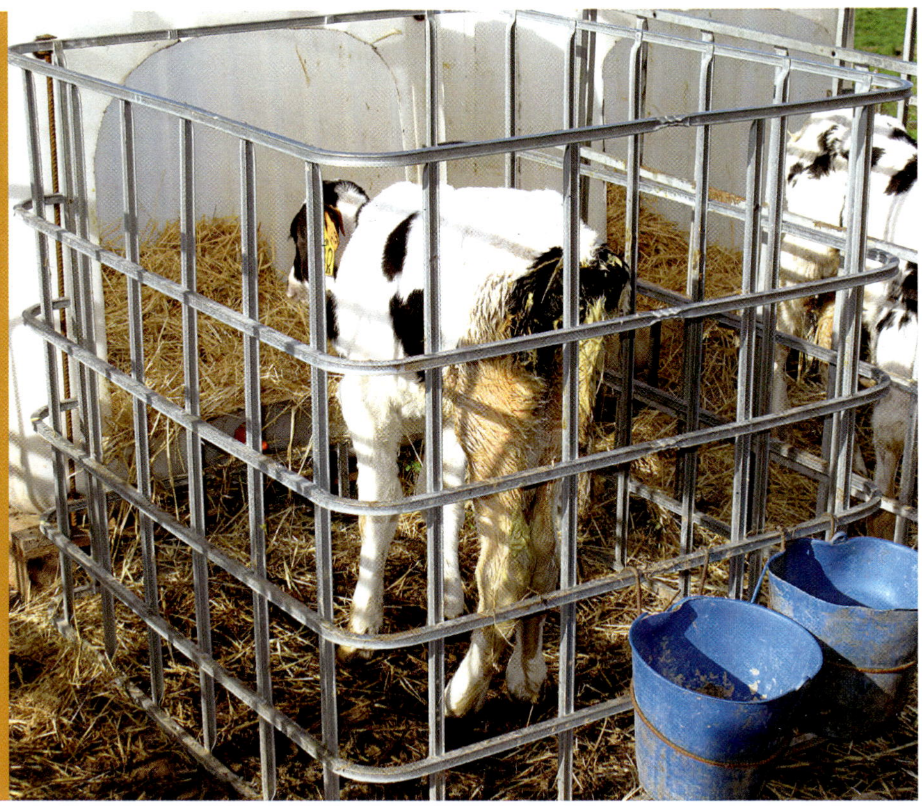

Image courtesy of Dr. J. V. González.

1 How are cryptosporidia maintained from one calving season to another?

Cryptosporidiosis affects both beef and dairy cattle. The main source of infection is faecal matter from diarrhoeal calves. An animal can eliminate between 10^6 and 10^7 oocysts per gramme of faeces during the diarrhoeal period, which multiplied by the daily faecal volume gives some idea of the scale of oocyst excretion. As such, the most dangerous source of infection for a newborn animal is the infected animals with which it shares the cowshed. If the number of animals per unit area is high, and hygiene inappropriate, conditions would favour outbreaks.

Although there appears to be no relationship between clinical cryptosporidiosis and natural or artificial feeding, a relationship has been found when feeding is incorrect.

If hygiene is deficient, the highest incidence usually occurs at the end of the calving season. The reason is very high contamination of the environment resulting from the fact that oocysts are highly resistant and can survive for several months at low temperature with sufficient humidity, thereby increasing the risk of infection. The fact that the calving season also usually occurs at cold and wet times of year may also aggravate the process both directly and also because keeping animals in closed sheds increases the likelihood of contagion.

Calves are receptive for at least their first three months of life and, although the immunity acquired after neonatal infection protects against reinfection, resistance also develops with age: the animals eliminate fewer oocysts and the clinical signs are less evident. Asymptomatic carriers have also been detected in the adult population.

2 How can calf deaths be avoided?

The management of a cryptosporidiosis outbreak is not simple as no drug is currently able to achieve a complete cure in sick animals.

In light of this, measures that are able to restore the physical condition of calves are of increasing importance. Symptomatic treatment may prevent high mortality rates and decrease morbidity-related effects to an "acceptable" level.

In order to apply support therapy, however, a good understanding of the fluid, electrolyte, hormone substrate and energy changes that occur as a result of the diarrhoea is required.

Restoration of the volume of extracellular fluids is vital to prevent shock and acidosis. An isotonic electrolyte solution containing glucose, amino acids, sodium, potassium

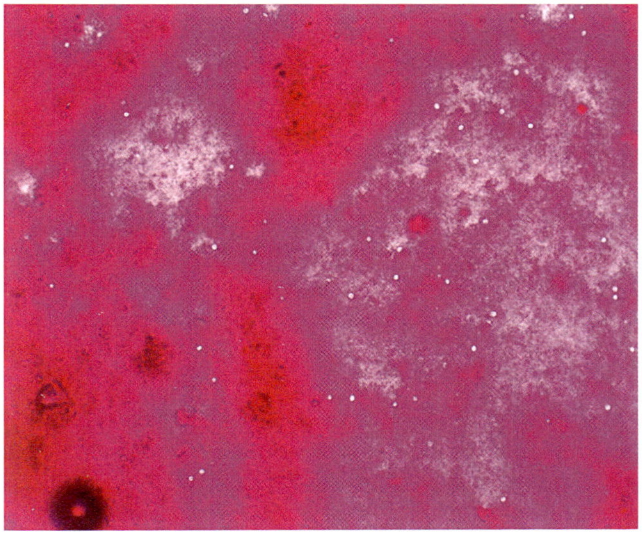

Cryptosporidium oocysts are infective from the moment they are excreted in the faeces and can survive for months in the environment as they are highly resistant. They are sensitive to drying and freezing. The main source of infection in domestic ruminants are faeces excreted by newborn animals with diarrhoea, although indirect transmission in contaminated feed and water is also possible (Heine negative staining method).

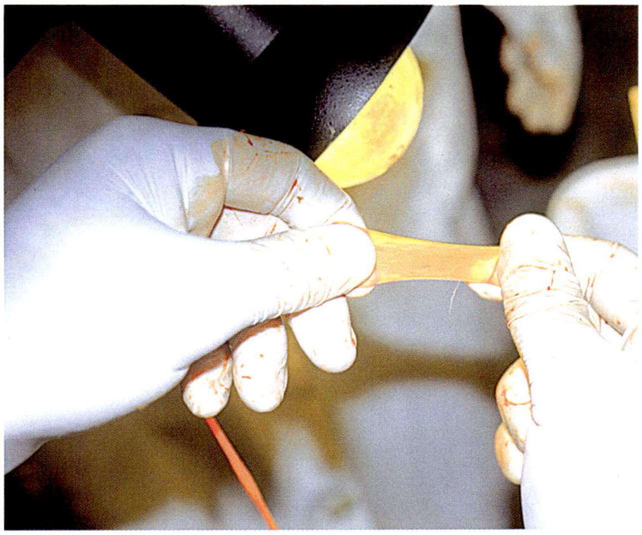

Infection of the enterocytes destroys the epithelial cells, which causes partial atrophy of the villi and the fusion thereof, clearly reducing the absorption surface. Malabsorption caused by these processes may become apparent even before atrophy of the villi occurs due to reduced enzyme binding to the membranes. This is aggravated by the passage of fluids from the villi into the intestinal lumen due to an increased osmotic pressure resulting from the accumulation of unabsorbed nutrients therein.

and chlorides should be administered endovenously to very dehydrated or moribund animals, ensuring that the initial potassium concentration is physiological due to the possible appereance of hyperkalaemia. As dehydration normalises, the potassium concentration can be increased. In the event of less severe dehydration, oral fluid therapy (generally with sufficient potassium and bicarbonate to replenish faecal loss of sodium and glucose) gives good results. The method of administration is important as absorption rates vary depending on whether therapy is administered via a gastric tube or orally. Oral hydration may be accompanied by the administration of some type of adsorbent.

Access of the animals to maternal or artificial milk must be restricted for an appropriate period of time. A reasonable practice involves administering electrolytes only for two days then gradually adding milk to the electrolyte solution (or allowing the animals to take milk from the mother).

The advisability of administering cholinergic antagonists and adrenergic agonists, which block secretion and prevent the entry of calcium into the crypts, or phenothiazine and prostaglandin inhibitors, remains unclear.

The administration of antibiotic to prevent secondary infections may be indicated.

As cryptosporidia are excreted in faeces, the main source of infection is faecal contamination of the environment by clinically affected animals. The possibility that carriers or reservoirs may also contribute to contagion should also be considered. Hygienic measures and disinfection of the installations, adequate ventilation, bedding, animal density and other basic measures are also particularly useful. The marked resistance of cryptosporidia oocysts to the majority of disinfectants should be noted.

Newborn animals fed on maternal milk are more resistant to infections than those fed artificially, irrespective of the absorption of immunoglobulins from the colostrum. This suggests that some components of the colostrum and milk that are not absorbed may play a specific protective role. Obviously, the other protective role is that provided by

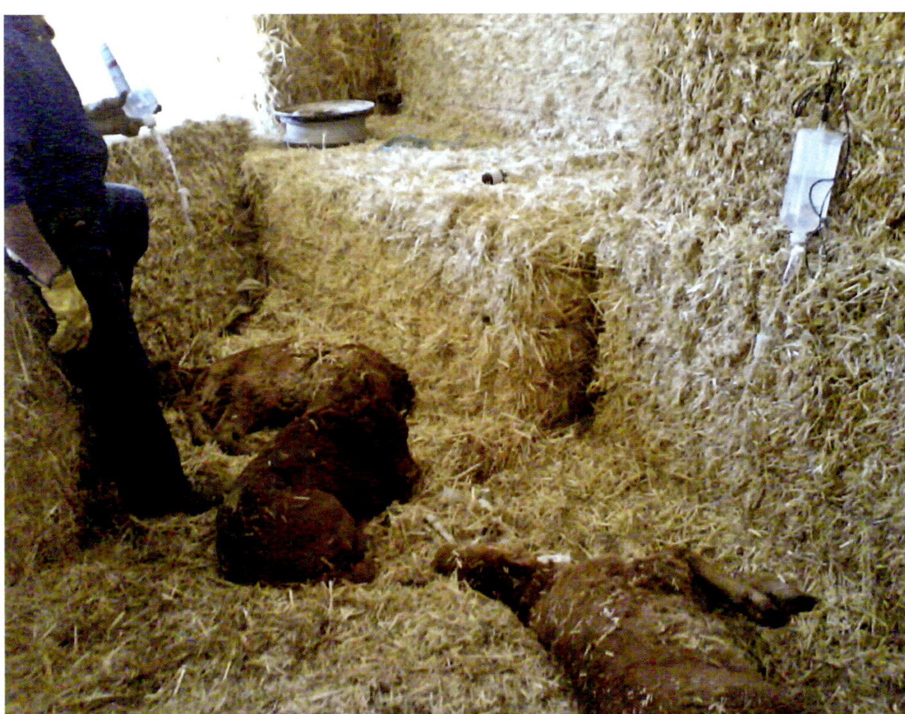

If the animals' condition is notably affected (highly dehydrated or moribund calves), the volume of extracellular fluids must be restored administering an intravenous isotonic electrolyte solution containing glucose, amino acids, sodium, potassium and chlorides. *Image courtesy of Dr. A. Diaz Guerrier.*

passive immunity by way of antibodies in the milk, which prevent the invasion of pathogenic microorganisms.

Although there is currently no drug which is completely effective, there are some compounds for the treatment of bovine cryptosporidiosis on the market.

Thus, halofuginone appears to reduce the diarrhoea, and therefore oocyst excretion, but does not provide a total cure. In calves aged 7-10 days, oral treatment with halofuginone (100 µg/kg) or decoquinate (2.5 mg/kg) did not affect the intensity of the diarrhoea, the dehydration, or the number of calves with diarrhoea or those excreting oocysts. However, after day 7, animals treated with halofuginone excreted significantly fewer oocysts and had a higher average daily weight gain than was observed in those treated with decoquinate.

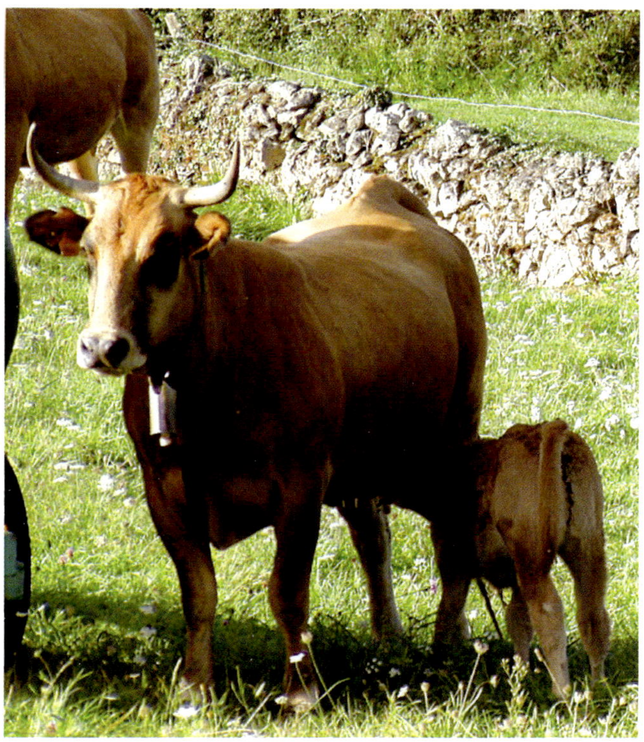

The colostral antibodies produced in response to a natural infection do not have a protective effect against infection in newborn calves. However, the hyperimmune colostrum produced by immunisation of the mothers may reduce the negative effects of infection by shortening the duration of the diarrhoea and oocyst excretion.

3 How is cryptosporidiosis diagnosed?

Although the clinical signs are non-specific, the epidemiology and symptomatology aid diagnosis. Thus, diarrhoea in animals aged up to three weeks, fever, dehydration, anorexia and weakness during the clinical examination help to establish a working diagnosis. However, an attempt should be made to establish an aetiological diagnosis.

Infected animals excrete large quantities of oocysts in faeces, therefore a faecal analysis is particularly useful. Various techniques, some of which are easier to apply than others and range from staining of direct faecal smears to oocyst concentration and immunological techniques, can be used to detect the parasite.

The first group comprises Giemsa stain, which is fairly non-specific, modified Ziehl-Neelsen stain, negative staining (Heine's technique) and other techniques based on the uptake of a fluorochrome by the parasite.

To increase the sensitivity, the oocysts present in the sample should be concentrated using solutions of different densities (Sheather's sucrose solution, zinc sulfate, sodium chloride) in which the cryptosporidium oocysts float and concentrate in the upper portion in the tube, or concentrating the oocysts by sedimentation in formalin/ether, formalin/ethyl acetate etc. Once concentrated, oocysts can be observed directly under a (phase-contrast or conventional) microscope.

The immunological techniques used to detect oocysts in faeces include latex agglutination test, immunofluorescence with poly-or monoclonal antibodies and immunocapture ELISA of parasitic antigens in faeces. Immunofluorescence is the most sensitive and specific of the more or less routinely used techniques.

In this case, it is vital to differentiate between cryptosporidiosis and other entities that progress with diarrhoea in newborns.

20 What are the repercussions of *Giardia* infection in bovines?

During the final year of the veterinary degree, and for the second consecutive year, the lecturers noted a significant drop in attendance at practical classes due to student illness. Most certificates of absence noted acute temporary diarrhoea, although some students had been hospitalised. A telephone survey of all students on the course concerned highlighted many more milder cases, such as soft stools or colic-type pain. All students were requested to submit stool samples to the microbiology and parasitology laboratory. *Giardia* trophozoites or cysts were detected in a high percentage of cases. All students involved had been in direct contact with different animals during feeding and handling dogs, and also when cleaning the stalls of ruminants.

1. Are the *Giardia* strains/genotypes that affect bovines zoonotic?
2. At what age is the risk of contagion highest?
3. What repercussions does it have on animal growth and how can these be avoided?

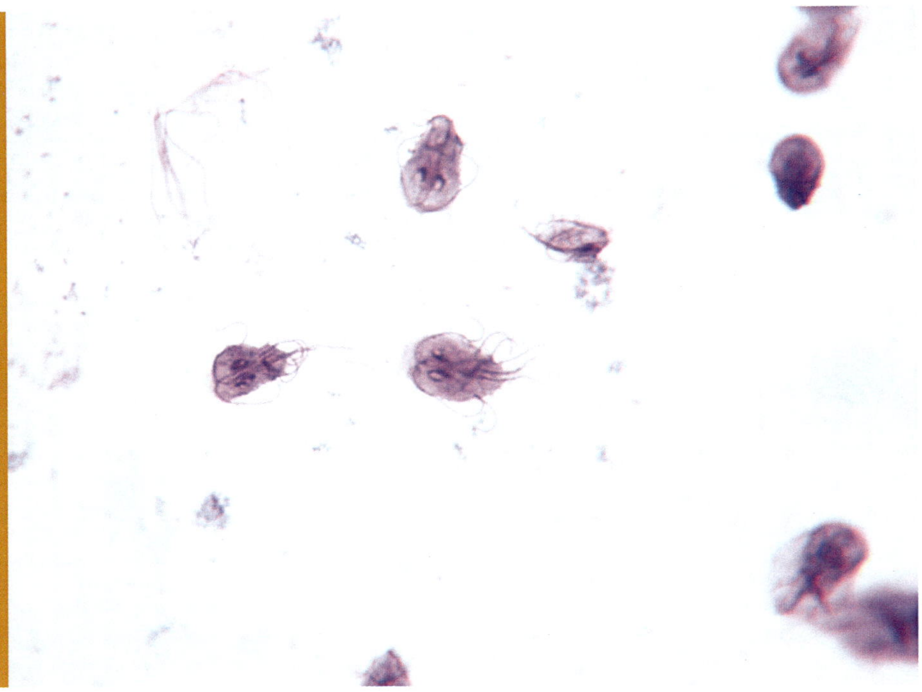

Image courtesy of Dr T. Gómez.

1 Are the *Giardia* strains/genotypes that affect bovines zoonotic?

On the basis of morphological and molecular studies, five species that infect amphibians, birds and various mammals have been accepted in the genus *Giardia*. The species *Giardia duodenalis* (= *G. lamblia, G. intestinalis*) is currently considered to comprise seven genotypes (A-G) with high host specificity. A new genotype (H) has recently been isolated from seals in the USA, although further studies are required to confirm this.

Of these, genotypes A and B have been isolated from ruminants and humans.

As such, in light of the origin of these isolates, the zoonotic nature of some genotypes must be taken into consideration. The table in the next page contains information concerning the hosts from which the genotypes identified to date were isolated.

Recent studies showed that, although zoonotic serotypes can be found in bovines, they are rarely found. Public health risk due to *Giardia* shedding in cattle faeces may be much lower than in other animals such as canids.

Giardia duodenalis genotypes and hosts from which they were isolated	
Genotype	Host(s)
A	Humans, primates, dog, cat, domestic ruminants, rodents, wild mammals
B	Humans, primates, dog, horse, domestic ruminants
C	Canids
D	Canids
E	Ruminants and other artiodactyla
F	Cat
G	Rodents

2 At what age is the risk of contagion highest?

Firstly, it should be noted that genotypes A, B and E are present irrespective of age. Genotype E is most commonly identified genotype in bovines. Genotype B has only been identified occasionally.

Some epidemiological studies have shown that the prevalence of *G. duodenalis* infection increases with age to a maximum of 93.1 % in animals aged 10 to 13 months, subsequently decreasing. However, other studies have reported that the highest prevalence occurs in animals aged 1-1.5 months, although the values observed up to two months of age are also high (approx. 61 %), remaining high in animals aged between three months and one year (32 %) and moderately high in heifers aged between one and two years (11.4 %).

As far as the presence of the most important genotypes is concerned, type A is rare in animals prior to weaning. Despite this, the prevalence in recently weaned animals can be as high as 7 % and up to 5 % in heifers.

As both genotypes (A and E) have been found to infect heifers simultaneously, the role of bovines as reservoirs of genotypes with a zoonotic potential for humans appears to be more important than thought until fairly recently.

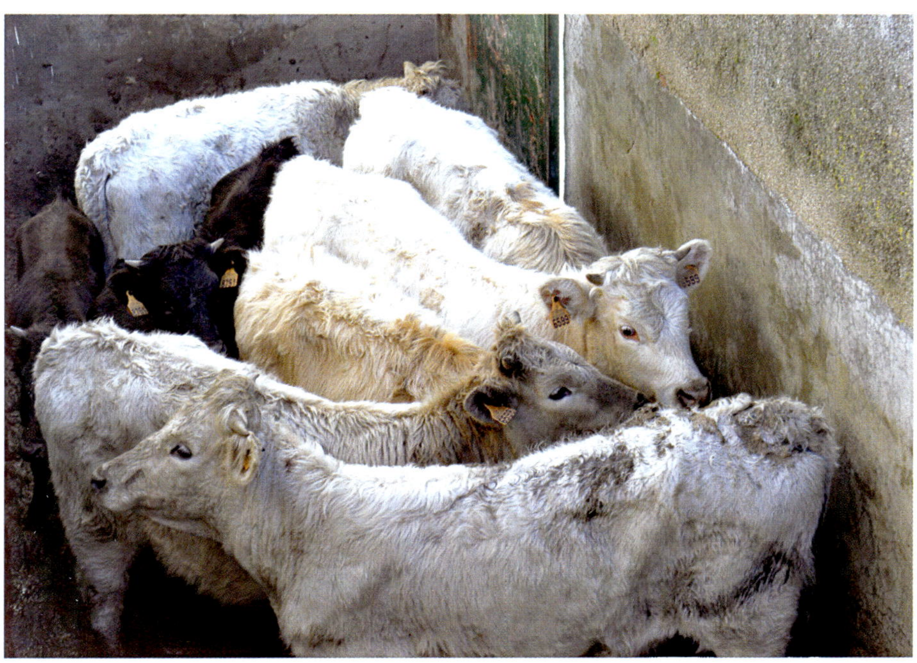

The source of giardiosis is usually a sick animal or an asymptomatic carrier, generally an adult animal, that excretes cysts. Pregnant cows excrete them at the end of pregnancy and during the first few days of lactation. The possibility that, given its poor host specificity, giardia may be introduced onto the farm by carnivores, rodents or even humans should also be remembered. The contamination of feed and drinking water may also be the cause of the disease.

3 What repercussions does it have on animal growth and how can these be avoided?

There is no clear relationship between genotypes and the clinical manifestations seen in hosts. However, even though infections do not always proceed with signs of disease, the pathogenic potential of the parasite has been clearly established.

Giardiosis is of great economic importance, especially in young animals in their growth phase.

Giardiae attach to the enteric mucosa (mainly the duodenum and jejunum) via a ventral disc and a mannose/lectin complex that binds to specific epithelial markers. This reduces the intestinal surface available for absorption and leads to a deficient absorption of fatty acids, vitamins, proteins and sugars, in other words the onset of malabsorption and more or less persistent diarrhoea with elimination of mucus in the stools, fever, dehydration, anorexia, abdominal swelling and, in some cases, death of the affected animals. In turn, the above leads to digestive disorders, growth retardation and significant economic losses, even in the event of subclinical infections.

If the cause of an outbreak compatible with giardiosis can be clearly identified, appropriate measures must be established to mitigate the effects of the parasite. Thus, the symptoms (diarrhoea, dehydration, etc.) must be controlled and attempts made to eliminate the agent.

Various molecules can be used for such treatment. Benzimidazole carbamates, especially fenbenzadole (5-20 mg/kg b.w. for 3 days), and paromomycin (50 or 75 mg/kg b.w. for 5 days), which achieve a marked reduction in cyst excretion and some clinical improvement by week 3, appear to give good results, although cyst elimination may recover shortly afterwards.

Nitroimidazoles, such as metronidazole, tinidazole and furazolidone, are also effective.

These measures should be accompanied by the application of basic hygiene and disinfection measures in the installations. 10 % ammonia improves the results, and the elimination of bedding with a high-pressure water jet, followed by drying and disinfection, is also effective. It should be noted that giardia cysts can survive for one week in faeces and up to seven weeks in the soil. Recent studies showed that although zoonotic genotypes can be found in bovines, they are very rare in cattle. Public health risk due to Giardia shedding in cattle faeces is much lower than in other animals such as canids.

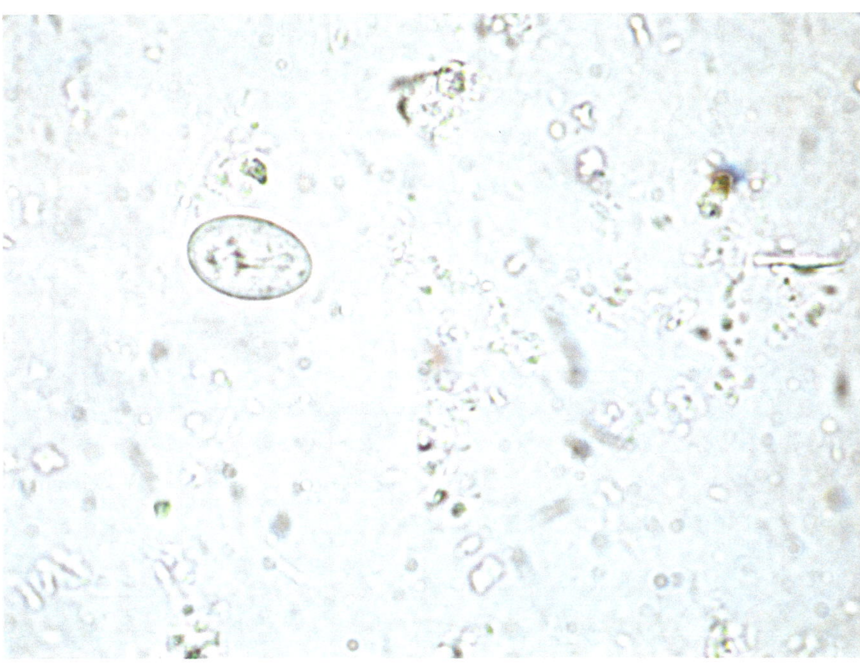

Diagnosis is performed by observation of the cysts using methods that allow oval structures 13.7 × 9.1 μm in size to be identified. As elimination is not constant, stool samples should be taken over several days to confirm the diagnosis. If diarrhoea is noted, the possible joint action of bacteria, viruses, other protozoa and helminths must be considered. *Image courtesy of Dr T. Gómez.*

21 How many species of *Eimeria* are there in bovines?

A coccidiosis with a faecal oocyst count of 1,320,000/g, which was identified as 100 % *Eimeria alabamensis*, is diagnosed in a 6-month-old calf with diarrhoea that had been grazing for only 3 weeks. Three further calves on the same farm aged only 5 weeks appear severely affected, with their hindquarters stained with bloody stools, their loins arched and their hair bristly. These animals barely produce stools when attempting to defecate and die rapidly. The necropsy confirms the presence of a large quantity of blood and clots in the caecum and colon. A generalised catarrhal enteritis, which is diphtheroid and necrosing in some regions, is observed in both the small and large intestine. The intestinal wall is thickened, congested and oedematous, with petechiae or diffuse haemorrhages. Yellowish-brown pseudomembranous layers and punctiform white or grey nodules are widespread. The intestinal lymph nodes are enlarged.

1. What is coccidiosis?
2. What does it mean that coccidiosis is self-limiting?
3. What factors affect the onset of coccidia-related diarrhoea?

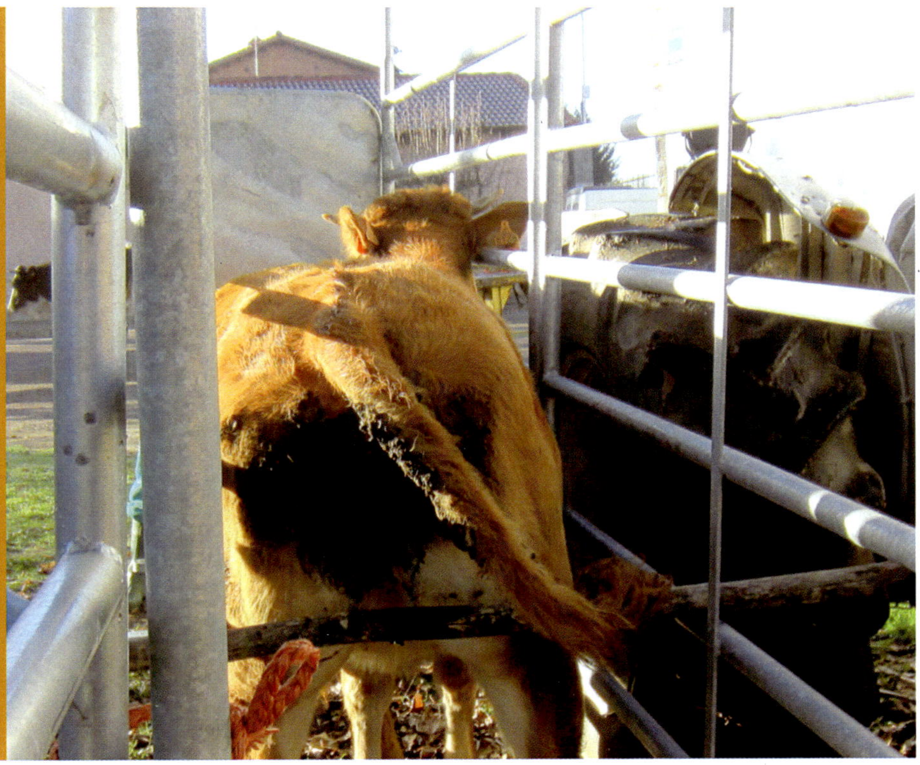

1 What is coccidiosis?

Bovine coccidiosis is an enteric parasitosis caused by more than ten species of coccidia, although *Eimeria bovis, E. zuernii* and *E. alabamensis* are considered to be the most important. It is most commonly found in animals aged between 6 months and 2 years, although it can also affect cattle up to 5 years of age. Clinical outbreaks occur with some frequency in cattle herds, although in recent years a continual increase in the incidence of this disease has been observed.

Infection may be subclinical, producing growth retardation, or, if the initial infective dose is high, it may lead to clinical signs mainly characterised by diarrhoea, which is sometimes haemorrhagic, bristly hair, weight loss and weakness. Nervous signs, such as tremor and limb movements, may also occasionally present. In the absence of other potential pathogens diagnosis is aided, a clinical history and pre-sentation of diarrhoea, tenesmus and melena, together with a finding of oocysts from the most pathogenic species in faeces and macroscopic and histopathological alterations.

2 What does it mean that coccidiosis is self-limiting?

Eimeria species have a self-limiting cycle, in other words if an animal were to suffer only a single infection it could remain free from coccidia as asexual development becomes increasingly difficult and finally leads to sporogony, which is propagative rather than multiplicative.

The biological cycle of all coccidia is basically the same. Thus, the oocysts excreted in the faeces need to undergo sporulation in order to be infective; if conditions are suitable spore formation can be completed in 48 hours. After being ingested, sporozoites are released and penetrate the intestinal cells, where they grow and multiply asexually to form schizonts. Growth of these schizonts leads to rupture of the infected cell, with the merozoites subsequently invading new cells and repeating the process. Finally, they differentiate sexually to form male and female gametes. Fertilisation leads to a zygote, which surrounds itself with a coating to form the oocyst, completing the cycle upon expulsion to the exterior. As noted above, infection is self-limiting, although animals normally become infected and reinfected several times.

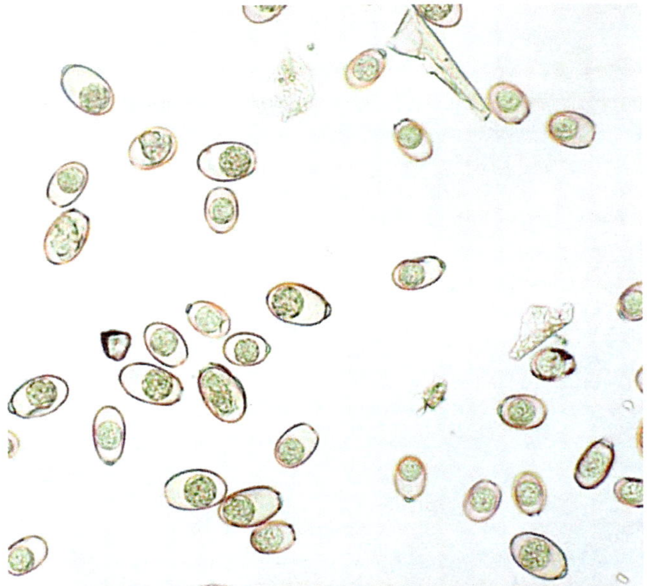

Clinical outbreaks rarely occur but it always results in decreased yields, especially on intensive farms. Coccidiosis is an intestinal infection produced by *Eimeria* spp. that mainly affects young animals and progresses with diarrhoea, which may be blood-stained, and dehydration.

Gamete conjugation produces a zygote surrounded by a strong membrane (oocyst), which is expelled to the exterior where it sporulates (sporogony) to form four sporocysts, each of which contains two sporozoites. This sporulated oocyst is the infective phase for a new host.

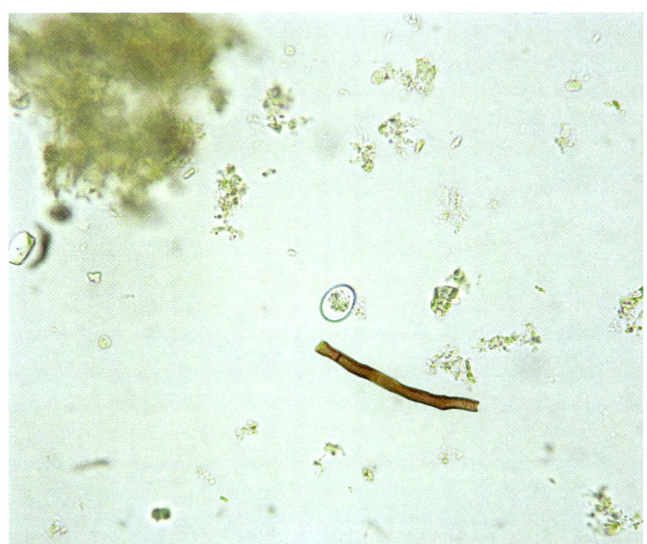

E. bovis is a highly pathogenic species. Schizont generation in the small intestine leads to breakage of the villi, whereas the sexual phases take place in the latter portion of the ileum, caecum and colon and are responsible for the pathogenic effects.

3 What factors affect the onset of coccidia-related diarrhoea?

Once they have formed spores, *Eimeria* spp. oocysts are highly resistant to environmental conditions. In some regions, they steadily accumulate and contaminate food and drinking water, thus meaning that animals can become infected with very high doses.

Coccidiosis is always acquired by the ingestion of sporulated oocysts with contaminated food or water. The disease is present all year round in humid and temperate regions, whereas in continental climates it is more common in spring or summer (if not very dry) and autumn, although the season may vary under some circumstances.

Concomitant causes that contribute to weakening the animal, such as colds, other parasitoses, infections, etc. affect the onset of the clinical process and its severity. Zootechnical practices also play an important role. In some regions, animals that return from grazing to be fattened under conditions that promote overcrowding become sick, whereas in others, such as northern Spain, animals fall sick after transfer to the extensive regime. When grazing large pastures or grasslands, the risk to herds belonging to the same owner is much lower than when the same animals are held in corrals or feedlots. In the north of Spain, each farmer normally possesses a limited number of animals that are stabled during the winter, thus limiting the spread of coccidiosis. However, once the animals begin to graze common pastures, the oocysts are readily disseminated and the disease spreads rapidly.

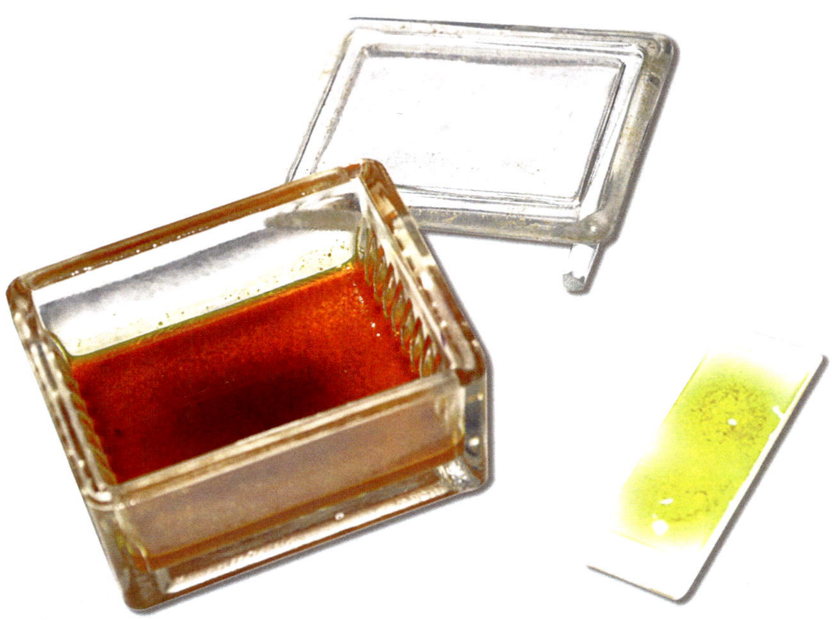

Microscopic stool analysis allows the presence of oocysts to be detected, although in hyperacute cases signs may appear some days beforehand. A specific diagnosis requires the identification of sporulated oocysts in faeces using a solution of potassium dichromate at room temperature over several days.

Biological cycle of coccidia

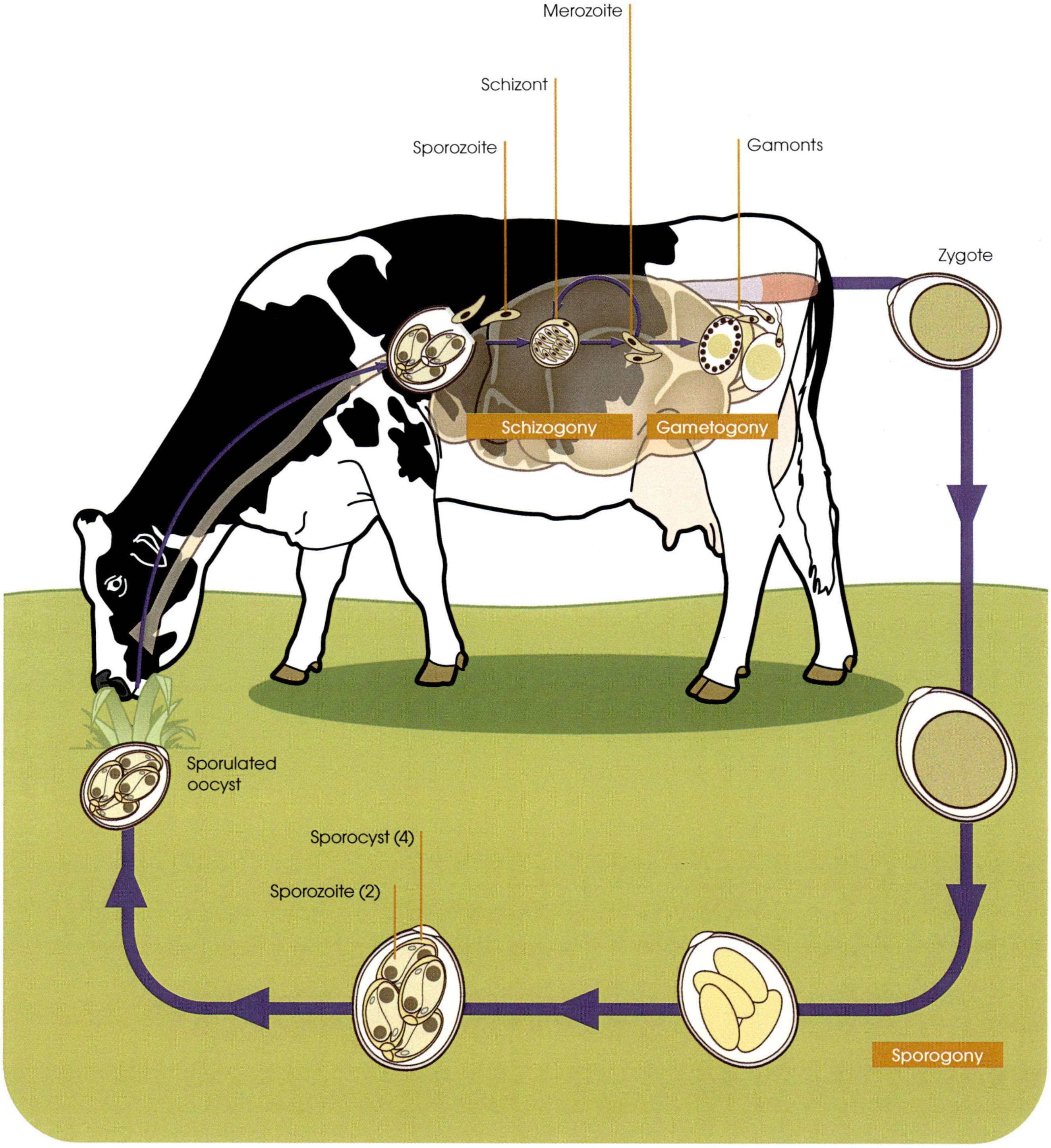

22 Why are some species of *Eimeria* more pathogenic?

In a particularly dry autumn, an outbreak of acute diarrhoea occurs in naturally grazed calves. The aetiological agent is identified as *Eimeria zuernii*. One calf from the group, aged 18 months and weighing 200 kg, presented nervous symptoms with erratic behaviour, distancing itself from the group, suddenly running in random directions, allowing itself to fall to the ground and suffering from convulsions for around two minutes, with limb spasms, nystagmus and rolling of the eyeballs, and whereas its nostrils remained dry it excreted abundant saliva from the mouth. The animal showed a magnified response to external noises (clapping of the hands) or to attempts to palpate the spinal region.

1. Why did a coccidiosis occur in grazing animals?
2. How does coccidiosis-related diarrhoea in calves occur?
3. How can the nervous signs be explained?

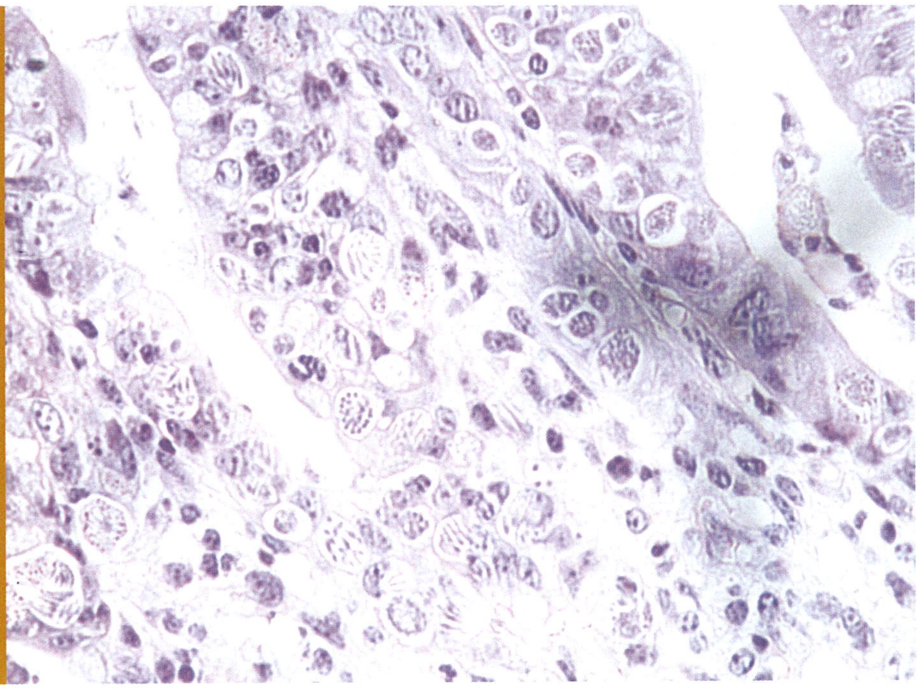

1 Why did a coccidiosis occur in grazing animals?

Bovine coccidioses tend to present in young animals. Adults generally behave as asymptomatic carriers.

Bovines are infected upon ingesting oocysts with food or water. The severity of the disease will depend on the number of oocysts ingested. Clinical signs are unlikely to be present if only a few are ingested, and repeated infections will lead to disease-free immunity. Ingestion of a large number of oocysts may cause disease and death, even in adult animals.

Overcrowding and lack of hygiene increase the risk of disease. The successive passage of coccidia from one animal to another often increases infection at a pathogenic level and leads to contamination of farms or pastures. This explains why severe coccidioses occur when calves are introduced to a pasture or farm that was previously believed to be free from infection.

Moderate temperatures (18-27 °C) and high humidity favour spore formation. They are inactivated within 4 days at 40 °C and die rapidly at higher temperatures. Some species can withstand freezing at temperature of between -19 and -25 °C for several months, thus implying the possible presence of viable oocysts in pastures during the winter. Hot and dry summers and direct sunlight are detrimental to the parasite. As such, climate conditions affect the development of oocysts.

2 How does coccidiosis-related diarrhoea in calves occur?

The pathogeny is due to destruction of the epithelial cells in various regions of the intestine, which depends on the number of oocysts ingested, the reproductive potential of the species concerned, the so-called crowding factor, and the exact location of the parasites. Thus, species that develop subepithelially cause more severe lesions, generally with haemorrhage, than those that infect epithelial cells.

The pathogenic action of coccidia can partially be explained from an understanding of the biological cycle and location in the host coupled with destruction of the host cell.

The parasites grow incredibly fast during the asexual phase, with a single schizont producing thousands of merozoites, as is the case with *Eimeria bovis*. On the other hand, the schizogonic phase lasts for several generations. In either of these cases the damage produced can be very significant even though the initial dose was not particularly high.

This traumatic action results in the production of numerous ulcers, which are initially microscopic but can become macroscopic if entire regions of intestinal villi lining cells or Lieberkühn glands are destroyed, leaving large areas free from these structures and revealing the underlying submucosal blood vessels, thus leading to enteric haemorrhages which on occasions can be significant. Such lesions lead to the haemorrhagic diarrhoea that often characterises clinical coccidiosis. Haemorrhages are very common in *E. zuernii* and *E. bovis* infections, although melena is not always constant.

These haemorrhages lead to anaemia, hypoproteinaemia and electrolyte loss. Moreover, the damaged mucosa can be colonised by bacteria, thus leading to secondary infections.

3 How can the nervous signs be explained?

The neurological syndrome in bovines may be due to *strictly* infectious, nutritional or metabolic causes or to toxins. Less often, it may be due to a type of coccidiosis first described in 1921, namely "nervous coccidiosis", in which affected animals also present intestinal coccidiosis. Despite being known for many years, there is as yet no agreement as regards the genesis of nervous coccidiosis.

Thus, according to some sources, this condition is not just a coccidiosis but a combination of stress factors, obviously including the damage caused by coccidia itself. The end result is decreased tissue magnesium and serum calcium levels, both of which lead to nervous signs. Intravenous and subcutaneous administration of calcium, magnesium, dextrose, electrolytes and sulfamides immediately after the onset of symptoms, when the animal is still able to remain upright, can give good results.

A further possible explanation is low copper levels in the kidneys of affected animals. It is also possible that this condition is due to the presence of a neurotoxin in the animals' serum which is not present in animals with intestinal coccidiosis alone.

Other hypotheses, such as a thiamine or vitamin A deficiency, hypoglycaemia, electrolyte (Mg, Na, K, P, Ca) imbalances, toxins produced by the parasites, etc., have also been proposed.

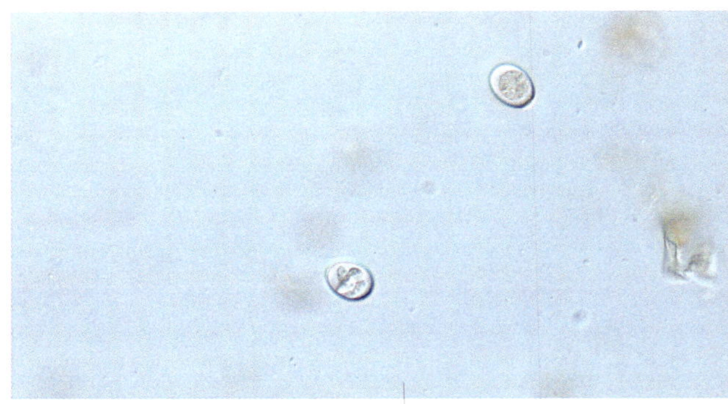

E. zuernii is the most common and most pathogenic species. The first schizogony occurs in the ileum and the second in the caecum and colon. The sexual phases occur in the lower part of the small intestine, caecum, colon and rectum.

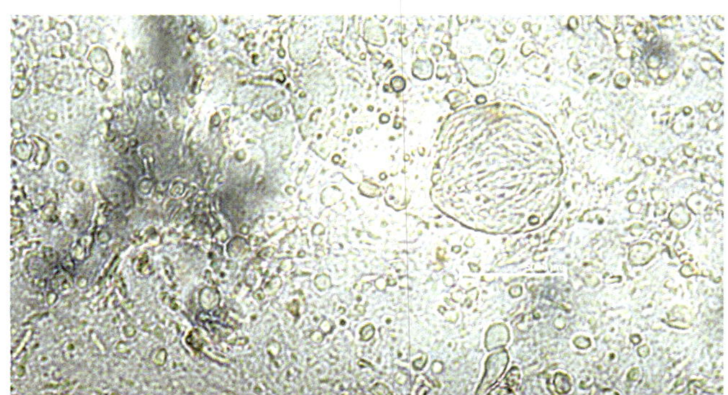

Infection commences with the ingestion of sporulated oocysts, which release their sporozoites upon the action of bile and trypsin. These sporozoites invade the epithelium of the small intestine, where they become rounded and form the trophozoite. The parasites divide asexually (schizogony) at this site to form schizonts. First-generation schizonts (macroschizonts or giant schizonts) may be large and contain thousands of merozoites, which invade new cells and, in most species, result in a second generation of smaller schizonts containing fewer merozoites. The last sexual phase in the cycle usually occurs between the end of the small intestine and the start of the large intestine. All phases in the endogenous cycle can be seen after scraping the intestinal mucosa.

23 How can coccidiosis-related losses be prevented?

During an outbreak of diarrhoea on a feed lot in Catalonia (Spain), 10 animals were examined. They presented with diarrhoea having mucus and streaks of blood in the faecal matter. Blood-stained diarrhoea, tenesmus and severe dehydration were observed in three animals. Faecal samples were taken and sent to the parasitology laboratory, which analysed the faecal matter, provided an oocyst count per gram (opg) and sporulated the oocysts in 2.5 % potassium dichromate at room temperature. The sporulation time was measured and the oocysts identified. All samples analysed contained coccidian oocysts, with minimum and maximum values of 5000 and 15,500 opg. The coccidia concerned were identified as belonging to the genus *Eimeria*, with *E. bovis* and *E. zuernii* being the most prevalent species (43 % and 56 % respectively). All oocysts sporulated within 48 hours. The morbidity in the feed lot was 100 % and the mortality 2 %.

1. What losses are associated with a coccidiosis outbreak?
2. How is coccidiosis diagnosed?
3. How can an animal with coccidiosis be cured and reinfection prevented?

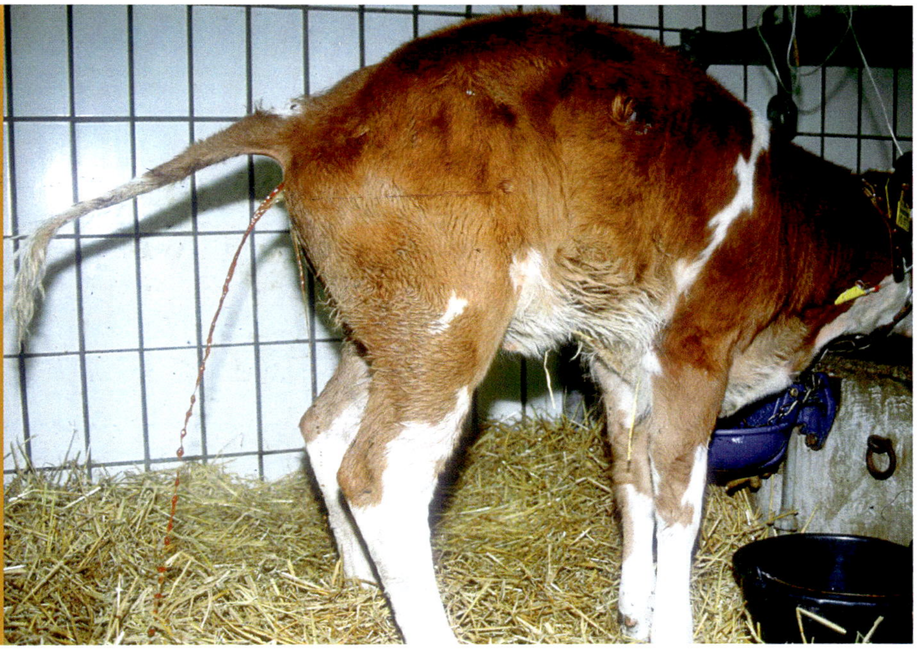

Image courtesy of Dr. G. Knubben-Schweizer.

1 What losses are associated with a coccidiosis outbreak?

Coccidiosis is characterised by haemorrhagic and mucus-containing diarrhoea produced by various species of the genus *Eimeria*, although the most important worldwide are *E. zuernii* and *E. bovis*.

The repercussions of these parasitoses arise due to the weight loss of affected animals, non-optimal feed use and the treatment required to control them.

The onset of disease is characterised by the appearance of diarrhoea. Liquid faeces mixed with mucus and small quantities of blood are initially eliminated. In any case, the hind third of the animals is completely stained, thus enabling affected animals to readily be identified. Depending on its severity, this diarrhoea can lead to dehydration and anaemia, anorexia, weakness and weigh loss. Some animals may develop nervous symptoms, with seizures and toxaemia.

Although the repercussions of coccidiosis are significant at any stage in an animal's life, they are much greater during certain phases of animal production. It is difficult to calculate the losses caused by this disease as indirect losses are more important than direct losses, which are much easier to determine.

However, feed wastage due to lack of appetite or anorexia of affected animals, the consequent weight loss and lowered immune response capacity against any other challenge are a very important factors that weighs heavily on the results of the farming enterprise.

Several publications in this respect refer to significant losses on a scale of several thousand dollars or euros, although these estimations by no means reflect the true scale of the problem.

2 How is coccidiosis diagnosed?

In light of the nature of the pathogens involved in diarrhoea in calves, there is no direct relationship between the presence of a pathogen in a sample and diagnosis of a disease due to that pathogen.

- Firstly, not all animals affected excrete the pathogenic agent, thus meaning that, irrespective of the sensitivity of the technique, a negative result does not exclude the possibility that this agent is responsible for the disease.
- Secondly, it should be remembered that various pathogens can be encountered in samples obtained from healthy animals.
- Thirdly, many outbreaks of diarrhoea (up to 75 % according to some studies) are multifactorial and may involve two or more pathogens simultaneously. In this case it should be considered that the results obtained from just a few animals may be of little use.

All these problems can be avoided by taking samples from an appropriate number of affected calves and their apparently healthy counterparts, although the price of the tests must also be taken into consideration.

Moreover, irrespective of the test used, faecal analysis for diagnosis is not conclusive for the majority of pathogens potentially involved in cases of diarrhoea, including coccidia.

A *post mortem* study of recently deceased animals is, however, of diagnostic value if macroscopic lesions can be analysed and histopathological studies performed.

It should be remembered at this point that, in coccidiosis, the absence of oocysts in the faeces of suspect animals is not indicative of an absence of disease.

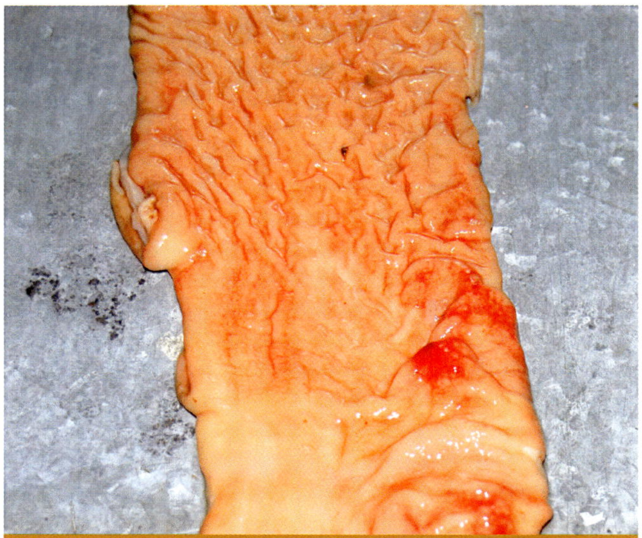

The pathogenesis is due to the destruction of intestinal epithelial cells, which depends on the number of oocysts ingested, the reproductive potential of the species concerned, the effect of overpopulation and the location of the parasites, with those species that multiply subepithelially being the most pathogenic.

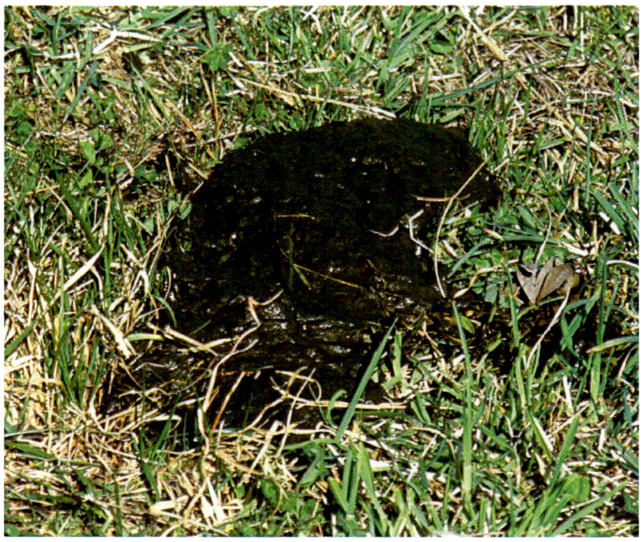

The diarrhoea in acute coccidiosis (red dysentery) is blood-stained, with abundant mucus and even blood clots. The animal's hindquarters may appear to be painted red. The diarrhoea may be accompanied by tenesmus, anaemia, weight loss and emaciation. Secondary infections, particularly pneumonia, are relatively common.

3 How can an animal with coccidiosis be cured and reinfection prevented?

The first measure to be taken during the treatment and control of coccidiosis should be the administration of antidiarrhoeal drugs and rehydration.

Sulfamides (or sulfonamides if preferred), such as sulfamethazine, sulfaquinoxaline or combinations of various such drugs, have traditionally been used to treat coccidiosis. Amprolium and ionophores such as monensin and lasalocid have also been used. As monensin is toxic, the dose must be calculated with great care. Its use as a growth promoter is forbidden. A similar situation is found for amprolium. In both cases, they should only be used as part of the "prescription cascade".

However, treatment success is limited if the animals remain in a contaminated environment, in which case efficacy is only temporary. Moreover, the majority of drugs have a coccidiostatic action but very limited coccidiocidal action. Coccidiostats are very useful when added to the feed or drinking water of animals exposed to the contagion but are less useful as a cure. Furthermore, care should be taken as the use of drugs such as amprolium may cause side-effects.

Prevention is the most effective method for preventing coccidiosis-related losses. Contamination of feed and drinking water with faeces must be avoided. Exposure to sunlight and a reduction in humidity (<25 %) are also good methods for destroying non-sporulated oocysts.

Although chemoprophylaxis is useful, it must be remembered that coccidiostats prevent disease but also inhibit the development of immunity, therefore severe outbreaks may occur if administration is stopped suddenly.

Appropriate management practices together with the use of drugs generally provides good results.

Continual exposure leads to the development of partially protective immunity. Schizogonic states are generally considered to be amongst the most immunogenic, which is why the coccidiostatic action of these drugs prevents the development of good immunity.

It should also be noted that adult animals are usually asymptomatic carriers and excreters of oocysts that contaminate the environment, occasionally to a very marked degree. The separation of animals by age, especially adults from young animals, and grazing in different areas usually gives good results.

Amongst other measures, the metaphylactic use of triazinones achieves good effects in terms of control and of some zootechnical parameters. For example, the administration of toltrazuril when diarrhoea first appears promotes weight gains in treated calves. Similarly, diclazuril produces marked weight gains with respect to untreated animals.

It should also be noted that oocyst excretion, and therefore environmental contamination and risks, are considerably reduced.

Hygienic measures are particularly useful. Sick animals can be isolated, with abundant dry bedding, in a scrupulously clean and disinfected area to prevent oocyst dissemination and they should be provided with copious amounts of feed that provides minerals and vitamins and administered rehydration therapy.

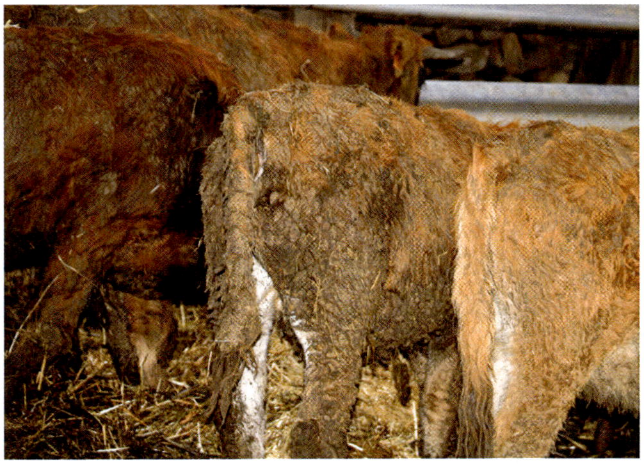

Winter coccidiosis is caused by *E. zuernii* and presents when temperatures are so low that oocyst sporulation cannot occur. However, the bedding provides sufficient warmth and humidity for sporulation, even in apparently clean stables.

24 Are any nematodes found in the oesophagus?

The presence of reddish, serpentine thread-like structures in the oesophageal wall is discovered during inspection of the carcasses in an abattoir. The vet impounds the oesophaguses and extracts the structures in the laboratory. These structures move under a hot lamp and present a vermiform morphology covered at the anterior end by cuticular plates, similar to flat warts, arranged in longitudinal rows under the microscope. A careful inspection confirms their presence in the pharynx and even free in the contents of the rumen in other animals.

1. How were the animals infected?
2. Can humans become infected?
3. Can they be differentiated from hypoderma larvae?

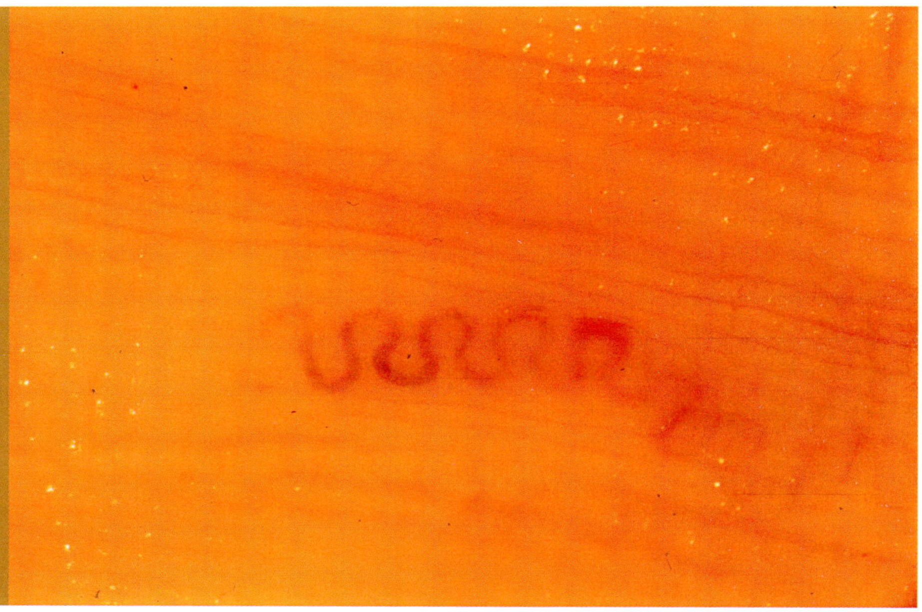

Image courtesy of Dr. M. Luzón.

1 How were the animals infected?

The characteristics of the structures described coincide with infection by a parasite from the spirurida group, the pathogenic role of which is very limited. In this case the organism concerned is *Gongylonema pulchrum*. Its presence in the oesophagus of animals has been linked to a chronic mild oesophagitis caused by the irritation produced at the sites where the parasites are attached.

Severe infections may lead to food rejection and oesophageal blockage due to nodule formation. It is localised in long, serpentine paths in the mucosa and submucosa of the oesophagus and rumen.

Adult gongylonema are filiform, average sized (3-14 cm × 150-500 µm), whitish or reddish in colour and present wart-like cuticular extensions arranged in long rows, which are highly characteristic and aid their identification, at the anterior end. Their eggs are thick-shelled, measure 75 × 35 µm and contain an embryo.

The biological cycle is indirect and infection of the definitive host occurs upon ingestion of the intermediate hosts that host the L3s. The larvae are released in the stomach or duodenum, where they migrate and attach to the oesophageal wall. They are covered by a pinkish or whitish-grey coating that may reach the size of a pea. Finally, the coating breaks and the adults attach to the mucosa and submucosa, forming the characteristic serpentine path.

The intermediate hosts that intervene in the cycle are coprophagous insects (coprophagous beetles and cockroaches) of various genera and species, which ingest the parasite eggs eliminated in animal faeces. The period between infection and formation of the infective L3s for the definitive host is about four weeks.

2 Can humans become infected?

Human infection is incredibly rare, although some cases have been reported in various European countries as well as in Asia, Africa and North America.

These generally occur due to "accidental" ingestion of intermediate insects infected with L3s or ingestion of food or water containing L3s released upon death of the insect.

Some clinical manifestations, such as lingual paralysis, chest or abdominal pain, bloody sputum and, occasionally, pharyngitis and stomatitis, are compatible with infections of this type.

3 Can they be differentiated from hypoderma larvae?

Gongylonema and hypoderma infections can coexist in the same animal and, at some point, alterations due to these different pathogens may appear in the same organ. In this sense, a difference must be made between hypoderma larvae and the alterations produced and the serpentine paths formed in the oesophageal mucosa and submucosa with a zig-zag shape. Once they have crossed the skin, the L1s follow different paths:

- *H. bovis* migrates to the epidural fat in the spinal canal via the ischiatic and radial nerves and the sacral, lumbar and brachial plexi over four months.
- Although the route followed by *H. lineatum* is not well known, it is known to rest in the oesophageal submucosa (its "winter camp"), which it reaches after around four weeks. Once there, it matures and grows for a further seven months then continues to migrate towards the dorsum, where it matures and moults twice, reaching L3 after one to one and a half months.

Recently hatched *Hypoderma* spp. larvae (L1) measure around 0.6-0.8 mm and are white, hyaline and almost circular in cross-section. The various segments are very similar in length and densely covered with tiny denticles. The most notable difference lies in the cephalic skeleton, in the so-called "buccal hooks". It grows and reaches a size of up to 17 mm prior to moulting to L2.

Even with little experience, it is difficult to confuse these two parasites when lesions occur in the same region.

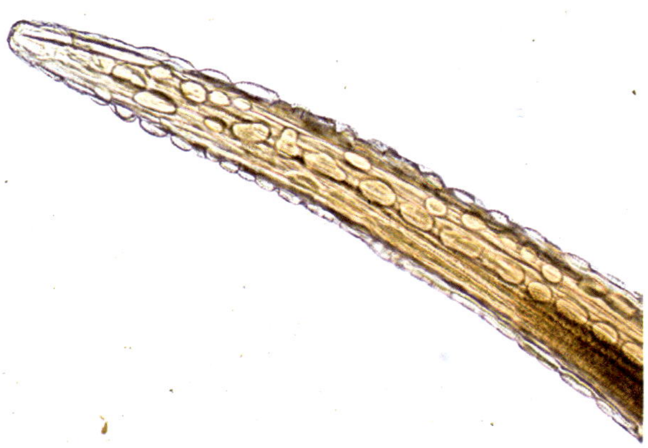

Spirurida are very thin white or pinkish worms located in longitudinal serpentine galleries in the mucosa and submucosa of the oesophagus and rumen. *Gongylonema pulchrum* presents cuticular plates, similar to warts, arranged in longitudinal rows at its anterior end. Although its pathogenic role is insignificant, human infections have been reported, probably as a result of accidental ingestion of live cockroaches or beetles infected with larvae or food or water contaminated with dead insects.

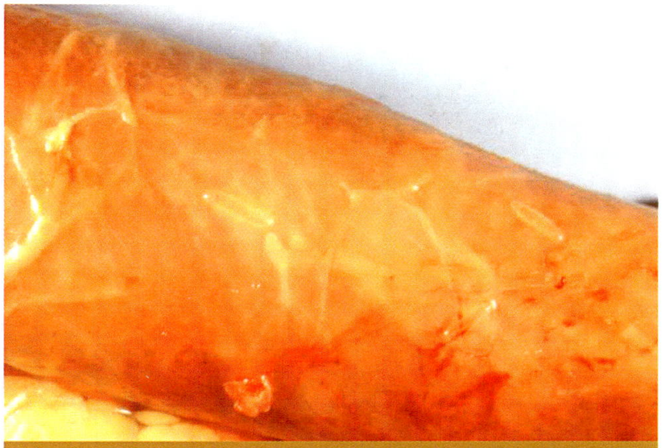

Hypoderma lineatum larvae may also occasionally be found in the oesophagus at necropsy or in the abattoir during so-called "winter camp". The tissue surrounding the larva may range from normal to oedematous, and may even contain congestive and haemorrhagic trajectories These are observed as cylindrical formations oriented along the longitudinal axis of the oesophagus.
Image courtesy of Dr. P. Morrondo.

2

Q&A

on endoparasites of the

respiratory system

Chapter 2

Q&A on endoparasites of the respiratory system

Introduction

This chapter describes and discusses clinical signs and problems produced by various endoparasites of the respiratory system which are mainly found in bovine bronchi and bronchioles. The respiratory system is not a particularly welcoming location for parasitic species of major importance for veterinary medicine in ruminants. However, some parasitoses described in this chapter stand out to a greater or lesser degree.

Dictyocaulosis, a process caused by bronchopulmonary nematodes that leads to disorders of some clinical significance in bovines, is perhaps the most important. Although the parasite species responsible (*Dictyocaulus viviparus*) does not represent a serious problem at our latitude, it can nevertheless produce disorders of some severity in young animals in certain regions and under certain circumstances. Dictyocaulosis is common in some parts of Spain, for example in more northern regions, where outbreaks with high morbidity and a mortality of up to 5-10 % occasionally occur. However, the relative importance of this parasitosis in the general context of respiratory disease, including other aetiologies, means that special attention should be paid to the diagnostic methods and techniques in order to establish appropriate therapeutic and prophylactic measures.

As is the case with other parasites whose biology is based on trophic predatory relationships, the Iberian peninsula is a "mini continent" that behaves as a species store. Its mountainous geography, size and varying climatology, as well as the abundance of wildlife, make it easy for any parasite to survive and propagate.

Echinococcosis (hydatidosis or hydatid disease), which is caused by *Echinococcus granulosus sensu lato*, spread throughout the world due to the export of Merino sheep. As such, it is likely that, together with the export of sheep to other countries, the gene pool comprising *E. granulosus s.l.* was also exported. This group of genotypes includes the bovine genotype (G5, currently *E. ortleppi*), which was probably present on the Iberian peninsula at some point. If that is the case, G5 leads to fertile cysts in cattle that would continue their biological cycle once the definitive hosts, namely dogs, intervene. The prior existence of G5 on the Iberian peninsula ensures its current presence, especially when considering the importance of cattle farming in some regions of Spain. Another possibility is that a G5 propagation phenomenon from central Europe occurred. The migratory flows of humans from northern and central Europe towards the southwest could easily have resulted in the "export" of genotypes, including G5, which could easily have become established amongst us.

The same clinical manifestations can appear in both domestic animals and humans although there are very few studies in this regard.

As the most commonly affected animals are sheep, goat and pig, the individual value of which is low, and the majority of clinical signs go unnoticed in animals, almost all the data available come from studies concerning species of greater individual value.

The most important parasites of the bovine respiratory system

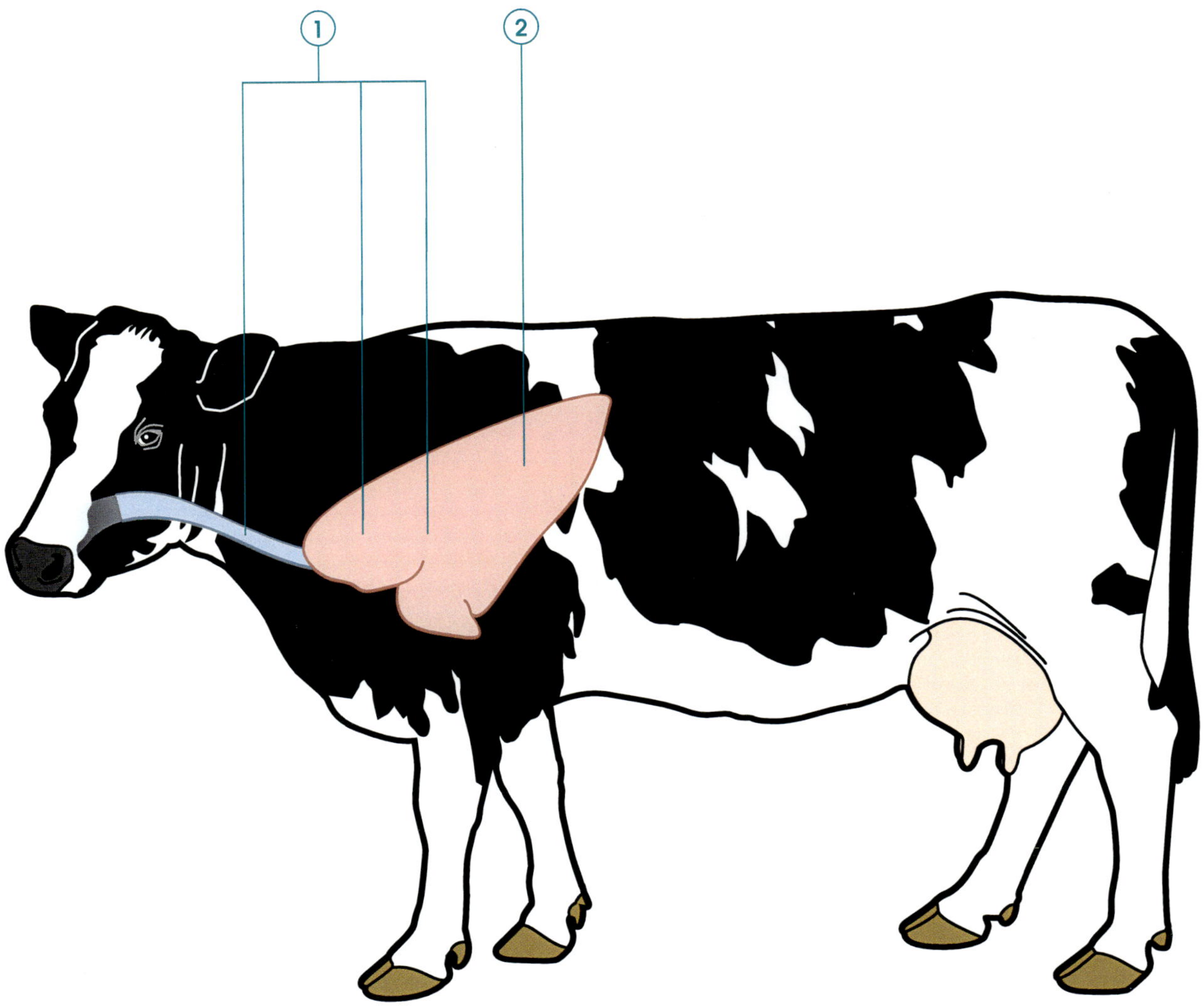

1. *Dictyocaulus:* trachea, bronchi and bronchioles
2. *Echinococcus*: pulmonary cysts

25 What are *Dictyocaulus* like?

In late summer, a group of 2 year calves on a beef farm in Asturias (Spain) developed a clinical presentation characterised by poor general appearance, dull and rough hair, continual dry cough and rapid weight loss. During his visit, the vet notes that some animals remain lying down and inactive, with clear signs of dyspnoea and weakness. The owner confirms the recent death of two animals with the same signs; long white worms were observed in the lungs on necropsy. According to the laboratory the animals were also suffering from a *Pasteurella multocida* infection.

1. What does *Dictyocaulus* look like and how is it transmitted to animals?
2. What is the risk population?
3. At what time of year does the greatest risk of suffering parasitic bronchitis exist?

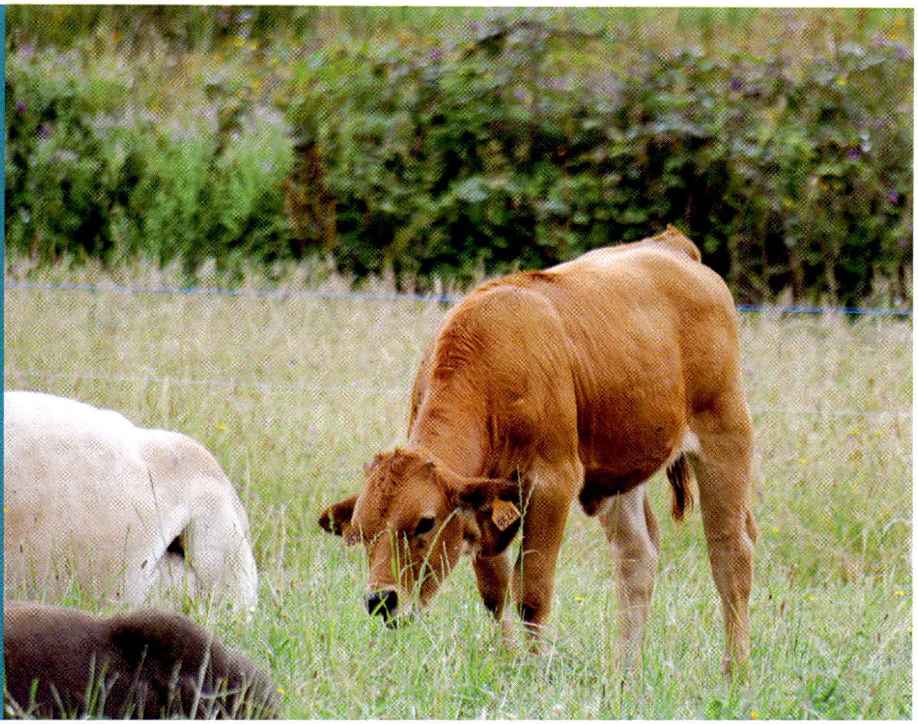

1 What does *Dictyocaulus* look like and how is it transmitted to animals?

These worms are found in the trachea and bronchi as adults. They are whitish in colour, thin and filiform. Males measure between 3.5 and 5.5 cm. They present a small copulatory bursa supported by ribs and short, thick, dark similarly sized spicules (approx. 200 µm) at their posterior end.

Females are twice as large as males (between 6 and 8 cm) and are oviparous. The vulva is located in the posterior part, and their posterior end is short and pointed. After copulation they lay eggs (approx. 55-85 µm in size) containing fully developed first stage larvae (L1).

L1 *D. viviparus* larvae measure between 390 and 450 µm in length and possess numerous intestinal cells and dark granules. Their oesophagus is rhabditiform, their anterior end is rounded and lacks a cephalic button. L1 larvae hatch in the bronchi, are rapidly released and ascend to the trachea with the help of the vibratory bronchial epithelia. Coughing fits allow the larvae to reach the nasopharyngeal space, from where they are swallowed with mucosal secretions or expelled to the exterior with the nasal flow. Egg hatching is completed in the digestive system and the L1 larvae exit the animal in faeces. The different larval stages develop in the environment,

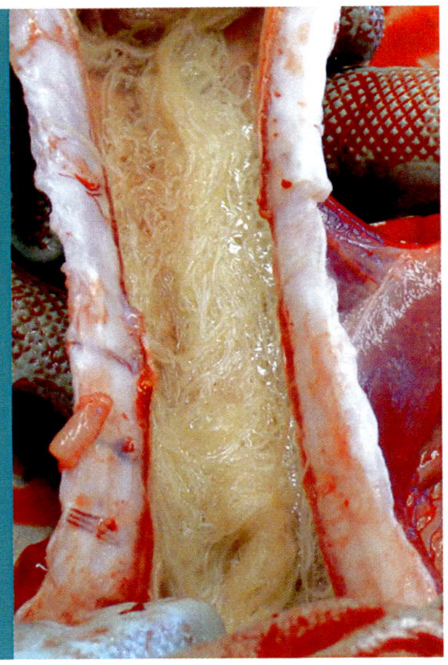

Trachea and bronchi with *Dictyocaulus*. During the initial phases of infection, the larvae migrate and block the bronchioles until the distal alveoli become obstructed. After around two weeks infected animals present polypnoea, dyspnoea and abdominal respiration as well as coughing fits and decreased appetite. They adopt a characteristic posture with the limbs separated, head extended, mouth open and nasal orifices dilated. The lesions mainly affect the respiratory tract. A large quantity of viscous, foamy and occasionally purulent mucus in which the parasites form balls that can block the lumen of the bronchioles and even that of the bronchi is observed.
Image courtesy of Dr. K. Steininger.

with this process taking 6-7 days under normal conditions, although it can last for several weeks. If both the temperature and humidity are favourable, the larvae moult twice inside the faecal mass and transform into L3, which is the infective phase for bovines. L3 larvae are between 0.9 and 2.7 mm in size, conserve the cuticle from the previous phase and clearly show intestinal cells. The larvae in this phase actively emerge from the faeces or make use of sporangia from fungi of the genus *Pilobolus* to move towards the grass.

Transmission normally occurs when the animals ingest L3 larvae with grass. Infected animals excrete L1 larvae in their faeces. Under suitable environmental conditions (temperature and humidity), they transform into L3 within 6 or 7 days, although this period may be longer (several weeks). L3 larvae normally abandon the faecal mass with the help of sporangia from the fungus *Pilobolus*, which grows in cow pats, thus helping the larvae to spread throughout the grass.

2 What is the risk population?

Individuals with no prior antigenic stimulus are at highest risk of suffering from dictyocaulosis, which is also known as verminous bronchitis. As a result, the disease is more common in young animals than in adults and normally presents in autumn, although outbreaks may also appear in winter in temperate and wet regions. Clinical outbreaks can occur at any time of year.

In the 1950s, and for several decades thereafter, dictyocaulosis began to be well-controlled in the UK using a vaccine based on irradiated L3 larvae. It is important, however, that the animals maintain some degree of immune protection after vaccination by natural exposure to the infection.

In the 1980s and 90s, the launch of long-acting anthelmintics resulted in a dramatic drop in sales of the dictyocaulosis vaccine as farmers began to use chemoprevention as the

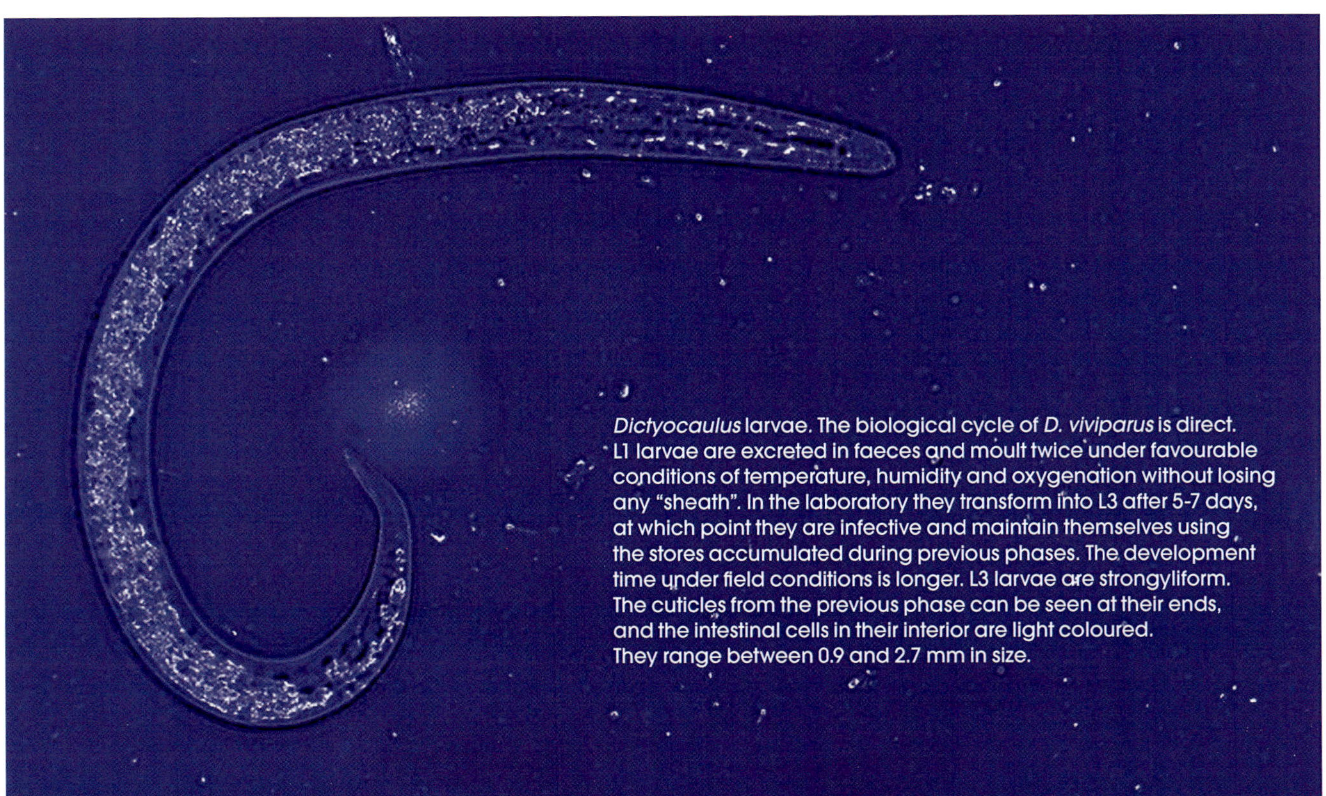

Dictyocaulus larvae. The biological cycle of *D. viviparus* is direct. L1 larvae are excreted in faeces and moult twice under favourable conditions of temperature, humidity and oxygenation without losing any "sheath". In the laboratory they transform into L3 after 5-7 days, at which point they are infective and maintain themselves using the stores accumulated during previous phases. The development time under field conditions is longer. L3 larvae are strongyliform. The cuticles from the previous phase can be seen at their ends, and the intestinal cells in their interior are light coloured. They range between 0.9 and 2.7 mm in size.

preferred control method. However, animals do not receive a sufficient antigenic stimulus to develop their own protection (insufficient exposure to the parasite) with this method, therefore they remain "receptive" to the disease when exposed to *D. viviparus* infection. This has been confirmed by an increase in the number of dictyocaulosis outbreaks in the UK over the past 20 years, especially in adult animals and those in their second grazing season.

3 At what time of year does the greatest risk of suffering parasitic bronchitis exist?

Bovine dictyocaulosis is most common in temperate regions with abundant humidity. These factors favour survival of a sufficient number of L3 larvae in grass for sufficient time, thus meaning that pastures contaminated in autumn remain a risk the following spring. This larval population is responsible for the infection of calves that are released to pasture for the first time.

After natural infection with L3 larvae, the animals develop some degree of protective immunity against reinfection. However, if the animals have not experienced an antigenic stimulus previously (by vaccination or contact with the natural infection) or if they receive an anthelmintic treatment that prevents the larvae ingested with the grass from becoming established, they will be susceptible to the disease.

The most important factors implicated in the appearance of clinical dictyocaulosis outbreaks in a herd include a history of verminous bronchitis on the farm and the presence of sufficient humidity to allow the migration of L3 larvae from the faecal mass to the grass (moist summers preceded by dry periods that also favour growth of the fungus *Pilobolus* in bovine faeces). The limited or non-existent migration of L3 larvae to the grass during drier months results in an "immune gap", which translates into a greater susceptibility of the animals in the following grazing season.

In conclusion, dictyocaulosis is more common in wet regions and when susceptible animals are introduced onto a farm in which the contamination levels in grass are insufficient to produce a clinical presentation in the original herd. Moreover, this latter situation triggers a high degree of grass contamination via faeces.

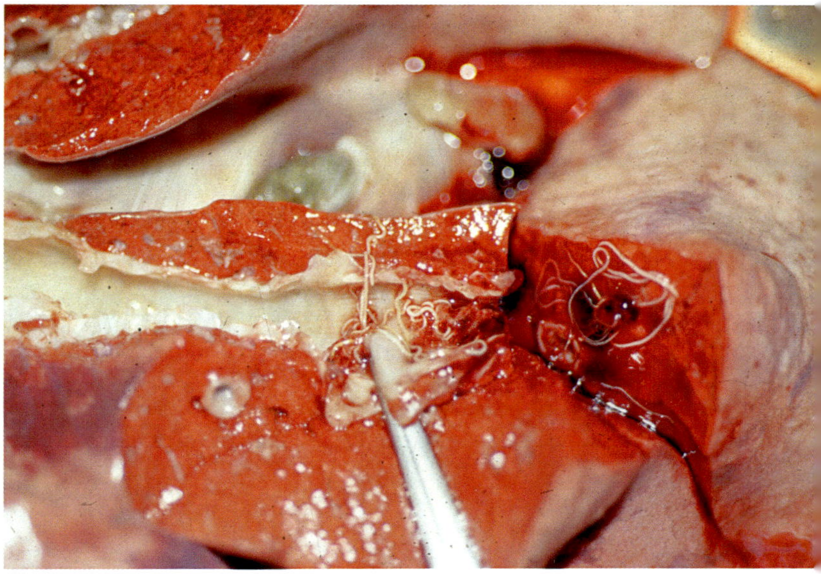

Adult *Dictyocaulus*. These are whitish, thin and filiform worms. The male measures between 3.5 and 5.5 cm and the female is larger (between 6 and 8 cm). The mouth is surrounded by four small lips and a small cavity with posterior chitinous ring. These nematodes have a small copulatory bursa.
Image courtesy of Dr. C. Novoa.

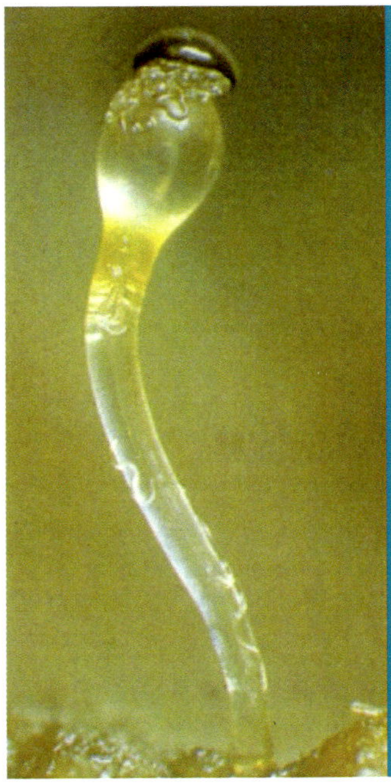

Pilobolus with *Dictyocaulus larvae*. The *D. viviparus* larvae present in the faeces can be spread by coprophilic *Pilobolus* spp. fungi, which often grow on cow pats. When the *Pilobolus* sporangium opens, the fungal spores, together with the *D. viviparus larvae,* are dispersed some distance. In the absence of *Pilobolus,* the contamination of pastures with *Dictyocaulus* larvae is considerably reduced. Wind, birds, manure spreading, vehicle tyres, footwear, etc. also contribute to larval dispersion.

26 Which parasite produces bronchitis with a constant dry cough?

A milk farm in the south of England has imported 20 high yielding cows from Spain. During the quarantine period these cows remain isolated in a field in which replacement calves from the previous year have been kept. By day 25 of isolation half the females present a high temperature as well as severe respiratory symptoms with a dry and continual cough that even prevents them from resting. The decrease in milk production is very noticeable.

1. What are the pathological repercussions of dictyocaulosis?
2. Is there a vaccine for preventing dictyocaulosis?
3. What happens to the dead worms?

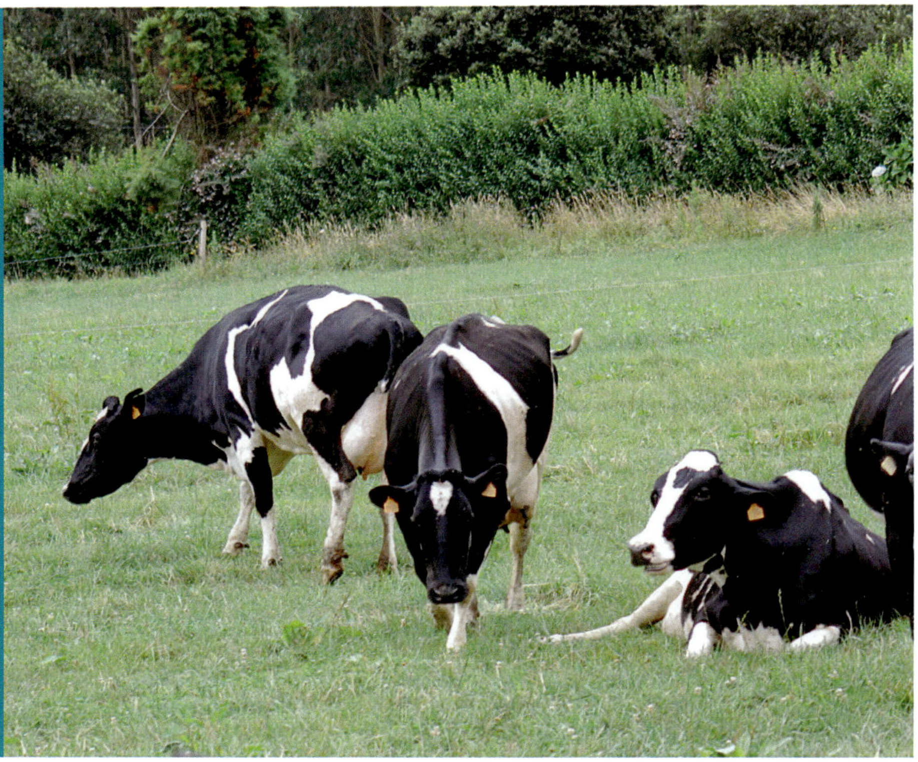

1 What are the pathological repercussions of dictyocaulosis?

As is the case for the majority of helminth-related infections, the severity and duration of the clinical manifestations in animals affected by dictyocaulosis mainly depend on the infective dose (number of L3 larvae ingested, animals' age and various environmental and management-related factors). Primary infections generally lead to chronic presentations, especially in calves aged 6-10 months. In contrast, the disease tends to be acute in the event of reinfection of young or adult bovines with a high dose of L3 larvae.

The clinical signs are usually related to the degree of infection, although they also depend on the age of the animals and the presence of other infectious or parasitic disease processes (ostertagiosis, fasciolosis, etc.). Sick animals present loss of appetite and weight loss. The manifestations vary depending on the phase of the infection, with cough appearing and breathing rate increasing as appetite decreases. These initial symptoms present at around 10-12 days post-infection and coincide with migration of the larvae and subsequent blockage of the small bronchi and bronchioles. Polypnoea, apnoea and abdominal respiration appear during this phase of the disease, with these symptoms gradually worsening until respiration becomes so tiring that the calves adopt typical postures (limbs separated, head extended) and a distressed expression.

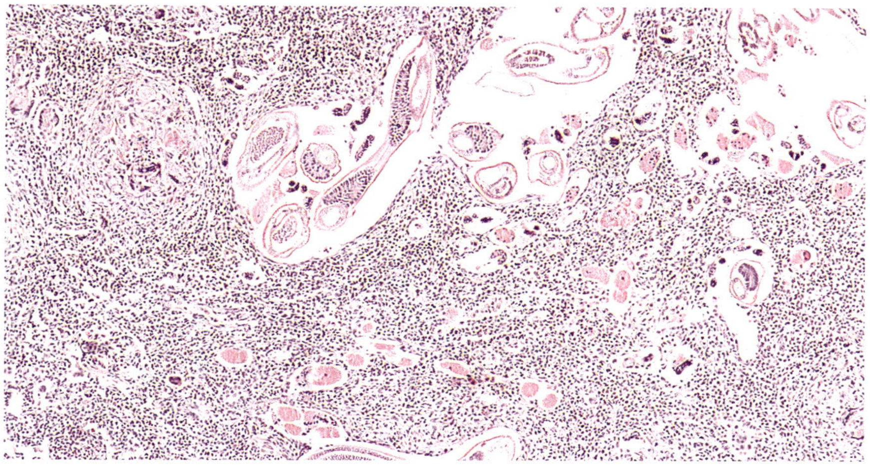

Histological section of an infected bronchus. The characteristic lesions of a chronic catarrhal tracheobronchitis with cellular infiltration (lymphocytes and eosinophils) and fibrin deposits can be seen. The inflamed bronchial mucosa acquires a greyish-pink colour and is swollen. Histologically, epithelial hyperplasia of the bronchi with loss of the vibratory cilia due to the irritant action of larvae that migrate towards the upper bronchi can be seen. Peribronchiolitis with regions of atelectasis and alveolar consolidation with lymphocyte infiltration and alveolar compression can also be seen.

In mild cases the cough usually presents when the animals exercise or are forced to do so. Although most animals affected in an outbreak recover, some (especially the younger ones) may develop severe respiratory symptoms that lead to death within a few days (1-4 days).

2 Is there a vaccine for preventing dictyocaulosis?

The prevention of dictyocaulosis is based on the development of immunity by the animals themselves either by vaccination or exposure to the natural infection provided this can be controlled using strategic anthelmintic treatments. Vaccination of dairy cattle prior to their first grazing season confers good and long-lasting immunity on the majority of animals. The immunity acquired, and the corresponding strategic planning of antiparasitic treatments, is a good tactic for controlling the disease, although mistakes can obviously occur. In this respect, errors as regards the treatment applied or the administration thereof at the wrong time pose the greatest risk of the clinical presentation of dictyocaulosis. Moreover, well-planned strategic anthelmintic treatments prevent mild infections in the first grazing season, although the animals may be "defenceless" when put out to pasture for the second time.

Although vaccination is a good prophylactic measure in high-risk regions, it must be accompanied by general preventive measures (prevention of grazing in hazardous regions and at certain times of year). Consequently, calves can be vaccinated at more than 2 months of age with a vaccine containing radiation-attenuated L3 larvae prior to being put out to pasture. This vaccine is administered orally in two doses separated by an interval of four weeks. During this period the animals must remain stabled to prevent infection prior to administration of the second dose. It should be remembered, however, that although the results of vaccination are good, this procedure does not prevent the development of some parasites still present in the pastures. In practice, this means that if the risk of a serious process is still present, the animals should be vaccinated annually. In non-endemic regions or in pastures with a low degree of contamination that does not pose a serious risk to the animals, vaccination makes less sense. In such cases strategic treatment with highly effective anthelmintics

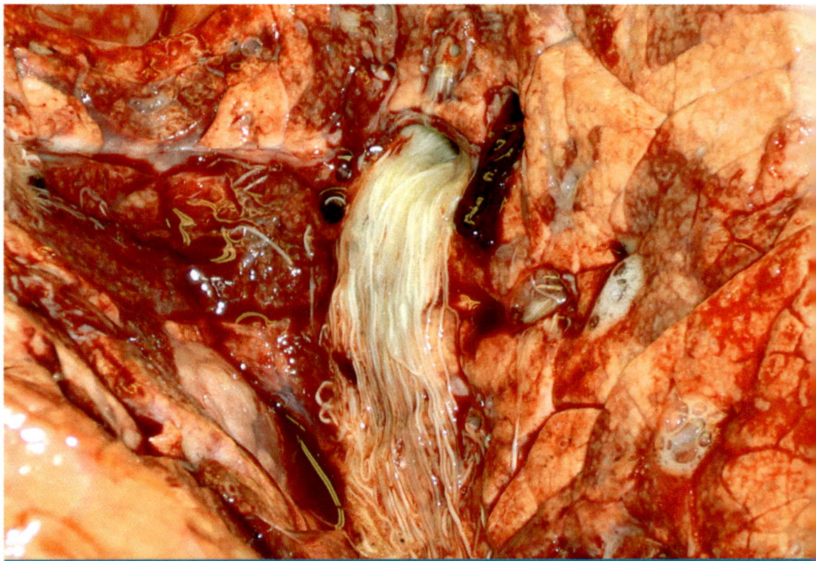

From an economic viewpoint, vaccination is applicable for dictyocaulosis control in endemic regions and those at high risk. Although immunity persists for around four months, mild reinfections, and therefore new stimuli that help the protective immunity to last longer, may occur if the animals subsequently remain in slightly affected pastures. Correct vaccination protects as required but does not prevent the development of a small number of nematodes that continue to contaminate the pastures, therefore it is advisable to vaccinate the herd each year.
Image courtesy of Dr. K. Steininger.

immediately prior to putting the animals out to pasture, or the administration of long-lasting drugs that reduce the number of treatments required for control, is more useful.

3 What happens to the dead worms?

A successful treatment depends on the correct choice of anthelmintic and the use thereof at the right time. Most animals recover after receiving a suitable anthelmintic, although some may present a slight growth retardation. It is recommended to treat animals with symptoms and allow the remainder to develop immune resistance. The majority of bovines affected overcome dictyocaulosis, especially after treatment, although a complete recovery may take several weeks. For some time, the animals become carriers and therefore the source of new infections.

As far as anthelmintic treatment is concerned, and irrespective of the clinical manifestations due to the presence of live worms in the respiratory system, the possible consequences of the accumulation of dead parasites in the tracheobronchial tree, should be considered, for example inhalation pneumonia, which may be significantly more serious.

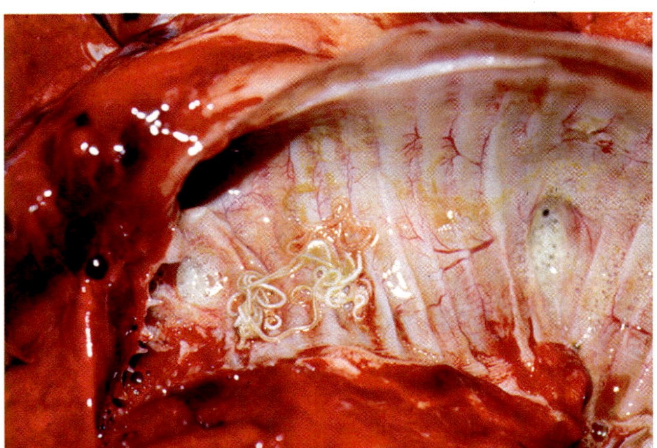

Adult *Dictyocaulus* in mucus. A *post mortem* diagnosis can be established upon identifying the pulmonary lesions| (purulent catarrhal bronchitis and bronchiolitis, reddish consolidation regions in the caudal lung lobes, emphysema and obstruction-related atelectasis). Eggs or L1 larvae can be seen upon examination of tracheal or bronchial epithelial scrapings. Adult worms are found in the tracheal lumen, bronchi and bronchioles surrounded by a large quantity of mucus. During pre-patent phases the immature forms can only be seen with a magnifying glass upon examining the mucus. Adult worms are no longer present in the post-patent phases of infections, although pulmonary damage allows an infection to be suspected.
Image courtesy of Dr. M. Castaño.

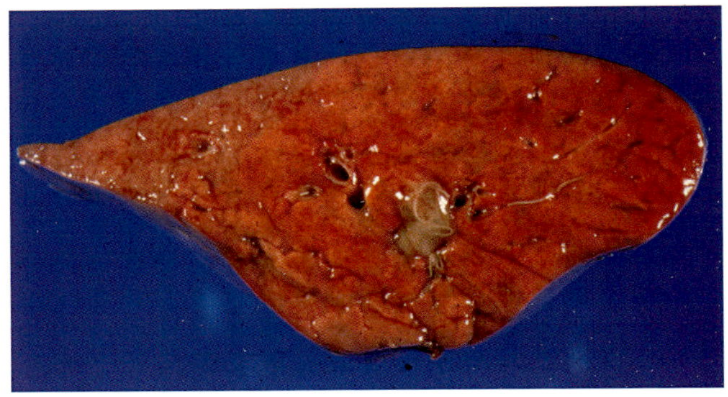

Parasitic pneumonia lesions in the lung. The differential diagnosis should take into account other sporadic processes inherent to colder months and which progress with acutely increased temperatures, although such processes normally present with less cough and dyspnoea. Some bacterial processes, such as pasteurellosis or pulmonary tuberculosis, or viral infections such as BVD, IBR, etc. often coincide with dictyocaulosis, in which case a specific diagnosis is required.
Image courtesy of Dr. M. Castaño.

As a result, it may turn out that some animals worsen or even die before an improvement is noticed.

Indeed, some antiparasitic agents, such as ivermectin, cause mass worm death, which carries with it the potential risk of anaphylactic shock, especially when the parasite burden carried by the animals is very high. If there is no need to worry about a period of milk suppression, and in severely infected cattle, the administration of an imidazothiazole, such as levamisole, which acts by paralysing the worms, is a good alternative.

In summary, the aim is to prevent a major build-up of dead parasites in the respiratory system. Once affected by the anthelmintic, most worms are paralysed and expelled as a result of natural organic defences (bronchial epithelium and cough), leaving the lungs parasite-free. If required, another anthelmintic from a different group can be administered one or two weeks after the first treatment to eliminate any worms that may have survived this initial treatment and prevent the worsening of sick animals due to large-scale worm death.

Biological cycle of *Dictyocaulus*

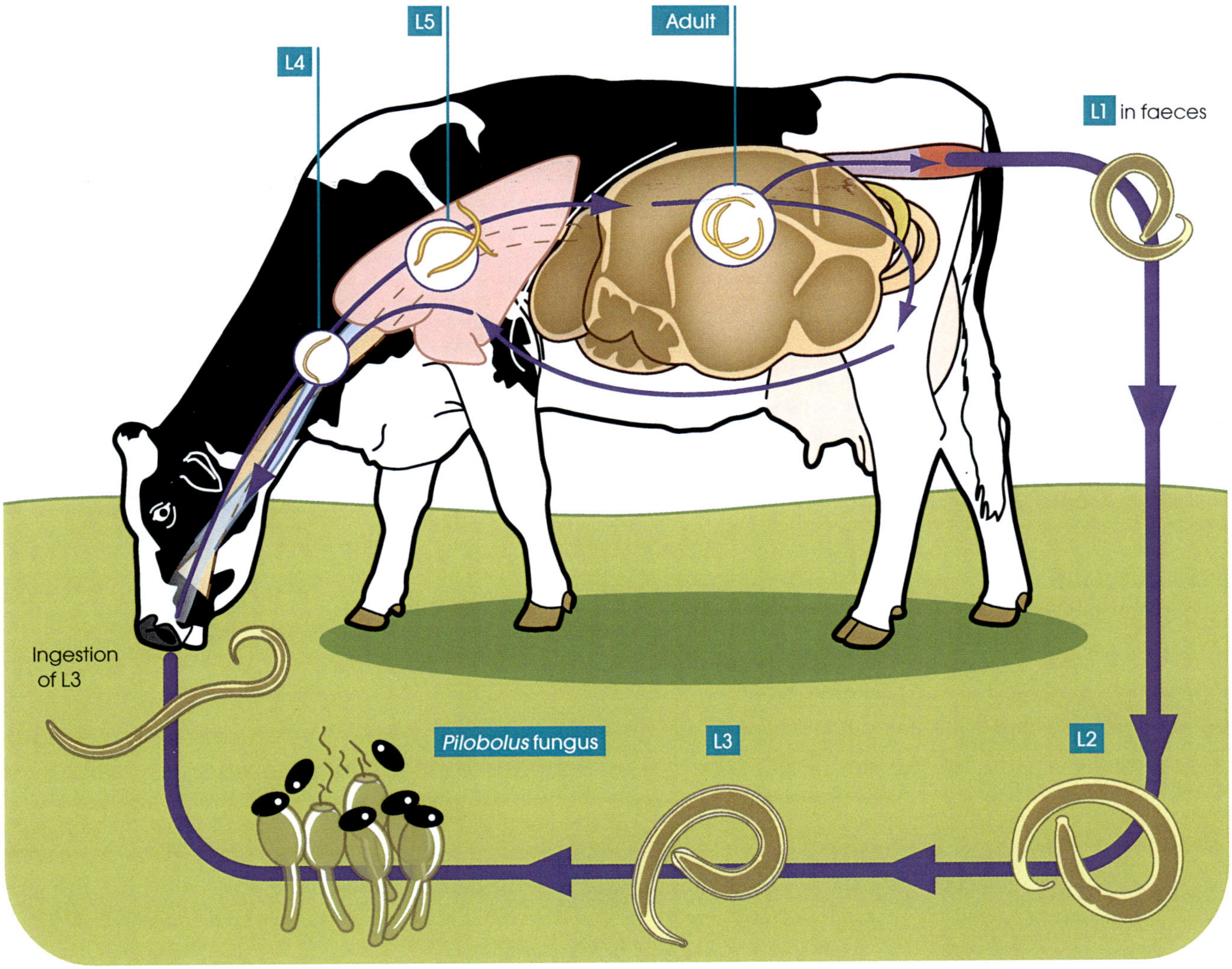

27 Are hydatidic cysts common?

During a regular medical checkup undertaken by staff at an abattoir in Zamora (Spain), the presence of cystic formations was detected in the lungs of three of the 20 employees. The history taking confirmed that they had previously shown non-specific respiratory signs such as dyspnoea, fever, chronic cough and even bronchospasm and haemoptysis. As they all smoked they hadn't considered these to be important as they considered them to be smoking-related. One of them reported that during a coughing fit he had coughed up something resembling uncongealed egg white with a salty taste. All were responsible for slaughtering cattle, including the removal of entrails such as lungs with echinococcal cysts.

1. What are the peculiarities of echinococcosis in Spain?
2. Is there a risk of transmission to humans in the abattoir?
3. How large are the cysts in bovine lungs and where are they found? And in humans?
4. When are cysts fertile or infertile?

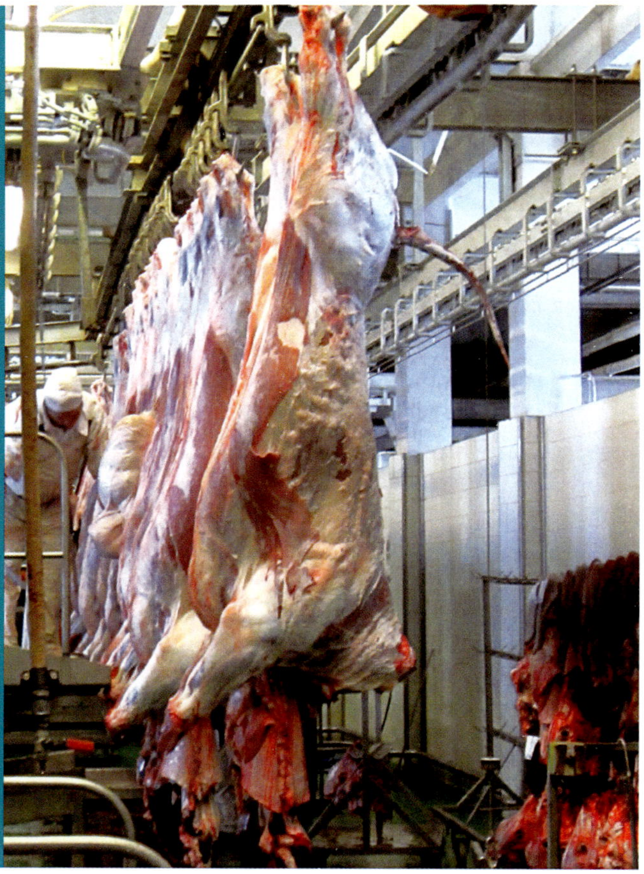

1 What are the peculiarities of echinococcosis in Spain?

Echinococcosis is a severe process whose prognosis depends on the location and type of cyst. One of the chief risks is rupture of the echinococcal cyst (hydatid cysts), which leads to vesicle seeding and the release of anaphylactic substances. Similarly, one of the most surprising characteristics of echinococcosis is the fact that the presence of large cysts may be completely asymptomatic. Moreover, no parasite produces lesions in as many organs as *Echinococcus granulosus*, with oncospheres being able to develop in the kidney, lung, liver, spleen, muscle tissue, brain, etc.

Echinococcosis was a notifiable disease in Spain between 1982 and 1996. Official Spanish data indicate that the incidence of human echinococcosis was 2.52 cases per 100,000 inhabitants in 1982. Control and eradication programs based on the routine treatment of dogs with praziquantel were launched in 1986 and remained in place for several years. The strict control of carcasses put into place due to the appearance of certain animal diseases, such as bovine spongiform encephalitis and catarrhal fever (blue tongue) in sheep, together with the treatment of domestic dogs mentioned above, resulted in a sharp drop in the number of cases of human echinococcosis to 1.01 per 100,000 by 1996. Since then the only cases of human echinococcosis recorded in Spain are those reported "voluntarily" by health authorities in the various autonomous communities, which in the opinion of some may pose a problem. A comparison of reported cases with hospital data shows that the number of cases of human echinococcosis in the past 10 years has been clearly underestimated. For example, the number of cases reported in the Autonomous Community of Castilla y León is 2.69 per 100,000, whereas calculations based on hospital records suggest that the actual incidence is four times higher.

Similarly, although the official prevalence of echinococcosis in domestic animals in 2000 was 0.98 % in sheep and goats, data obtained by staff from the various control programs indicate a rate some 20 times higher in sheep from some regions of Spain, such as La Rioja. Official data show that bovine echinococcosis decreased from 0.97 % in 2000 to around 0.5 % in 2008. In any case, prevalence rates are higher in animals farmed extensively than in those farmed intensively.

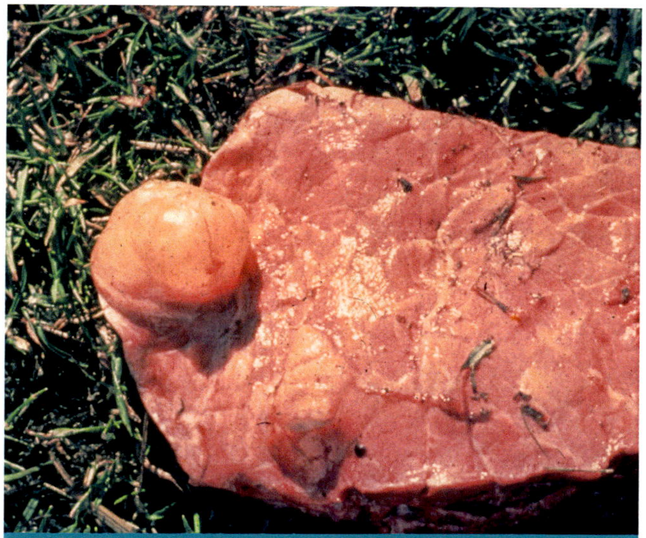

Echinococcal cyst. The *E. granulosus* metacestode is normally unicameral and sub-spherical in shape. It grows expansively by concentric lengthening at a rate of between 1 and 5 cm per year, depending on the strain, host species and severity of the infection. The *E. granulosus* cyst comprises two elements: the vesicular larva and a fibrocellular coating produced by the host (white adventitious membrane of varying thickness, depending on the inflammatory reaction). From a structural viewpoint, this is a large parasitic granuloma consecutive to an initially sub-acute inflammatory process that subsequently becomes chronic. *Image courtesy of Dr. M. Castaño.*

2 Is there a risk of transmission to humans in the abattoir?

People working at an abbatoir are not in risk of infection from the animals coming from the slaughterhouse. Species from the genus *Echinococcus* have an indirect biological cycle in which both definitive and intermediate hosts participate. The definitive hosts (carnivores) become infected upon ingesting echinococcal cysts containing viable protoscolices. The vesicles are released by chewing and by the action of pepsin in the stomach. At around six hours post-infection, most of these protoscolices (around 85 %) evaginate and attach to the epithelium of the small intestine, where they reach the adult phase. Egg production commences at 30 days post-infection. Each *Echinococcus* produces between 34 and 58 eggs per day, with the majority of these (around 70 %) being released in the intestine and subsequently eliminated in the faeces.

The intermediate hosts, including humans, become infected upon ingesting parasite eggs with contaminated food or water. The oncosphere found inside the egg is released, evaginates and penetrates the crypts between the villi in the jejunum and upper ileum until it reaches a small blood or lymphatic vessel, from where it passively reaches various organs. Most oncospheres are retained in the liver, whereas others reach the lung and some can be found in the kidneys, spleen, muscle tissue, brain, bones, etc. At 10-14 days post-infection the parasite begins to rearrange itself to form the echinococcal cyst. After ingestion of the eggs by a suitable intermediate, only approximately one out of every 70 oncospheres becomes established and only one out of every 250 manages to survive and develop to form a cyst. When the cysts break, either spontaneously or secondary to trauma or surgery, seeding and the formation of new cysts (multiple secondary echinococcosis) may occur and the hosts may become infected or suffer an anaphylactic reaction.

Humans only become infected upon ingestion of food or water contaminated with parasite eggs or upon close and careless contact with infected dogs. As a result, most infections tend to occur in infancy.

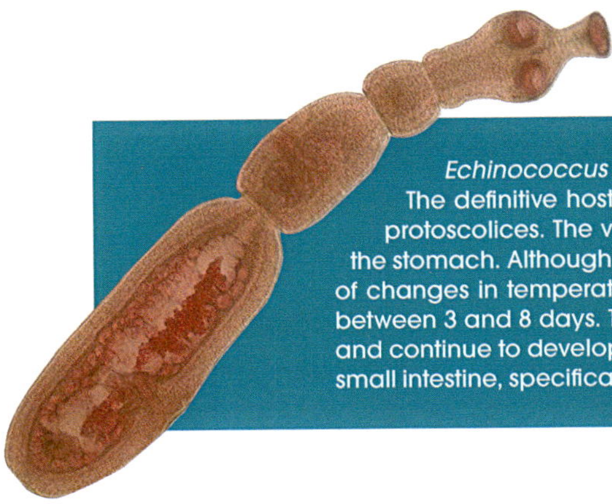

Echinococcus granulosus. Species from the genus *Echinococcus* have an indirect biological cycle. The definitive hosts (carnivores) become infected upon ingesting echinococcal cysts containing viable protoscolices. The vesicles are released by chewing and subsequently exposed to the action of pepsin in the stomach. Although the exact stimulus that induces evagination remains unknown, it could occur as a result of changes in temperature and osmotic pressure or stirring phenomena. Complete evagination may require between 3 and 8 days. The protoscolices then attach to the intestinal epithelium using their suckers and hooks, and continue to develop until they reach adulthood. Adult forms tend to be restricted to a specific region of the small intestine, specifically the Lieberkühn crypts, due to its unique nutritional significance.

3 How large are the cysts in bovine lungs and where are they found? And in humans?

Studies show that adult animals present a larger number of cysts in offal than younger ones and that they are normally larger in size. The preferred pulmonary location of echinococcal cysts in young animals has no logical explanation as the oncosphere larvae first pass through the liver. The reason for the relative size increase of liver cysts in older animals is also unknown.

Cysts with a diameter of less than 10 mm have been found in 67 % of younger animals but not in adults. Indeed, cysts larger than 10 mm have been found in all adult animals and in 33 % of younger animals. The discovery in some studies that all small cysts in young cattle were infertile confirms the hypothesis that echinococcal cysts generate protoscolices once they reach a size of between 15 and 20 mm, which occurs at 5 or 6 months after ingestion of the cestode eggs. As a result, cysts with a diameter of less than 10 mm are always considered to be infertile. The fact that older animals do not present small cysts could be due to the development of immunity against the parasite, which means that constant reinfection, and therefore the formation of new cysts, is avoided.

The largest cyst and highest accumulation of cysts reported in humans may well be the case of a farmer from the Otago region in New Zealand. When aged 6 he fell onto a large rock, which almost certainly broke the echinococcal cyst inside him as he was seriously ill for several weeks thereafter, although he slowly recovered. However, after 2 or 3 years his abdomen slowly began to grow and increased substantially in size over the next 30 years. By 39 years of age he weighed 108 kg and his abdominal girth was 145 cm. His physical status slowly worsened to such an extent that he required a surgical intervention during which various cysts of different sizes, with a total content of 50 litres, were removed. He was diagnosed with a further two cysts around 2-3 years post-surgery, and these cysts were surgically removed 13 years later when their size had increased to that of the head of a human foetus.

As far as cyst development is concerned, the most notorious case is probably that of an 11-year-old English child who had an abdominal echinococcal cyst removed at St. Bartholomew's Hospital in London in 1882. He subsequently moved to the USA and, aged 67 (56 years after the first surgical intervention), again underwent surgery for the removal of two hepatic cysts.

Hepatic echinococcosis, which affects the two lobes of the liver equally, is by far the most common form in humans, although some authors have reported that it affects the right lobe more than the left (54-90 % vs. 29-40 %, respectively).

The size of echinococcal cyst is important for various reasons. Thus, irrespective of the relationship with the disease that may occur, the size, shape and location of cysts has a marked effect on treatment success. As far as size is concerned, it would appear that the highest therapeutic success is achieved when cysts are 5 cm in diameter or smaller, whereas only 20 % of those measuring more than 12 cm are resolved.

4 When are cysts fertile or infertile?

Fertile and viable cysts have live protoscolices on the proligerous membrane or in their interior, and contain hydatid sand in the hydatid fluid. In order to determine whether the protoscolices are alive, their structural integrity, ability to spontaneously evaginate or, in the presence of ruminant bile, movement of the protonephridian cilli or solenocytes and temporary exclusion of vital dyes, such as methylene blue, must be checked.

Echinococcus egg. When eliminated in the faeces, most eggs are already embryonated, are spherical or elliptical in shape and range in size between 30-50 µm/22-44 µm. The main layer, known as the embryophore, comprises 54 cells that provide physical protection. The vitellin layer (external coating) detaches from the egg prior to its release. The embryophore is relatively thick and impermeable and is formed by polygonal blocks made from a protein similar to keratin. After the ingestion of viable eggs by a suitable intermediate host, the embryophore coating dissolves in the stomach and intestine as this process requires the action of proteolytic enzymes (although it does not depend on any specific enzyme). Activation of the oncosphere and release of its membrane then occurs. The oncosphere evaginates its three pairs of hooks and penetrates the crypts between the villi in the jejunum and upper ileum, using its penetration glands (which smooth the tissue whilst protecting the parasite from the host's digestive enzymes) and rhythmic body movements, until it reaches a small blood or lymphatic vessel, from where it reaches various organs passively.

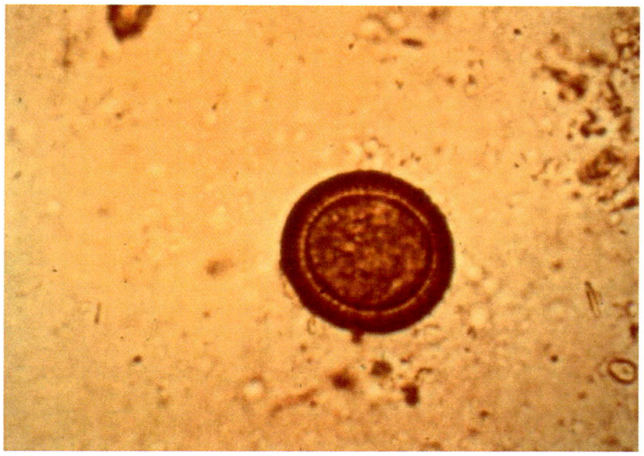

Layers in the cysts (b) and hydatid sand (a). Fertile and viable cysts have live protoscolices, known as "hydatid sand" on the proligerous membrane or in their interior, as well as in the hydatid fluid. Echinococcal cysts comprise three membranes (adventitious, laminar and germinal). The adventitious membrane is fibrous in nature and comprises three layers that form as the result of the host reaction during the initial phases of oncosphere development. Proligerous vesicles form inside the cysts after about 5 months as a result of asexual proliferation of the germinal layer. The asexual gemmation process is repeated in their interior and leads to the formation of thousands of protoscolices, which remain viable for up to 6 years.

a

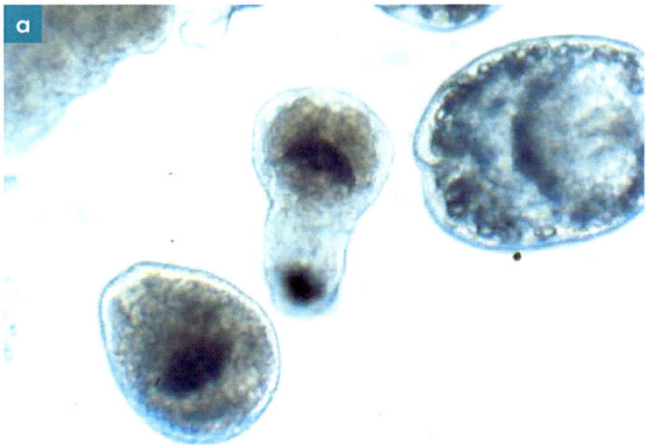

b

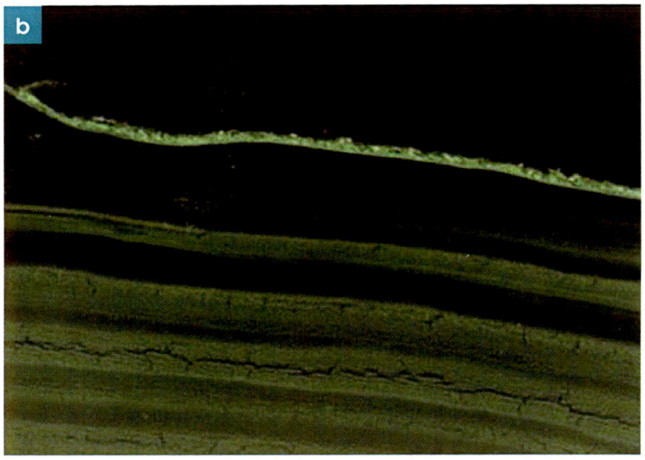

Infertile cysts, which are also known as acephalocysts, lack protoescolices. They may be young cysts that are developing in a suitable host or cysts from a non-specific strain which, irrespective of age, develop in unsuitable hosts.

The number of fertile cysts in cattle is generally quite low (prevalence 15 % in animals aged more than 5 years), with some authors reporting even lower values (3.3 %). The most common location is hepatic, followed by pulmonary, with approximately 20 % of echinococcal cysts in cattle being pulmonary. Various authors have also reported that the liver is more commonly infected than the lung (34 % vs. 25 %, respectively). Almost all clinical studies of bovine echinococcosis come from countries in which this animal species is of major importance to rural economies. Severe echinococcosis (numerous cysts in the lung and liver and adherences between the pleura, lung, chest wall and pericardium), with some complications (tympanites, etc.), may appear in animals older than 8 years. Moreover, in mass infections cysts may develop at other sites (spleen, kidney, heart, brain, bones, etc.). It should be noted that a single case of prenatal echinococcosis in a calf has been reported.

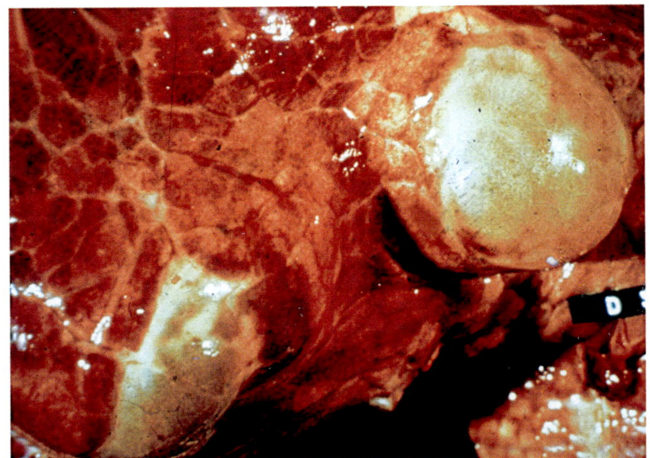

Large echinococcal cyst. Development of the echinococcal cyst is slow up until the fifth month, at which point it begins to take shape, measures 1 cm in diameter and two membranes can be distinguished in its wall. Growth is much faster after this point, and round about the seventh or eighth month it can be several centimetres in size, remaining active and viable in humans for up to 50 years. The development of cysts in the human lung leads to an asymptomatic presentation or signs such as cough, fever, pain, expectoration, nausea and vomiting. One of the most common complications is cyst fracture, which produces an anaphylactic reaction and the formation of daughter cysts. Further important risks include secondary bacterial infection and, finally, calcification of the cyst. Although mass infections occur in the lung and liver, echinococcosis is generally asymptomatic or presents with non-specific symptoms in domestic animals. The only major sign is a marked drop in yields.
Image courtesy of Dr. M. Castaño.

3

Q&A on **systemic** endoparasites

Chapter 3

Q&A on systemic endoparasites

Introduction

The parasitic problems included in this chapter are, by definition, very varied. The term systemic refers to "general things" that can compromise various organs, systems and functions. However, the systemic condition of a process does not necessarily mean that it is not more closely related to a specific organ or function, simply that, as it may also affect other parts of the body, it cannot be ascribed exclusively to a single apparatus or group of diseases, like those related to reproduction for example.

Similarly, as is the case in other animal species, the bovine parasitoses covered in this chapter are of particular significance as they also affect humans. Indeed, most of them are more important as a result of their zoonotic condition than for their ability to cause clinical problems.

Fortunately, some of these parasitoses are not as prevalent as in the past, whereas others have never been especially important at our latitudes. Despite this, there is currently a greater likelihood that diseases which were traditionally restricted to specific geographical regions can spread more easily.

As processes with other aetiologies have become better controlled, some diseases which currently cause significant problems in cattle on both intensive and extensive farms have acquired greater protagonism. In light of the fact that most of these have been known for some time, although perhaps not fully understood, their current situation means that they can be considered to be emerging or re-emerging. Others have been sufficiently well understood since instruments and devices that allow microscopic organisms to be observed were first developed. Although their relative importance has varied over the years, they should nevertheless not be forgotten.

"Piroplasmosis", a term that is incorrect but is nevertheless proving very difficult to eradicate, deserve special attention. Infections caused by *Babesia* and *Theileria* have been, and indeed continue to be, sufficiently important to be included here without further explanation. In the same manner as in other animal species, such as equids, the epidemiological model for these "vectorial diseases", which are transmitted by ticks, is changing in line with the environmental changes affecting the biology of their vectors.

We have also considered that a small section of this chapter should be dedicated to various infections currently considered to be "minor", at least in our setting. Infections caused by trypanosomes, some "filaria", schistosomes, etc. complete the section dedicated to "systemic" diseases.

Agents for systemic parasitoses in cattle

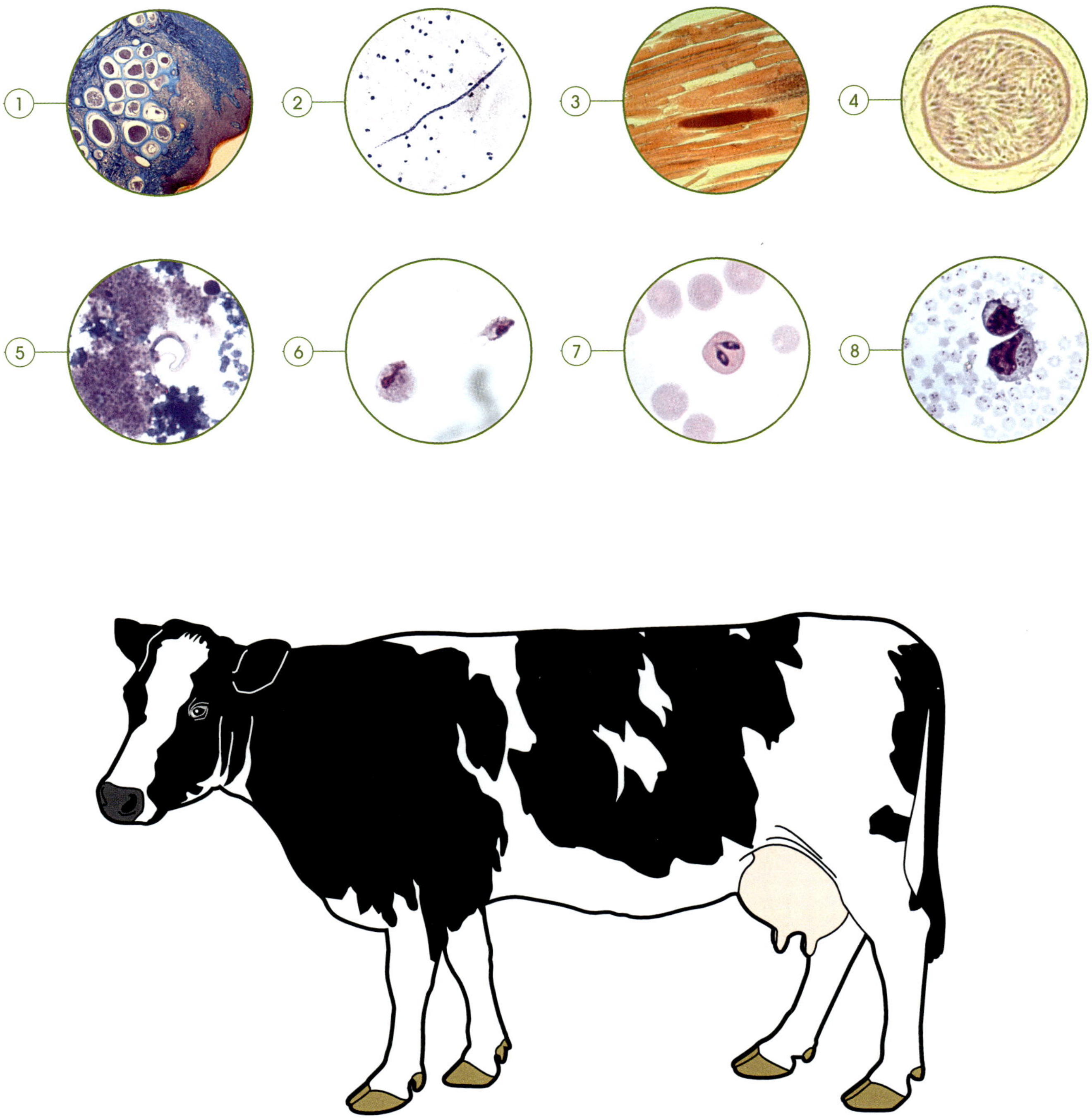

1. *Besnoitia*
2. Microfilaria
3. *Sarcocystis*
4. *Neospora*
5. *Trypanosoma*
6. Tricomonas
7. *Babesia*
8. *Theileria*

28 Can piroplasms be fatal?

After observing abnormal behaviour in an adult non-domesticated cow grazing on an estate in the Sierra de Guadarrama, Spain (the animal was more aggressive and faltered when walking), the breeder returned the following day to find the animal had died. A *post mortem* study revealed the presence of more than 200 ticks, subsequently identified as *Rhipicephalus*, and that the visible mucosa were pale and yellowish coloured. Haemolytic anaemia and jaundice, especially in the liver and kidney, with obvious lesions, as well as in the digestive mucosa and serosa, were observed upon opening.
This was not the first case of sudden animal death and the breeder was aware of the possibility of an outbreak of piroplasmosis in years with high tick numbers, especially in adult animals. Blood tests performed on other affected animals showed only 5 % *Babesia* parasitaemia not related with the acute anaemia.

1. Which piroplasm species is related to nervous signs?
2. What clinical signs are caused by babesiosis?
3. Why do mainly adult animals die on beef farms in endemic regions?
4. Is climate change affecting tick populations?

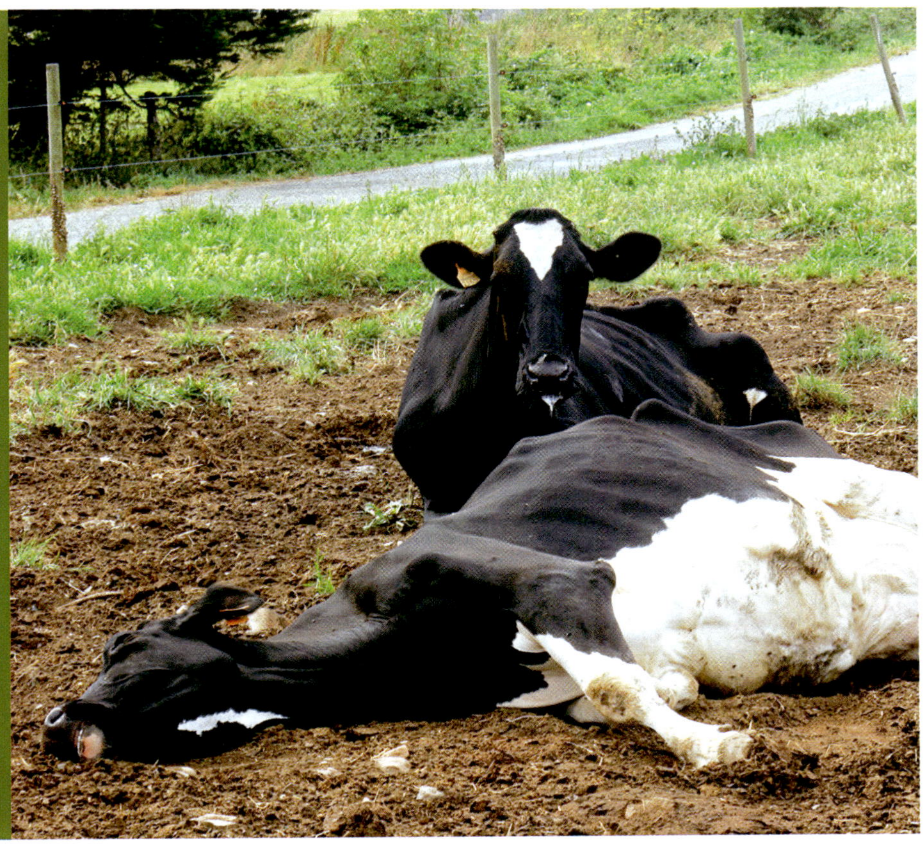

1 Which piroplasm species is related to nervous signs?

Babesia bovis is considered to be the most pathogenic of the species that affect cattle. Although classical signs such as fever anaemia and haemoglobinuria are observed, this disease is characterised by the fact that the anaemia is disproportionate to the number of red blood cells infected. Nervous clinical signs, which are clearly related to the presence of red blood cells attached to the cerebral endothelium in this species, and the onset of hypovolaemic shock, are also common. Some animals infected with *B. bigemina* also present a cerebral form of babesiosis that results in lack of motor coordination, paralysis of the hind third, seizures and coma. Despite initiating suitable treatment, these animals normally die.

The adherence of infected red blood cells to the vascular endothelium has been particularly linked to *B. bovis*. The reason for this is partly the appearance of button-shaped protuberances on the surface of these red blood cells, the number of which is directly related to the virulence of the parasite strain.

The direct consequence is blockage of local circulation, especially in organs such as the brain, thereby mostly explaining the nervous symptomatology associated with some forms of babesiosis. A build up of parasites in the agglutination zone also occurs, with localised release of substances with an enzymatic or toxic action by the parasites.

Similarly, the release of proteolytic parasitic enzymes is associated with activation of the kallikrein-kinin system. These enzymes favour the transformation of prekallikrein (naturally present in the blood) to kallikrein. As well as its hypotensive and capillary permeability enhancing properties, plasma kallikrein acts indirectly on haemostasis by releasing (parasympathomimetic effect) bradykinin and activating clotting factor XII, which activates intravascular coagulation.

The consequences of this mechanism include peripheral vasodilation with increased vascular peripheral, haematic stasis and hypotension-related shock due to activation of vasoactive substances and complicated by the presence of microthrombi in organs such as the lung and brain.

2 What clinical signs are caused by babesiosis?

Once an animal becomes infected, multiplication of the parasites reaches a peak that coincides with the onset of clinically detectable haemolysis within a period of between 7 and 20 days. This haemolysis leads to anaemia, jaundice and haemoglobinuria. Death occurs due to anaemia-related anoxia. If the animal survives, it becomes a carrier in which subclinical, symptom-free disease maintained by an immunological balance between the parasite and the host's antibodies develops. This type of disease is found with *B. bigemina* and *B. divergens*. In contrast, some acute *B. bovis* infections lead to severe haemostatic alterations with low parasitaemia a few days post-infection. *B. major* is only slightly pathogenic and rarely causes clinical signs.

Depending on the factors governing the pathogenicity, typical clinical manifestations appear a few days post-infection. The most common clinical form of babesiosis is acute, which proceeds with high morbidity but relatively low mortality.

The incubation time for field infections ranges between 2 and 3 weeks. *B. bigemina* and *B. bovis* produce clinically different symptoms including the sharp onset of fever (41 °C), anorexia, depression, weakness, suspension of rumination and decreased milk production. The animals present tachypnoea and tachycardia and their mucosa rapidly become pale. In the terminal phases, severe jaundice is observed and the urine presents a dark red to brown colour with persistent foam. Severely affected animals die at this point, a mere 24 hours after onset of the disease. The febrile period in surviving animals can last for up to a week, with the clinical presentation lasting for up to three. Pregnant females may abort. Surviving animals recover slowly and soon recover their appetite, although anaemia is an inevitable aftermath. Young animals may present a subacute form with fever but without haemoglobinuria. Actually so many different signs can be observed in babesiosis that it is difficult to name a symptom that cannot appear. The process commences with a general state of despondency, asthenia and anorexia. Affected animals isolate themselves and a hyperthermia of up to 41 °C or higher is observed from the onset, especially in babesiosis produced by *B. bovis*.

Other signs include jaundice and diarrhoea, which alternates with periods of constipation. A state of anaemia, with haemoglobinuria (more marked in *B. bigemina* infections), tachycardia and tachypnoea, slowly becomes established. Abortions may occasionally occur. In the case of *B. bovis* infection the animals become more aggressive, stagger and present seizures and sialorrhea.

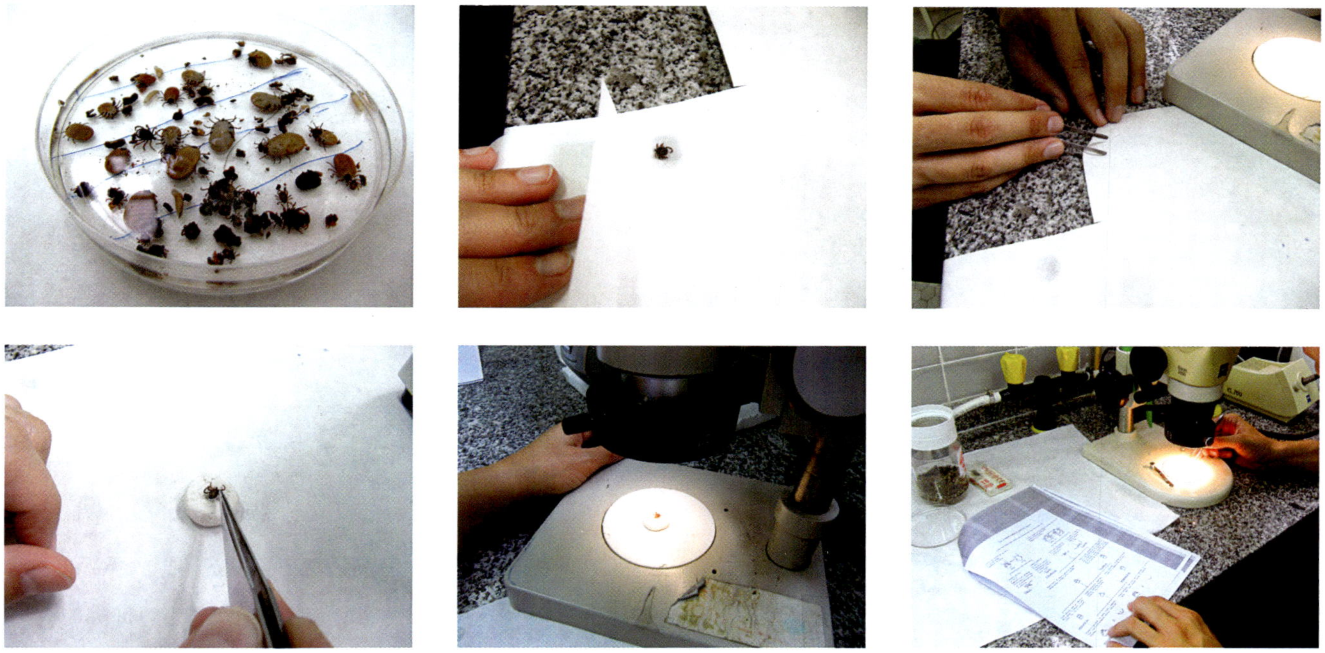

Ticks can be identified using a series of clues that allow the individuals collected in the environment or from animals to be characterised at a species level. Thus, the dorsal surface of the body of ixodes has a shield that covers at least the anterior half, with rigid protective palps. The shape of the anal groove, the presence or absence of eyes, the length and breadth of the face, the colour of the shield and other characteristics help to identify the most important genera. *Image courtesy of Dr. A. S. Olmeda.*

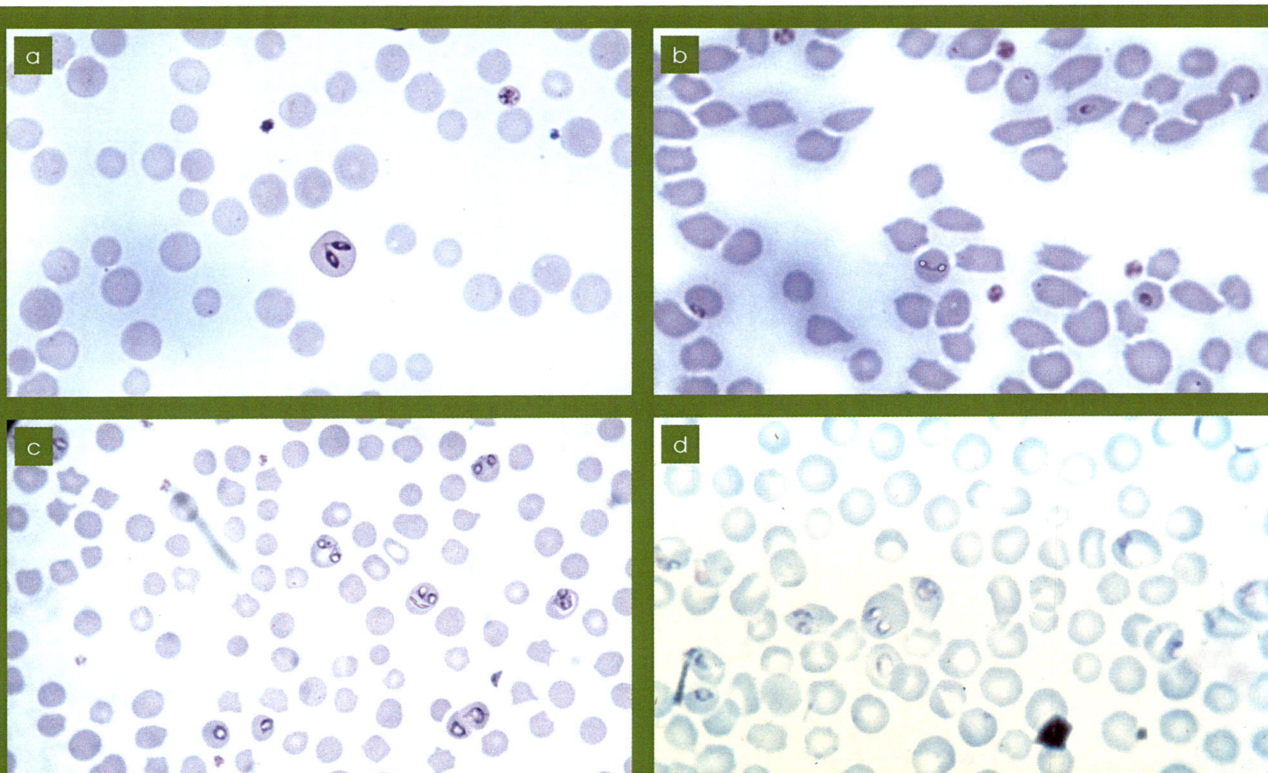

B. bigemina (a), *B. divergens* (b), *B. bovis* (c) and *B. major* (d). Classically they have been classified into two large groups: the large (2.5 to 5 µm) and small babesia (1 to 2.5 µm). *Babesia bovis and B. divergens* are small, whereas *B. bigemina and B. major* are large. Moreover, the position in the red blood cell and the angle they form, the number of parasites and other characteristics allow their identification. They are currently performed by molecular identification, antigenic characteristics or enzymatic patterns. *Images courtesy of Dr. A. S. Olmeda.*

3 Why do mainly adult animals die on beef farms in endemic regions?

Babesiosis-related mortality in endemic regions is generally low due to the resistance of animals being repeatedly in contact with the parasite. This results in an "unstable equilibrium" due to non-sterile immunity that can be displaced for several reasons. Death often occurs in infected animals from disease-free regions or in immunodeficient individuals (chemotherapy, surgery, unsuitable nutrition or with concomitant infections). The mortality may be high in such cases.

Once the host-parasite equilibrium has been displaced, *Babesia* may reach other vital organs, producing irreversible alterations and death.

The pathogenic action is related, amongst other factors, to some peculiarities of the host, such as age. Indeed, the pathogenicity is higher in adult animals than in younger ones (up to 6-8 months, approximately) living in endemic regions due to the immune memory transferred via the mother's colostrum.

Calves exhibit strong "innate" immunity against *Babesia bovis*. Various *in vivo* studies have shown that the rapid appearance of interleukin-12 (IL-12) and interferon-γ (IFN-γ) in the spleen plays a key role in the response of young animals to virulent strains of *B. bovis*. Moreover, its been shown *in vitro* that IL-12 and IL-10 are important immunoregulatory cytokines. However, IL-12 and IFN-γ expression in the spleen has been found to be very delayed in adults animals that have died as a result of this infection, with no blood antibodies being detectable prior to death.

In short, it can be stated that babesiosis tends to be more serious in adults, often proving fatal, while young animals are less affected clinically.

4 Is climate change affecting tick populations?

It seems clear that an increase in tick-related diseases is occurring in Europe. It has been proposed that climate change could be affecting the biology of these vectors, their geographical distribution and therefore the infections they transmit.

It is also possible that climate change is responsible for changes in the distribution of certain tick species, such as *Dermacentor reticulatus*. The greater activity of some tick species during the winter months appears to be related to the fact that winters are getting milder. Retrospective studies suggest that very hot summers change the dynamics and seasonal activity model of these vectors, thus leading to higher tick activity towards the end of the year. Some studies suggest that as many as eight tick species are likely to colonise more northerly regions than where they are currently found.

However, the complex ecology and epidemiology of some tick-transmitted diseases makes it difficult to directly relate climate change to the increased prevalence of some parasitoses. Further climate-model studies are therefore required in order to better understand the processes involved in the abundance of vectors and pathogen transmission, and therefore able to predict the risks and other aspects of these infections.

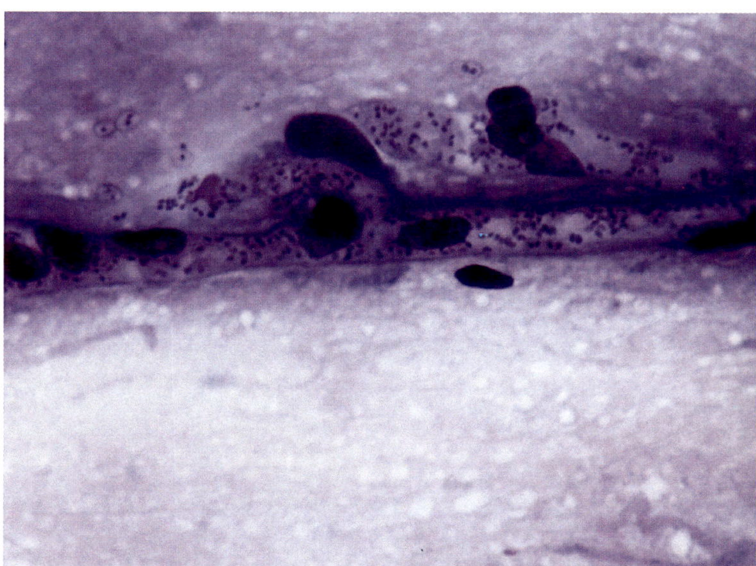

B. bovis infection causes infected red blood cells to adhere to the vascular endothelium, which can be partially explained by the growth of protuberances on the surface of these red blood cells. These protuberances probably comprise antigens from babesia or autoantigens produced after the action of various proteins and esterases released by the merozoites in red blood cells.

Biological cycle of *Babesia*

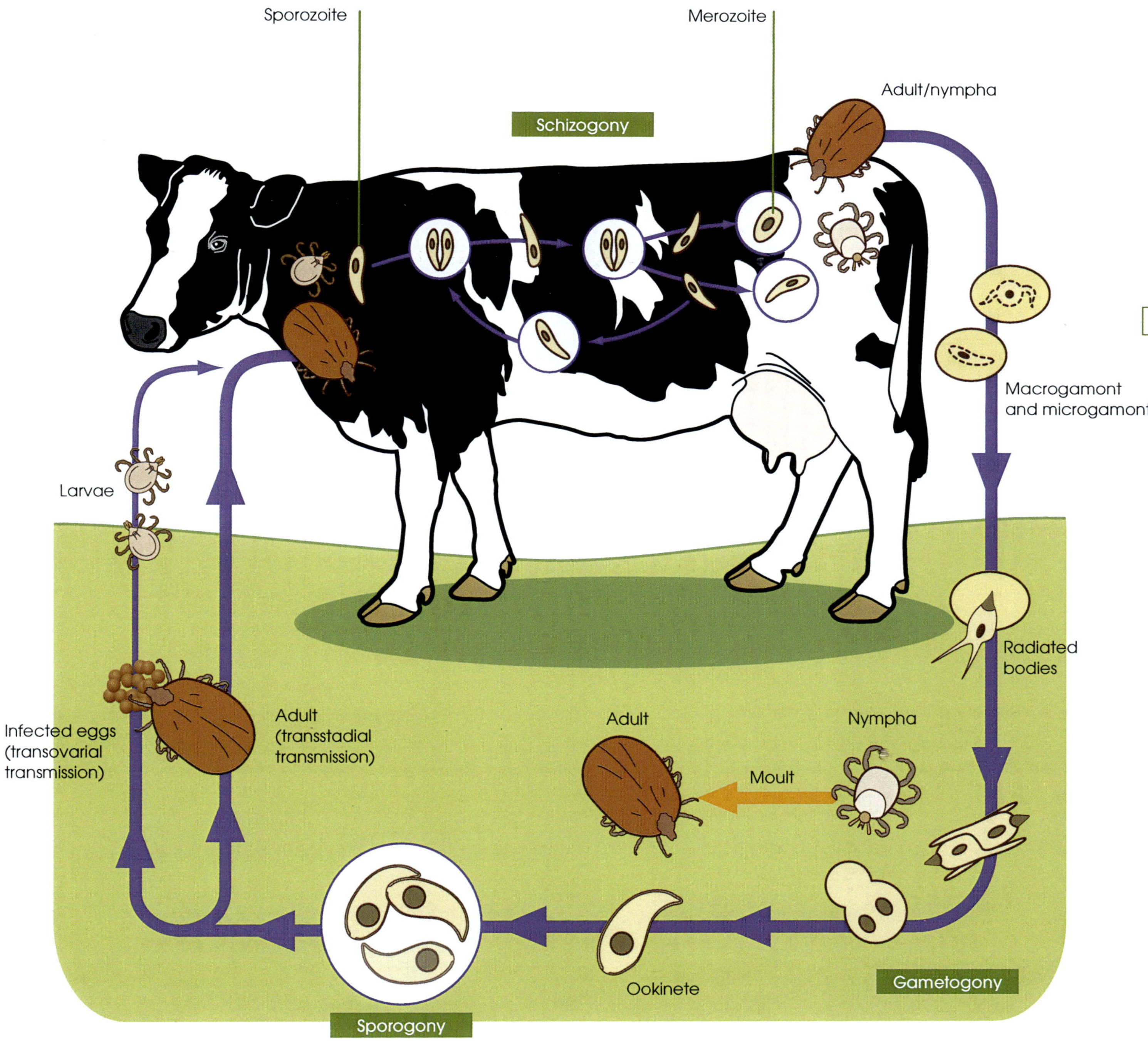

29 How is piroplasmosis diagnosed?

An outbreak of piroplasmosis occurs annually on a dairy farm in Cardeñosa (Ávila, Spain). The traditional system used on the farm comprises taking the cows out to graze for 4-8 hours on nearby pastures between the morning and evening milkings. The animals are provided with a mixture in the cowsheds, which is available at all times. The farm is in a dry region with granite outcrops in which the winters are very cold and the summers very hot. It is a pre-mountain region with pastures and shrubs and a large variety of small fauna such as rabbits. For antiparasitic control, a pour-on macrocyclic lactone that has no withdrawal period for milk is usually applied to the herd in May.

The disease usually presents in young animals, especially first-birth heifers and during the stress and immunosuppression period that occurs during the puerperium. Production falls sharply and the animals present fever (40.5-41 °C). The vet notes enlarged, easily examinable superficial lymph nodes, along with mild diarrhoea in some animals and varying degrees of mucosal pallor with dyspnoea. The orange colour of the faeces in some animals, which readily stains clothing, is notable. Jaundice or haemoglobinuria are rarely observed (not even using urine reagent strips).

Some years the process presents in older animals, namely in cows with 3 or 4 previous births, but is usually accompanied by other diseases (ketosis, steatosis). The mortality in affected animals is very high. As is the case every year, laboratory tests indicate the presence of piroplasms and anaplasma.

1. Which methods have been used to identify these agents in the laboratory?
2. What medical treatment is recommended in such cases?
3. Is the use of an autogenous vaccine recommended?
4. What other recommendations would you give to the farmer?

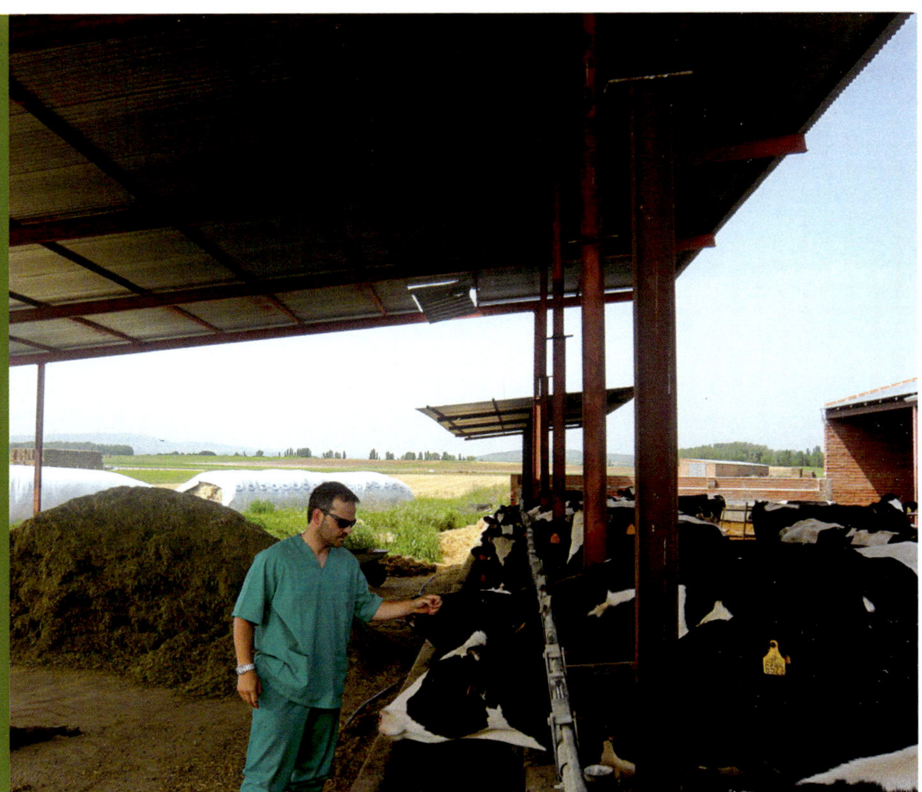

1 Which methods have been used to identify these agents in the laboratory?

Babesia can be identified in an analytical laboratory using various methods.

Thus, the parasite can be observed in thin blood smears stained with Giemsa, which allows the parasites to be seen inside red blood cells. This method has the drawback that the parasitaemia is usually low and that *Babesia* can easily be morphologically confused with other microorganisms (*Anaplasma* or *Theileria*) or with artifacts (stain on the surface of the red blood cell). Moreover, *Babesia* can only be found in peripheral blood in the first few days post-infection. Despite this, the low cost and speed with which this method can be performed, together with epidemiological and clinical findings (which requires a great deal of practice and an understanding of ruminant disease), are a great help for diagnosis.

Immunological methods are very useful and widely used. Although various such techniques, such as agglutination, haemagglutination, precipitation and complement fixation, have been used, the most commonly used currently are indirect immunofluorescence (IIF) and ELISA, both of which are highly sensitive and specific (>97 %), especially the latter.

Molecular biology techniques are currently used, such as the different PCR techniques, which are highly efficient but more expensive and currently restricted to specialised laboratories.

2 What medical treatment is recommended in these cases?

Two aspects should be taken into consideration as regards treatment. Firstly, specific treatment with a babesicide and, secondly, the need to initiate support therapy, such as blood transfusions and fluid therapy without forgetting the administration of antipyretics.

Although various babesicides are known, the most widely used and effective are imidocarb dipropionate, which markedly reduces the parasitaemia, and aromatic diamidines such as diminazene aceturate. Imidocarb is highly effective and not especially toxic at a dose of 1 mg/kg b.w. It can be used as a chemoprophylactic at twice the dose, providing good protection for around six weeks. Higher doses are required for parasite sterilisation, although this must be suitably evaluated as it suppresses any possible natural immunisation in the animal.

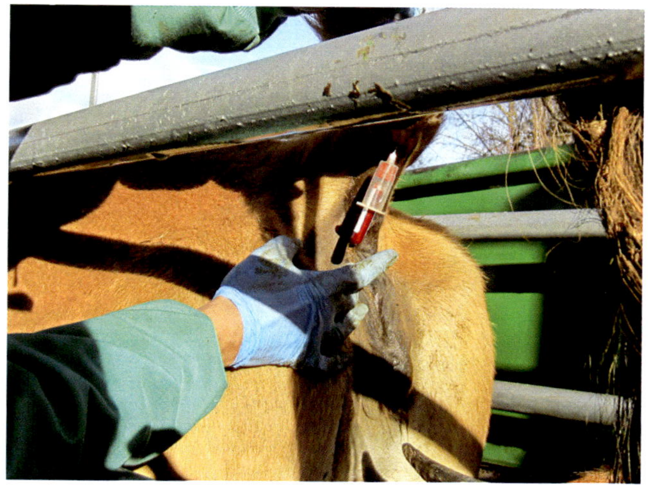

Irrespective of the technique(s) used to confirm the diagnosis, taking of a blood sample is an essential prior step. A small blood sample allows a smear to be performed and subsequent staining with vital dyes (Giemsa, etc.) for observation under a light microscope to detect intraerythrocytic forms. The rest of the sample can be used for techniques such as agglutination, hemagglutination, complement fixation, indirect immunofluorescence and ELISA, etc.

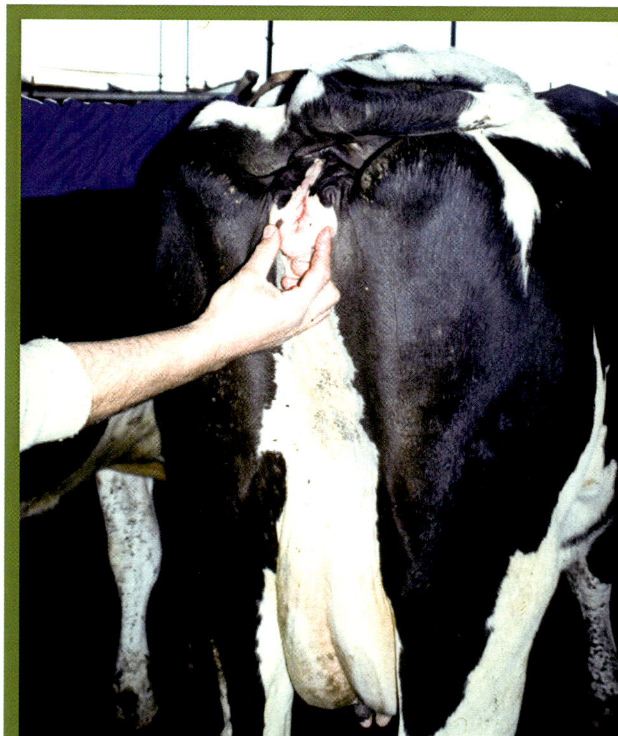

The symptoms of babesiosis vary widely. The initial symptoms include asthenia, anorexia, hyperthermia and diarrhoea, which alternates with intestinal constipation. Other alterations (haemoglobinuria, tachycardia, tachypnoea, abortion and anxiety attacks, tremor, seizures and sialorrhea) may also present. Anaemia, which can easily be seen from the pallor of the external mucosa (vulva, ocular conjunctiva, etc.), is a constant sign in babesiosis.

Babesiosis often presents together with *Anaplasma* infection, and antibiotic therapy with oxytetracycline is very effective in such cases.

Support therapy is always required, although more so in severely affected animals. Haematopoiesis stimulating factors (iron, copper, etc.) should be administered and liver functionality should be supported with liver protectors and vitamin B12. Cardiotonics and diuresis activators are also of great use.

Blood transfusions produce good results. Around five litres of blood is obtained from a healthy cow, mixed with an anticoagulant and immediately transfused into the recipient animal.

3 Is the use of an autogenous vaccine recommended?

Although the first immunoprevention trials date back as far as the late 19th century, very little progress has been made in this respect. This may be due to the fact that the antigen variability of babesial organisms allows them to avoid the body' immune response.

Since then, immunisation has been attempted using blood containing irradiated merozoites or by performing controlled infections in an attempt to provoke premunition. However, all these procedures have some degree of risk.

Vaccines containing attenuated live *Babesia* have been developed in some countries by repeated passage in splenectomised animals.

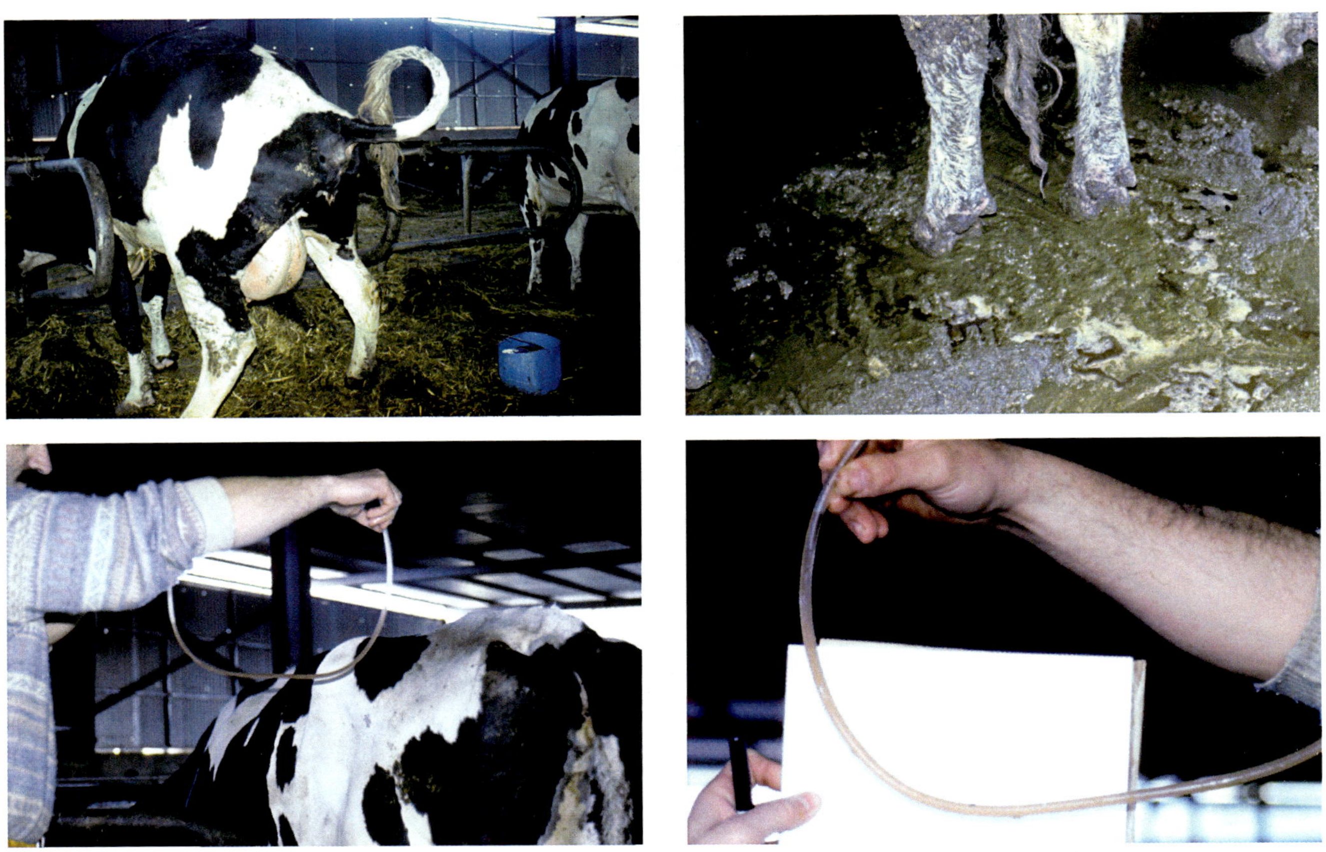

Multiplication of babesia concludes with destruction of the red blood cells, which causes fever, haemoglobinuria and anaemia. If red blood cell destruction is intense, the haemoglobin may not be completely transformed into bile pigments in the liver, exceeding the renal threshold and being eliminated in urine, thus producing haemoglobinuria ("red urine" for farmers).

Manufactured autogenous vaccines have led to a difference of opinion, but can also be used. Thus, although some farmers remain sceptical as regards their worth, experience has shown that, at least partially, they provide results that help to control babesiosis.

4 What other recommendations would you give to the farmer?

First of all, it should be stressed that successful control is unlikely without the collaboration of the farmer.

As spread of the disease should obviously be prevented, rapid and correct identification of affected animals is essential in order to isolate them from the rest of the herd. Furthermore, animals should be separated by age in light of their different sensitivities towards the disease. In this regard, measures that help to strengthen the immunity of young animals (administration of colostrum, etc.) in order to achieve satisfactory premunition are of particular interest.

Special attention should also be paid to immunosuppressed animals, attempting to avoid any factors that reduce the body's response to *Babesia*.

Measures to combat the ticks that act as vectors are also important, although their success cannot always be guaranteed. Thus, the application of acaricides in dips, sprays, pour-on, topical use, etc. is recommended and usually gives good results. Biological methods (use of hormones, male castration, predators) may also be of use.

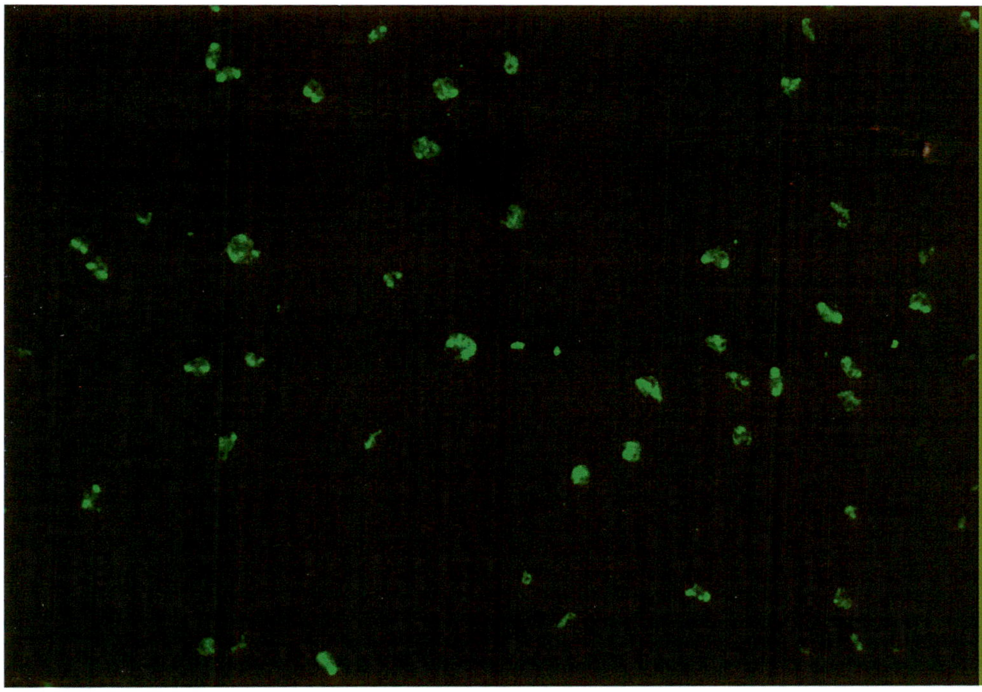

Methods that demonstrate the presence of the parasite or contact with the host should be used to confirm the diagnosis. Although various techniques, including agglutination, hemagglutination and complement fixation, can currently be used due to their high sensitivity and specificity, the two techniques most commonly used are indirect immunofluorescence (IIF) and the immunoenzymatic ELISA technique, which can detect the antibodies produced to combat specific *Babesia* antigens.

30 Can a theileriosis be transmitted without ticks?

This case concerns an average sized dairy farm producing around 20-25 litres of milk per animal per day which has recently been transferred from the farmer to his sons. Since they purchased a new group of animals, the sons have noticed that most cows have developed a very high fever, many have died and dark urine has been observed in others. The animals have been treated with a tetracycline and those that survived appear to have improved, although the lower milk production remains. Some of these animals have lost weight and slowly develop anaemia, whereas this is not the case in others. On the farm, the vet notes some animals with anaemic mucosa, dyspnoea and tachycardia. Various animals present catarrhal symptoms with tearing and abundant nasal flow and, most significantly, a generalised and very marked lymphadenomegaly that allows a presumptive diagnosis to be established. A careful observation of the surroundings allows the vet to note the presence of a bottle of oxytocin with the needle of a syringe inserted on a windowsill.

1. What results would you expect to find in a blood test?
2. How can the lymphadenomegaly and catarrh be explained?
3. How can infection be explained if the animals have no contact with ticks?
4. What measures would prevent this process from reappearing?

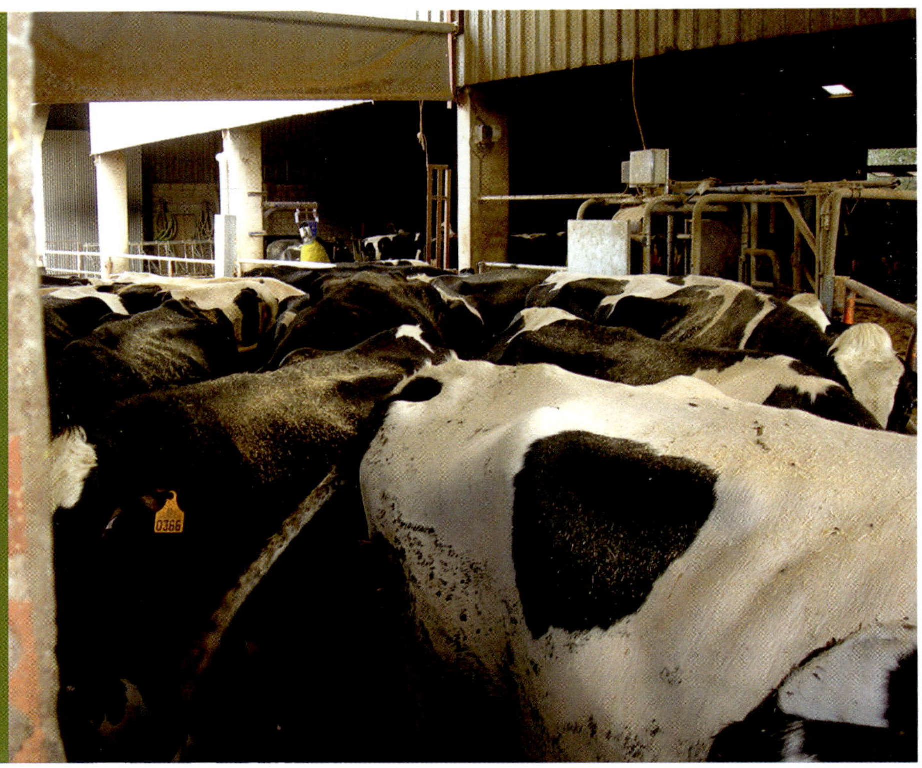

1 What results would you expect to find in a blood test?

The signs are relatively specific and infection can be confirmed by observing parasites (piroplasms) in red blood cells or schizonts in impression smears performed using material obtained from lymph node biopsy and stained with Giemsa. Peak parasitaemia levels are achieved at around 10-12 days post-infection.

Morphologically, *Theileria* found in red blood cells have various shapes. The most common shapes for *Theileria annulata* are rounded, although ovoids or rings, as well as commas or bars, may also be seen. Their size ranges between 0.5 and 6 µm in diameter (2-5 µm for rings, 1-6 µm for rods and 0.5 µm for commas). When stained with Giemsa, their eosinophilic cytoplasm presents a basophilic chromatin granule at one end. They can be present alone, in pairs or in quadrads (Maltese cross).

Blood tests show anaemia, a marked decrease in haematocrit, and leukopenia, which can convert into leukocytosis at the end of the process.

2 How can the lymphadenomegaly and catarrh be explained?

Lymphoproliferation, initially in the lymph nodes closest to the inoculation site, commences a few days (5-7 days) post-infection. The ticks attach to various parts of the body, including, depending on the tick species concerned, around the ears. As a result, the lymph nodes in that region are the first to become enlarged. After invasion of the parasite, synchronic division of the parasite and host cell occurs. This leads to a series of transformations in which the cells resulting from the division are infected. The size of the lymph nodes, especially the parotid, but also pre-scapular and precrural nodes, which are easy to examine, increases markedly.

Panleukopenia, which normally coincides with the detection of parasite forms, develops during this phase of the disease.

Lymphoid atrophy and necrosis and infiltration of infected lymphoblasts, which is very clear from the interstitial lung tissue and causes severe oedema, occur in subsequent phases of the infection. Tearing, nasal discharge, dyspnoea and diarrhoea are also common. Shortly prior to death, the animal experiences a decreased body temperature, marked dyspnoea and prostration. Nasal discharge is usually evident. These symptoms are compatible with alterations caused by pulmonary oedema and asphyxia, which leads to death within 18-24 days, although some animals succumb sooner (14-15 days).

3 How can infection be explained if the animals have no contact with ticks?

The main route of contagion is via the specific invertebrate host or mechanically (via surgical instrumentation). The presence of a syringe with its needle inserted into a medicinal product suggests frequent needle reuse without basic health precautions. Information obtained regarding the purchase of a new batch of animals, which may be carriers, may also help determine the source of the infection.

The clinical cure of sick animals does not necessarily imply elimination of the parasite from the host's body, especially

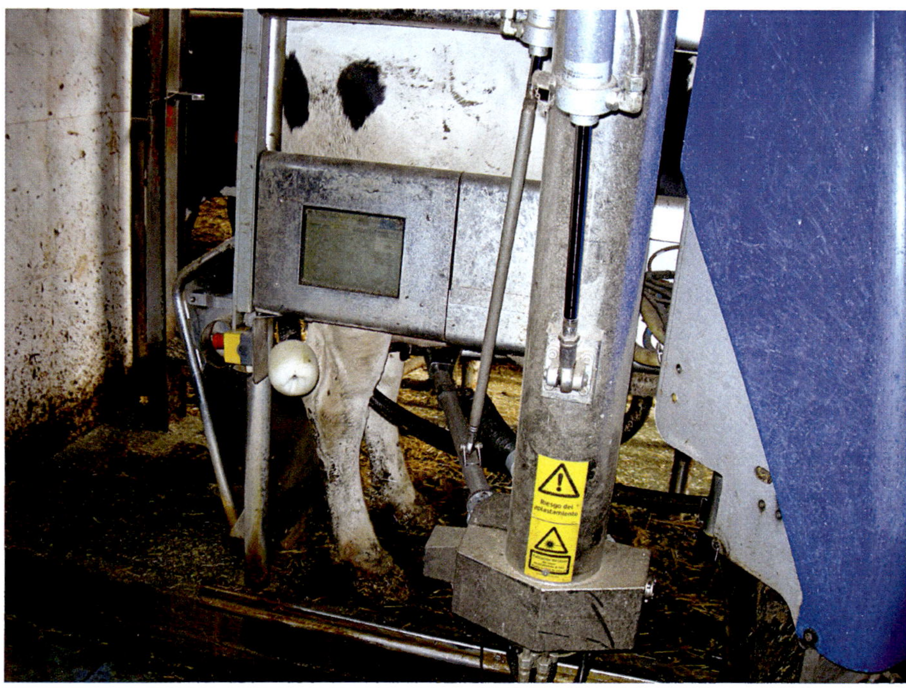

Apart from the medical consequences of theilerioses, the effects of these parasitoses are also economic due to the important loses resulting from decreased productions (mainly milk), abortions, impoundments, deaths and medical and veterinary bills.

when considering that *Theileria* "colonises" organs in the mononuclear phagocyte system, somehow protected from the pharmacological action of the products used during therapy. This situation has been termed "endemic stability", which refers to an epidemiological state in a population in which the clinical process is the exception despite there being some degree of infection in the host population. This concept was developed precisely to describe models for bovine infections transmitted by ticks.

4 What measures would prevent this process from reappearing?

One of the premises is to prevent iatrogenic transmission by taking the appropriate measures. Moreover, chemotherapy is vital to control an outbreak. Some chemotherapeutic drugs and products can be used prophylactically in *Theileria* spp. infections. This is the case for chlortetracycline, which has been shown to be moderately effective against the phases that infect leukocytes. Other products, which are always indicated due to their ability to control other infections (anaplasmosis, babesiosis, bacterial infections), can also be used. The specific antitheilerial drugs known to exhibit good efficacy include naphthoquinones (parvaquone and buparvaquone), which destroy the lymphocytes and help high percentages of animals to recover (80-94 %) but do not destroy the parasite completely, thus meaning that the animal becomes an asymptomatic carrier.

Immunoprophylaxis can also be put into practice. The inoculation of stabilised macerates produced using sporozoite-containing ticks and subsequent treatment with specific drugs has allowed animal breeding to continue in some regions as there is often a severe risk when selected animals are introduced into some countries. In any case, "vaccination" creates asymptomatic carriers, with their resultant problems. These problems can be avoided by immunising the animals with vaccines prepared from purified sporozoite or schizont proteins, the results of which appear highly promising.

Other infection-prevention measures involve control of the vector populations in both the environment and the animals themselves. Actions undertaken in the former are complex and the results are not always as expected. It should be remembered that ticks use several hosts, including wild animals, thus complicating their control.

Special attention should be paid when introducing animals from infection-free regions into endemic regions. Protection of a herd should take into account all epidemiological factors involved in the maintenance and transmission of *Theileria* in the host populations.

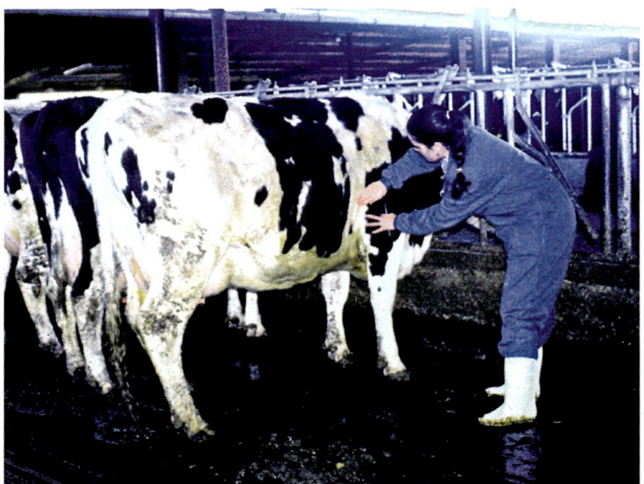

One of the signs that almost always appears in theileriosis is enlarged, readily examinable lymph nodes, especially the prescapular nodes, which tend to be painful upon palpation. This enlargement presents shortly after infection (8 days) and reaches a maximum at around 13-15 days post-contagion. This lymphadenomegaly coincides with the presence of schizonts inside the lymphocytes.

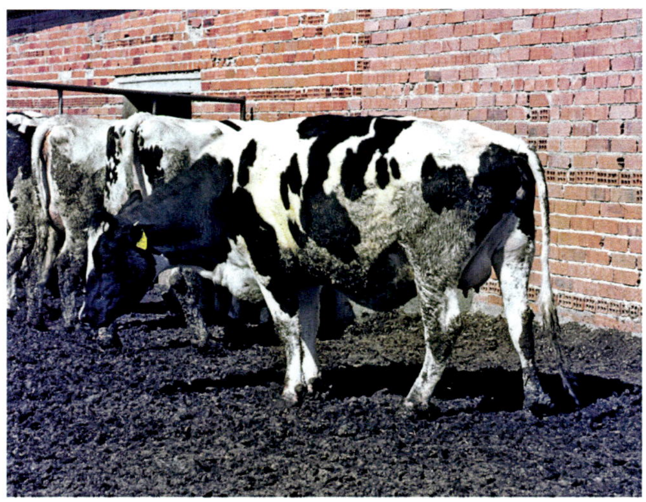

The subacute form of the disease typically found in endemic regions is characterised by fever with hyperthermia, general weakness, marked loss of appetite and ruminal asthenia. Other signs that may appear include tearing and abundant nasal secretion.

31 Do animals remain infected but asymptomatic after a piroplasmosis?

Around 15 days after the introduction of a group of Charolais cows onto a recently purchased 450 ha estate in Salamanca province (Spain), over half of the animals have died or are very weak. The vet diagnoses acute piroplasmosis. A total of 132 Morucha cattle from the previous owner are maintained on the estate on the same fields that have always been used when weather conditions allow, with some being used in winter and others in summer. There is no contact between the animals, but a large number of ticks is observed on all the animals. The previous owner states that there have been no problems with either native breed-cows or calves for many years, although the serological tests performed some years previously showed that many were positive.

1. Why have only new animals died?
2. How is infection maintained in the absence of obvious parasitaemia?
3. What measures can be taken to facilitate the introduction of animals with no prior exposure to infection into an endemic region?

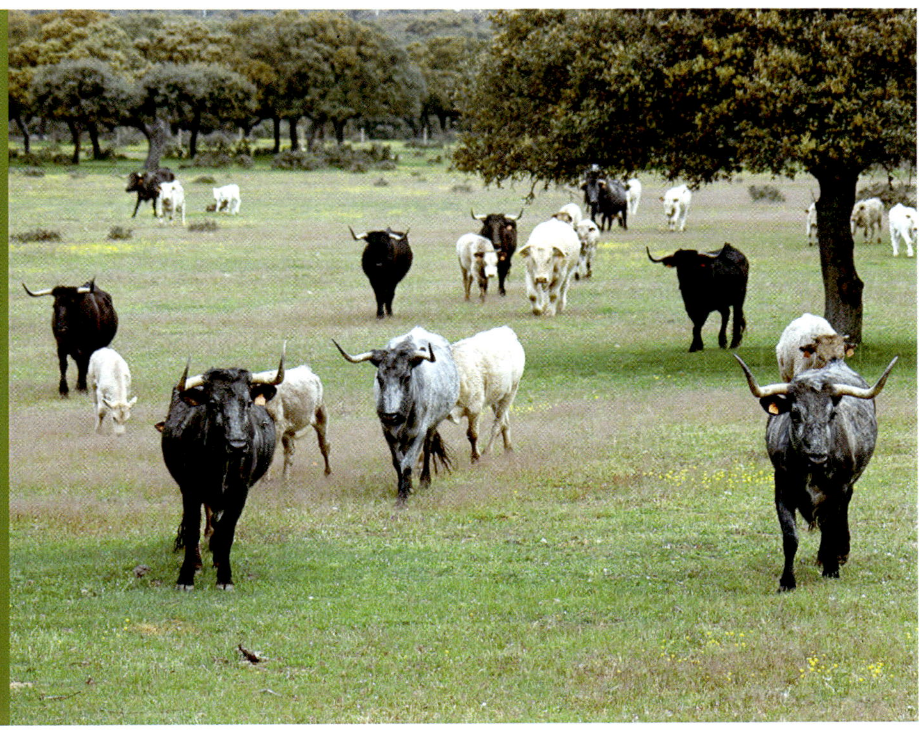

1 Why have only new animals died?

The first link in the epidemiological chain comprises sick animals, healthy asymptomatic carriers or wild animals. Environmental factors that govern vector populations, which also play a key role, and can be considered the second link. The final link involves receptive animals.

The morbidity in animals living in endemic regions, the "natives", is low due to the antibodies developed against these parasites as a result of repeat contact, thus meaning that infection remains at low levels due to non-sterile immunity or premunition. The end result of this is that clinical disease can occur when the host-parasite equilibrium is disturbed due to external factors. If receptive animals from regions in which they have had no contact with *Babesia* spp. are introduced into enzootic regions, the newcomers suffer a severe process that can occasionally prove fatal.

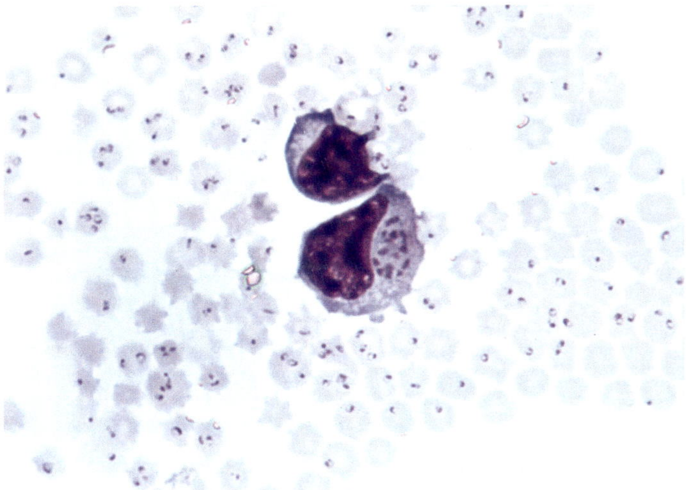

After penetrating bovine lymphatic cells, the sporozoites begin to reproduce asexually to form schizonts (macro- and microschizonts). The schizonts, which are also known as Koch's blue bodies or spheres, measure between 2 and 12 µm in diameter.

2 How is infection maintained in the absence of obvious parasitaemia?

When an infected tick bites an animal it first of all injects anticoagulants and vasodilators together with the sporozoites found in its salivary glands. These penetrate the erythrocytes and start to multiply indefinitely, thus meaning that it is common to observe red blood cells containing one, two or four merozoites. From this point the infected cell splits and releases the parasites, which penetrate new cells. This process is repeated until the disease remits due either to self-limitation of the process or antiparasitic treatment.

Imidazole derivatives (imidazole carbamate) are effective treatment alternatives. Although injection is painful due to the irritation produced by the excipients that accompany the active substance, these compounds can even be administered to pregnant cows, although their meat or milk should not be consumed for 28 days or 2-4 days, respectively. In most cases the animals improve clinically within 36 hours post-injection.

Much higher doses must be administered if the animal is to be completely freed from parasites, injecting 2-3 mg of imidocarb with the above-mentioned characteristics. However, this process should be considered carefully as it prevents the important natural immunisation of the animal that arises due to the presence of parasites (non-sterile immunity).

Drugs act against dividing parasites, which are therefore the first to disappear, with the pyriform types in peripheral blood following shortly afterwards. All parasites have disappeared from peripheral blood within 9-45 hours.

As is the case with other species of *Babesia*, this disappearance may only be temporary —small numbers of parasites appear and disappear as the animals begin to recover. There is still however some uncertainty remaining regarding this process. For example, it is not known exactly how long after treatment blood can contain *Babesia* after an apparent recovery. Similarly, it is also not known whether the parasites present in recovered animals have a different virulence and whether they are able to infect ticks.

3 What measures can be taken to facilitate the introduction of animals with no prior exposure to infection into an endemic region?

There are a series of guidelines which can be of great help when it comes to introducing susceptible animals from disease-free regions into an enzootic zone.

The first such measure involves allowing the new animals to become immunised by facilitating a natural infection (similar to a "natural vaccination"), which generates an immune response whilst the contact between host and parasite lasts.

No other measures need to be taken until approximately one week (5-7 days) after introduction of the animals into the zone. After this time, administration of a drug that is able to control the infection is recommended in order to avoid possibly undesirable clinical effects. This allows the new animals "to keep the infection under control". The same drug should be administered again one month later to control infections due to other haematozoic pathogens.

Serological analyses should be performed in order to confirm the efficacy of the two treatments administered, which should protect all animals in the herd. If the level of protection turns out to be inadequate, the animals should be re-exposed to the infection.

In order to facilitate contagion ("natural vaccination"), substances that are active against ticks should not be applied. Acaricidal drugs should obviously be applied to control tick populations but they should not be used to eradicate them completely.

Other measures, such as the injection of infected blood into the new animals, have also been suggested. However, this method is very dangerous and, if used, must be applied in such a manner as to ensure that the "artificial infection" is very well controlled to avoid acute infections and other undesired effects.

Another method is vaccination. It should only be used to protect fully susceptible animals that are to be transferred to regions where the disease is enzootic and to protect animals in such regions when the tick population is insufficient for them to be infected naturally during the first few months of life, when they are still relatively resistant. A series of measures must also be taken in this case, with one of the most important being vaccinating the animals prior to sending them to the enzootic region (at least 30 days beforehand) to ensure that they arrive at their destination with a strong immunity.

If vaccination is performed in the new region, strict tick control measures should be put into place during the adaptation period. In any case, only clinically healthy animals aged 4 to 10 months in a good nutritional state should be vaccinated.

In light of the stress caused by transport, and other stress factors, the new animals should be provided with food and water *ad libitum* and shaded rest areas in the new region, and should not be used for reproductive purposes for 30 days following their arrival.

The large-scale presence of ticks should be monitored and the animals should be checked daily: if they present compatible symptoms an effective drug should be administered.

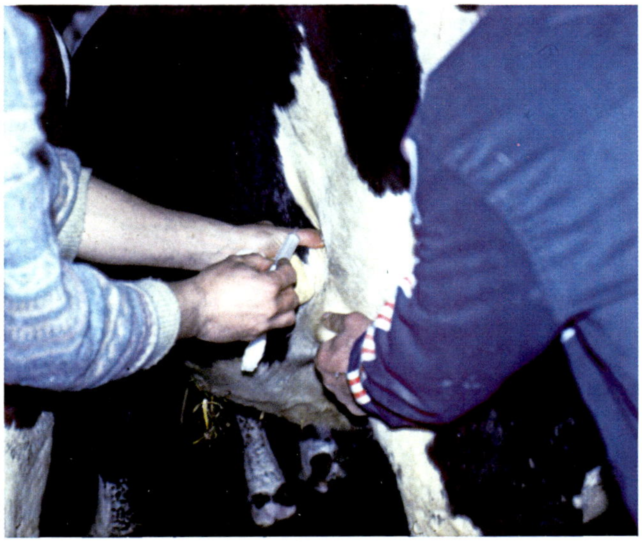

In most cases epidemiological and clinical data are insufficiently valid to confirm the diagnosis. As such, methods that allow the parasite or its components to be located and identified should be used. Direct parasitological methods include lymph node puncture to obtain material that can be used to perform smears or footprints, which allow the parasites to be observed after staining with Giemsa-type stains.

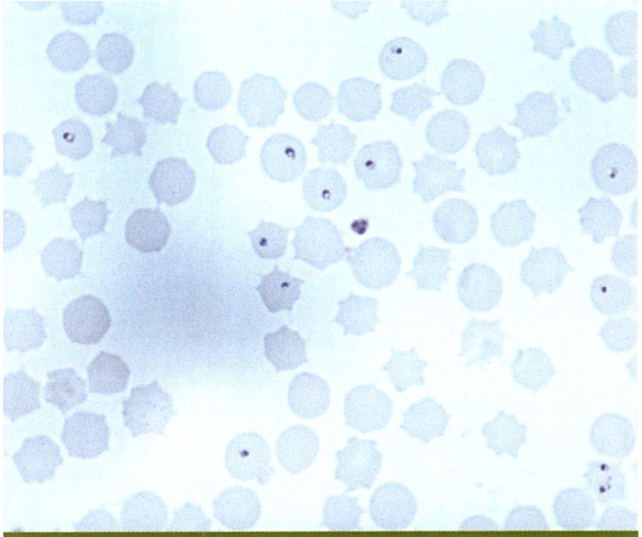

Theileria species can be differentiated on the basis of their antigenic characteristics, cross-immunity assays between species or strains, detection of differences in their DNA sequence, types of protein found in the schizonts, etc. However, their morphological characteristics when present inside the erythrocytes, which are rounded, ovoid or ring-shaped, such as in *T. annulata*, can also be used for identification purposes.

32 Are *Sarcocystis* infections common?

After collecting two dogs from a shelter, the farmer notes that young calves are listless, weak and have no appetite. The animals have been sharing the cowshed since they arrived more than a month ago. The calves have lost weight and the distal parts of their limbs and tail have lost hair. They cannot walk properly and present lesions of various types on both the carpus and tarsus, and even interdigitally. Some present fever, anaemia and neurological disorders such as nystagmus and opisthotonos. A coprological test of dog faeces shows sporocysts of sarcosporidia.

1. Which species can be involved in bovine sarcosporidiosis?
2. What pathogenic mechanisms occur in sarcosporidiosis?
3. Is there any specific treatment?

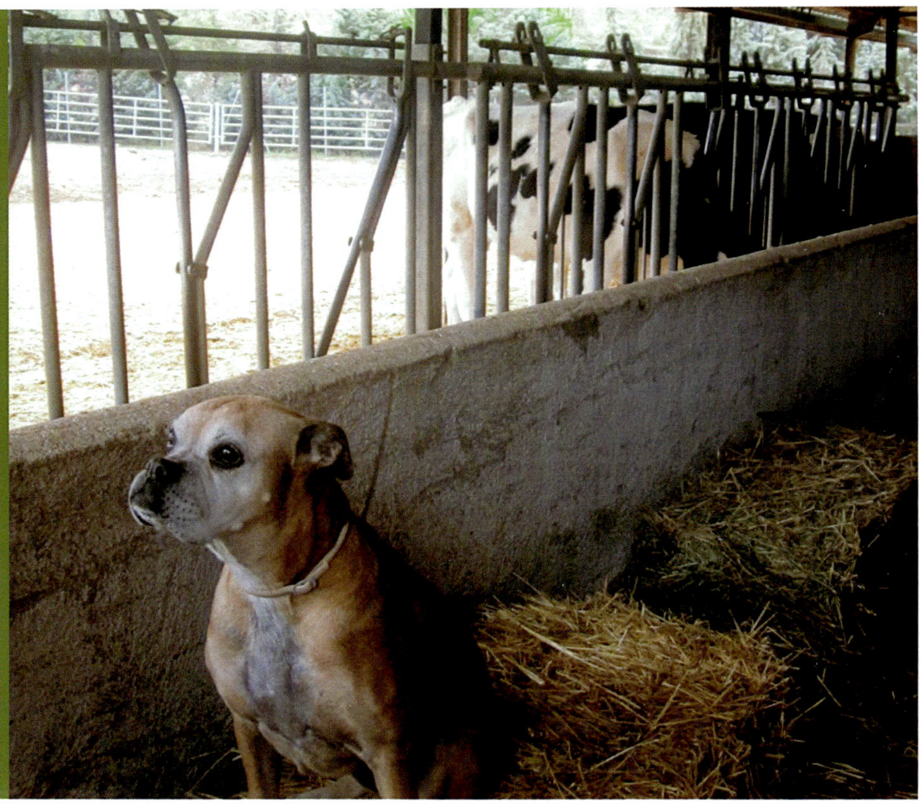

1 Which species can be involved in bovine sarcosporidiosis?

Sarcosporidia are parasites in whose biology predatory species, in this case carnivores (dogs, cats, humans), are involved as definitive hosts and their "prey" (herbivores) as intermediate hosts for *Sarcocystis* species. These become infected when the oocysts expelled in the faeces of the definitive hosts are ingested with contaminated water, food, etc.

The oocysts have a very thin wall which is readily broken to release the sporocysts. These are approximately 12-16 µm × 9-11 µm in size, sporulated and contain the infective forms: the sporozoites.

The following species affect cattle:

- *Sarcocystis cruzi* (= ***S. bovicanis***), which is the most pathogenic and whose cycle involves dogs and bovines.
- *Sarcocystis hirsuta* (= ***S. bovifelis***), which infects bovines and cats.
- *Sarcocystis hominis* (= ***S. bovihominis***), which is a bovine and human parasite.

In light of the definitive hosts that participate in the cycle of these sarcosporidia, the prevalence is highest in regions in which contact between the definitive and intermediate hosts is closest and in which hygiene is poor.

2 What pathogenic mechanisms occur in sarcosporidiosis?

The pathogenic action depends, amongst other factors, on the parasite species responsible for the infection and its ability to multiply, the location of the merogonies, the prolificacy of the schizonts and the likelihood of reaching the CNS. The infective dose and reinfections must also be taken into consideration as some genera, such as *Sarcocystis*, are able to develop protective immunity. Stress, pregnancy, a deficient nutritional status and lactation predispose the host to infection.

During the proliferative phase, sexual multiplication of the parasite in endothelial cells results in rupture of the host cell, which causes endarteritis and increased capillary permeability, thereby favouring the outflow of fluids, blood and mobile cells. Vacuolisation and leukocytic infiltration in the tunica media, especially in mid-sized vessels, occur in some cases. The remnants of broken cells that remain in the artery walls, as well as those released into the bloodstream, trigger an increase in blood pressure, and therefore oedema and haemorrhage, in smaller vessels and capillaries by obstructing their lumen.

To repair this endarteritis, thrombocyte fixation and the blood clotting system are activated, thereby stimulating microthrombi formation and slowing down the blood flow. Vasoactive substances that increase capillary permeability and activate fibrinolysis, thereby initiating the complement cascade, some of whose components also have chemotactic and vasoactive activity, are also produced during this process, thus contributing to the appearance of oedema and haemorrhage.

When infection occurs in gestating cows, the parasites multiply in the placental cotyledons, myoepithelial cells and, very occasionally, in the foetal annexes, with areas infiltrated with mononuclear cells (monocytes and lymphocytes) and necrotic tissue. These trigger foetal death and abortion usually towards the second half of pregnancy.

In cystic phase, eosinophilic myositis related to high IgE levels and granulomas can be observed, as well as perivascular infiltration of mononuclear cells and in apparently healthy infected muscle fibres. The reaction occurs in degenerating cells, with open cysts in which neutrophils and mononuclear cells are abundant.

These processes evolve towards the formation of giant cell granulomas or fibrosis and calcifications that hinder muscle contraction. Depending on the location, the final clinical outcome is the onset of chewing, movement or cardiac functionality problems. A non-purulent meningoencephalitis that causes neurological alterations has been observed when the cysts are located in the CNS.

It has been found that the intravenous administration of substances obtained from bradyzoite extracts (sarcocystine) produces haemorrhage, paralysis, oedema and even death.

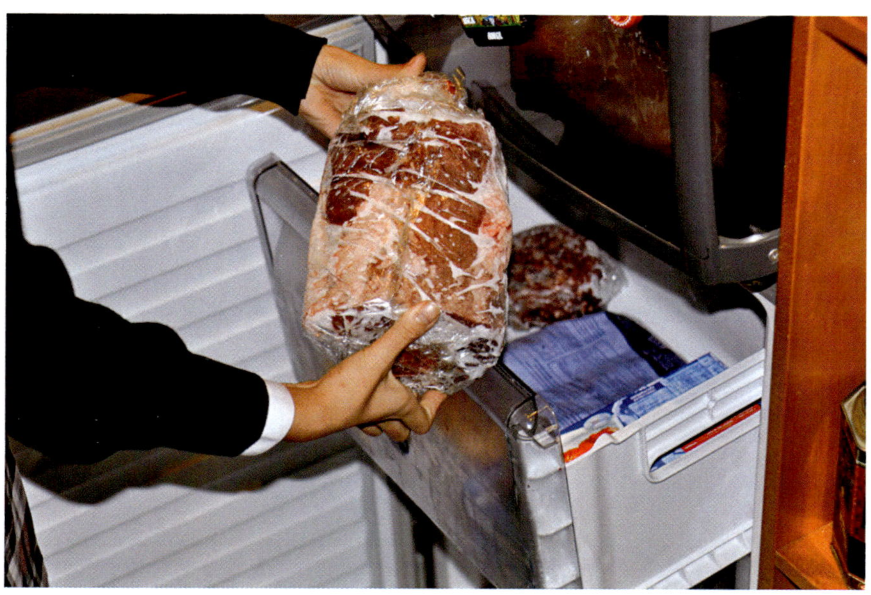

The cysts lose their infective ability after storage in a domestic freezer (-20 °C) for 3 days. Upon refrigeration at 2 °C, the cysts remain viable for almost 15 days. Heat inactivation of the cysts is directly related to the thickness of the piece of meat. Complete inactivation requires temperatures of 65-70 °C for 10 minutes to ensure bradyzoite death.

3 Is there any specific treatment?

Although treatment of these processes makes little practical sense, if required, drugs that are known to be effective against coccidia, such as amprolium or salinomycin for two weeks, halofuginone for four days, or oxytetracycline, can be used.

However, measures that reduce the risk or prevent infection are highly recommended. Control is based on preventing the biological cycle of sarcosporidia from reaching completion, especially at those points in the epidemiological chain at which it is easiest to act. For example, measures that prevent dogs and cats from becoming infected by correct treatment of impounded carcasses and preventing these animals from accessing meat remnants and ruminant bones are of particular importance. Similarly, the infection of intermediate hosts should be prevented. Control of the dog and cat populations and basic hygiene measures to prevent the spread of oocysts in drinking water, feed, hay, etc., or in feed storage bins are of great utility.

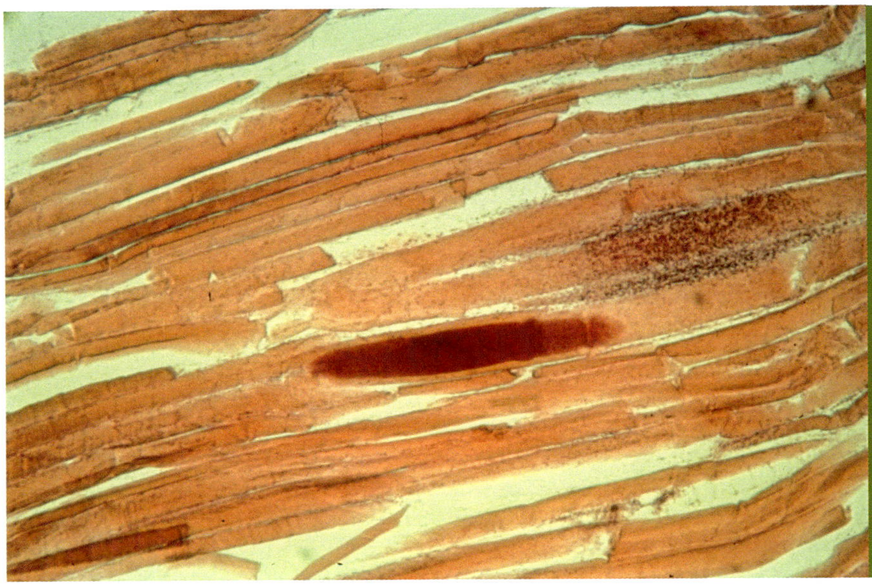

The cysts wall may be either thick or thin and usually presents highly characteristic digitated, pallisade, or fringe-type structures, etc., which can be used for morphological identification provided that the histological section is appropriately orientated or the cyst has been removed from the surrounding muscle. Septa filled with numerous bradyzoites can be seen internally. *Image courtesy of Dr. C. Novoa.*

33 How is a *Sarcocystis* infection detected?

The carcasses from an organic farm in Lleida (Spain) have been impounded for the third consecutive time. The vet's report indicates that they present numerous thin and twisting intermuscular cysts some 3-4 mm in length and that their possible identification as *Sarcocystis bovihominis* has been confirmed upon compression. Samples have been sent to a laboratory to confirm their aetiology and if confirmed, will begin using the appropriate prophylactic measures on the farm.

1. How is a *Sarcocystis* infection confirmed?
2. What measures should be taken to prevent carcasses from being impounded?
3. Can muscular cysts withstand the cold?

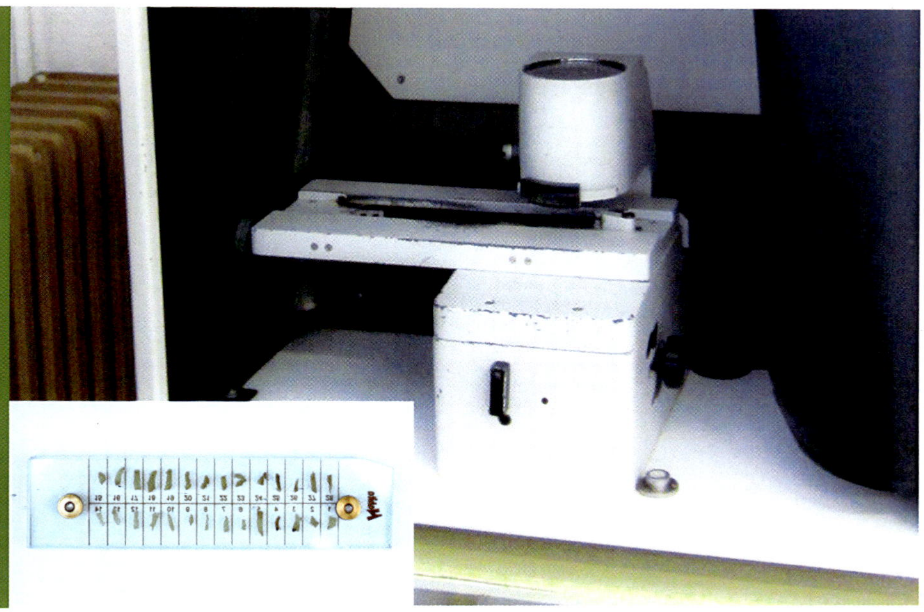

1 How is a *Sarcocystis* infection confirmed?

An *in vivo* diagnosis of sarcosporidiosis is difficult as the clinical manifestations are very non-specific and can also present in other diseases. Epidemiological data may serve as a guide and are normally useful if the results of coprological analysis for cats and dogs are available.

The *post mortem* diagnosis is based on the observation of macroscopic lesions, which have already been described in the corresponding section, together with a histological study of samples preferably obtained from the mesenteric lymph nodes and kidney.

Muscle infection is almost always diagnosed *post mortem* and is based on the macro- or microscopic observation of cysts, which can be seen at necropsy or upon inspection of the carcasses in the abattoir.

Thin, twisting, macroscopic cysts with a length of 1.5-4 mm and width of 0.3-0.7 mm are indicative of *Sarcocystis bovifelis*.

Their microscopic counterparts, which can be obtained from small portions of muscle placed between trichinoscope plates, can readily be observed under a stereo microscope. The cysts should not be pressed too hard as they may burst and release the bradyzoites, although they can also easily be seen moving in the fluids around the pressed tissue..

Histological sections or artificial digestion with trypsin, which has the advantage that whole cysts can be obtained for subsequent study and identification, can also be used. This is performed by dissolving the muscle tissue samples in artificial digestion solution (0.13 g of trypsin in PBS -phosphate-buffered saline-, pH 7.2), incubating at room temperature for 15-20 minutes then filtering the digestion fluid through a double gauze. Finally, a few drops of the resulting sediment are placed between a microscope slide and cover-glass and observed under the microscope.

2 What measures should be taken to prevent carcasses from being impounded?

Preventive measures are of the utmost importance. Actions targeting the definitive hosts are able to reduce the infection levels in intermediate hosts in the medium term, thereby preventing carcasses and entrails, etc. from being impounded.

As the cycle for sarcosporidia requires a predator-prey relationship, efforts should be made to prevent the cycle reaching completion. The infection of definitive hosts is, on most occasions, due to human negligence, therefore the actions of those people who come into contact with, or are responsible for, these animals can either be a guarantee of success or can ensure that the cycle continues.

As is the case for other models with the same characteristics, population-based health education is of particular importance, especially in rural regions. It is impossible for the definitive hosts, in this case dogs, cats, etc., to become infected if they are prevented from eating entrails, organs or tissue from animals containing macro- or microscopic cysts. As such, it is theoretically very simple to prevent the sarcosporidia cycle from continuing.

As far as the intermediate hosts are concerned, both extensive and intensive cattle breeding and farming help to prevent the links in the epidemiological chain from being completed, especially the intensive one.

Similarly, the infection of intermediate hosts should be prevented. Dewormings, control of the dog and cat populations and basic hygiene measures to prevent the spread of oocysts in drinking water, feed, hay, etc., or in feed storage places are of great utility.

3 Can muscular cysts resist the cold?

As is the case for the cysts from other protozoa of the *Apicomplexa* type that develop in various organs, entrails, etc., sarcosporidia cysts are fairly resistant, although the standard treatments to which tissue and organs for human consumption are subjected are sufficient to ensure their destruction. Normal cooking destroys them and, if present in muscular tissue, the time required to ensure the safety of the meat depends on both the temperature used and the size of the pieces subjected to heat treatment.

The organs and other remnants destined for animal use, which are not normally treated and can therefore contain live forms that are able to continue the cycle, pose a different problem.

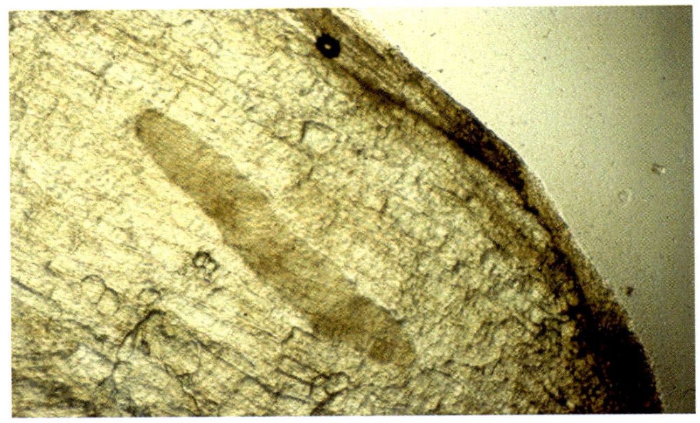

The detection of *Sarcocystis* cysts is basically *post mortem* during the macroscopic and microscopic observation of cysts, which are mainly seen during necropsy or inspection of the carcasses in the abattoir. Muscle cysts are mainly spindle shaped and microscopic, and are present in large numbers.

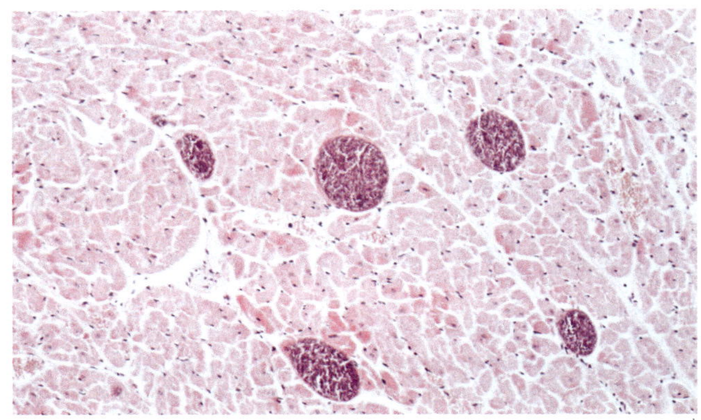

A degenerative myopathy and multifocal myositis occur in affected muscular tissue. Granulomas in spaces between degenerated fibres and large regions of eosinophilic infiltration are also common.

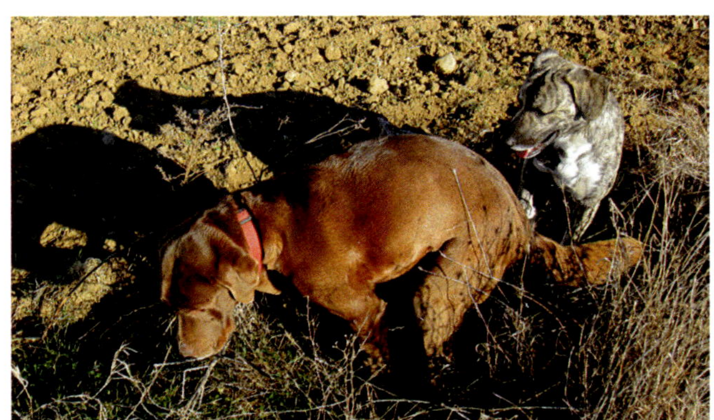

The dog, which is the definitive host, completes the biological cycle upon ingesting tissue from intermediate hosts with bradyzoite-containing cysts. The enteric phase finishes with the formation of isosporoid-type oocysts (containing two sporocysts). As sarcosporidiosis normally goes unnoticed during the veterinary inspection, meat cuts and food remnants, etc. may accidentally reach dogs or other definitive hosts.

34 In which organs can echinococcal cysts be found?

After a radiographic study of an adult cow with progressing lameness in its right leg when walking, a radiolucent image with sclerotic borders consistent with a primary bone tumour is found in the right iliac wing of the pelvis. The pelvis also showed a large osteolithic lesion with a disordered displacement of bone fragments compromising the right iliac bone, and the presence of a liquid-like tumoral lesion up to 6 cm in diameter. Biopsy of the tumoral lesions resulted in the emission of abundant whitish hydatidic membranes together with a transparent "rock water"-type fluid compatible with pelvic hydatidosis. The blood count showed an increase in eosinophil levels (5 %) and the serological study for hydatidosis was positive for IgG and negative for IgE. The diagnosis was completed with an abdominal ultrasound and chest X-ray, which showed numerous structures compatible with cystic lesions.

1. Which organs can host hydatid cysts in cattle?
2. How important are cattle in the transmission of the infection to humans?
3. What control measures should be taken on the farm of origin of the animal affected?

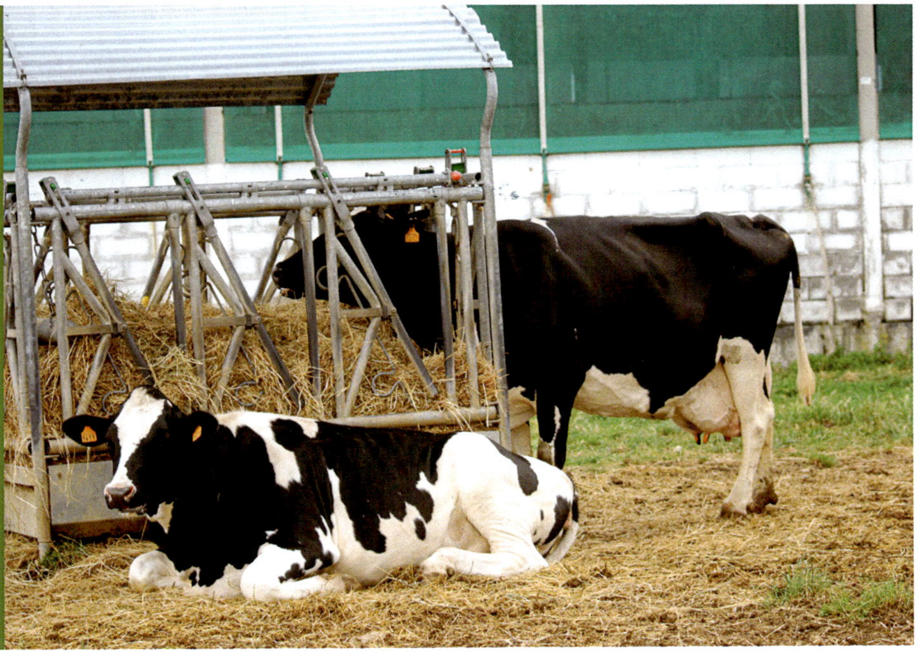

1 Which organs can host hydatid cysts in cattle?

After infection of the intermediate hosts, the embryophore cover dissolves, releasing the oncosphere into the stomach and intestine. Once it reaches a small blood or lymph vessel, it is passively transported to many different organs. Almost all organs and tissues can become infected and host hydatid cysts.

Some oncospheres die or are destroyed, whereas others begin to develop and transform into hydatid cysts. Most are retained in the liver, whereas other pass into the lungs and some can be found in many other organs and tissues such as kidneys, spleen, muscular tissue, brain, heart, bone tissue (mainly the spine, pelvis, femur, ribs and other long bones), etc. Shortly after reaching their final destination, the embryos measure 40 µm, and after 10-14 days they begin to reorganise to form an hydatid cyst.

Although cysts can develop in numerous organs, they tend to be found in the liver and lungs in animals.

Cysts act by compressing the organs in which they settle, therefore their effects vary depending on their location and size. A growing cyst initially causes atrophy, followed by necrosis due to compression of surrounding tissue, although as this growth is slow the cysts may be present for some time before it affects a vital structure.

The presence of echinococcal cysts at the most common sites in animals (liver and lung) either does not normally cause clinical manifestations or leads to non-specific signs that are difficult to diagnose. Disorders may be produced at other sites (brain, bones, heart) depending on their nature (seizures, bone fractures, embolism and blockages). The only notable effect is a decrease in production, mainly as regards meat production, and changes to the composition of milk.

2 How important are cattle in the transmission of the infection to humans?

Echinococcus ortleppi (previous *E.granulosus* G5) may be transmitted from cattle to humans. Recently, *Echinococcus* species have been validated using molecular techniques by way of a compromise solution that agrees better with the biology of this genus. The genetic differences between "isolates" and "strains" in this genus permit the equine and bovine "strains" to be added to *E. granulosus* and therefore to be considered as a species, namely *Echinococcus equinus* and *Echinococcus ortleppi*, respectively.

As is the case with other parasites whose biology is based on trophic predatory relationships, the Iberian peninsula is a "mini continent" that behaves as a species store. Their geographical characteristics and varying climate, as well as the abundance of wild animals, mean that any parasite which arrives finds it relatively easy to become established.

Hydatidosis caused by *Echinococcus granulosus sensu lato*, spread throughout the world due to the export of Merino sheep. It is possible that the genetic heritage of *E. granulosus s.l.*, which includes the bovine genotype (G5, currently *E. ortleppi*), which was probably present on the Iberian peninsula at some point, will also be exported in a similar manner. If that is the case, G5 leads to fertile cysts in cattle that would continue their biological cycle once the definitive hosts, namely dogs, intervene. The prior existence of G5 on the Iberian peninsula ensures its current presence, especially when considering the importance of cattle farming in some regions of Spain. In any case, *E. ortleppi* (formerly the G5 strain), which has been reported in some countries, is infective to humans.

However, the most important animal species in the epidemiological chain for hydatidosis in Spain is sheep, which, in combination with dogs, form the ideal pair through which *E. granulosus s.l.* circulates and is maintained. Humans represent a dead-end as it is very difficult for the definitive hosts to access the entrails (mainly the liver and lung) of humans infected with hydatidic cysts.

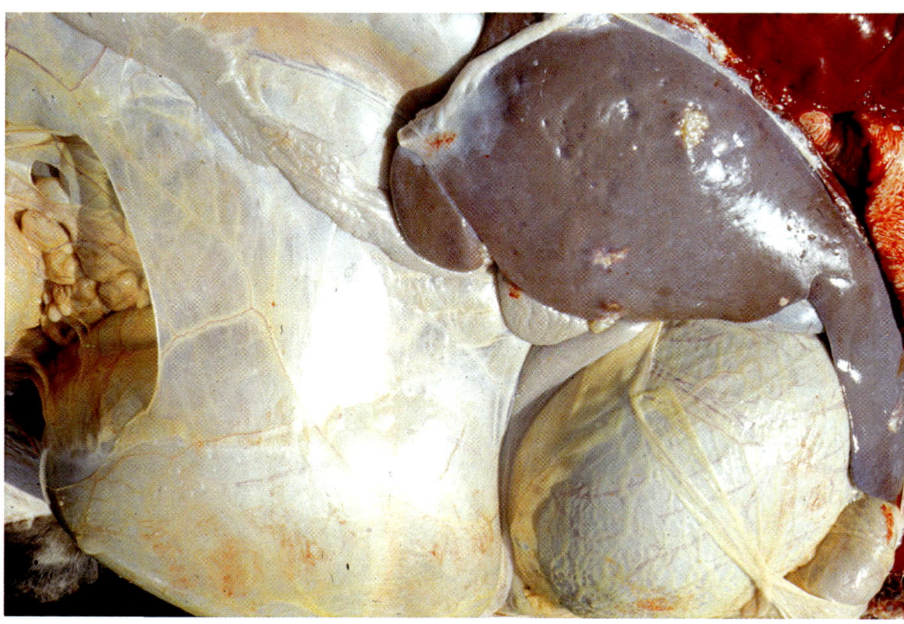

Once a cow ingests viable parasite eggs, the oncospheres penetrate the crypts of the jejunal and ileal villi, from where they reach a large number of organs, in which they commence vesicular evolution into echinococcal cysts, via the blood or lymphatic circulation. The embryos measure 40 µm within a few days and form a cavity inside the infected organ. Within 10-14 days post-infection they reorganise and form a central cavity, develop germinal and laminar layers and form the echinococcal cyst, which is typically unilocular and subspherical in shape.
Image courtesy of Dr. P. García Palencia.

3 What control measures should be taken on the farm of origin of the animal affected?

As almost all the biological and epidemiological characteristics of hydatidosis are known, numerous official guidelines and recommendations have been published, and should be followed, to ensure that this disease is controlled. Incorrect human behaviour therefore helps to maintain hydatidosis.

Firstly, an accurate and up-to-date canine census must be available and any stray dogs picked up from the streets. A parasitological study should subsequently be undertaken in these sacrified animals to determine the prevalence of infection.

As far as the definitive host dogs are concerned, the parasitic biomass should be reduced by administering effective anthelmintics (praziquantel or epsiprantel) every 6 weeks, destroying the faeces of dewormed animals and disinfecting using physical and chemical disinfectants (sodium hypochlorite, ethanol or benzalkonium).

The only chance for dogs to become infected is by eating raw entrails containing echinococcal cysts. As such, all measures should aim towards preventing this, thus meaning that the entrails produced in abattoirs and butchers shops should be inspected and those containing echinococcal cysts impounded and destroyed in septic tanks, landfill sites or salt baths (20-30 % or saturated sodium chloride solutions). The optimal solution would be to sterilise the entrails. Coking for 40 minutes or freezing at -18 °C for at least 48 hours destroys the cysts. Fermentation of infected entrails also ensures destruction of the protoscolices. Likewise, the measures required to prevent farmers from feeding dogs with raw entrails, and putting an end to the custom of abandoning dead animals or their entrails, should also be put into place.

All such measures share a common aspect, namely health education, which is one of the basic pillars for the control and prevention of hydatidosis.

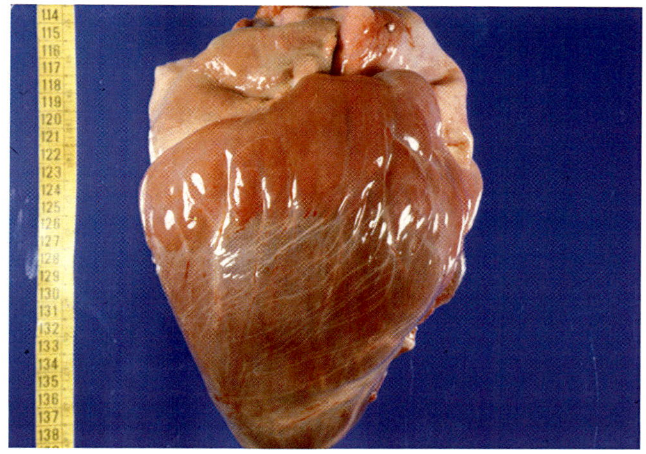

Although echinococcal cysts can theoretically develop in a wide range of organs, they prefer the liver, lung or both. Hydatid cysts located in the heart, kidney, spleen, thyroid, brain or bones are much less common. They can also be found in subcutaneous connective tissue, the peritoneal or thoracic cavities or muscular tissue, in which case they are secondary cysts.

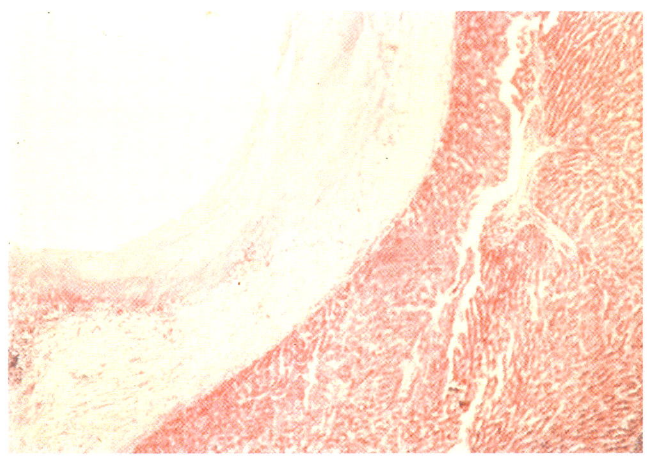

The cyst has three layers: the external or adventitious, which comprises modified host cells and inflammatory cells and represents the dense fibrous response of the host; the middle or laminar layer, which is acellular and is formed by a mucoid polysaccharide secreted by the parasite; and the internal or germinal layer, which is the membrane where the scolex and daughter capsules or proliget vesicles that remain attached to the germinal membrane via a pedicule develop.

35 Which species of cysticerci are parasitic in bovids?

After arrival of a zebu stud of great economic value from Ethiopia, the animal was diagnosed with a cardiac arrhythmia with discrete dyspnoea that increased with exercise. The echocardiogram showed the presence of multiple intramyocardial cysts in the interventricular septum, with mild obstruction of the left ventricle outflow tract. Between six and seven non-septated cysts of different sizes and with a non-echogenic content were counted; some of the cysts had an amorphous echogenic morphology.

1. How long do cysticerci survive?
2. How can a *Taenia saginata* infection occur in a country with an adequate sanitation network?
3. How can degenerated cysticerci be identified in muscle?

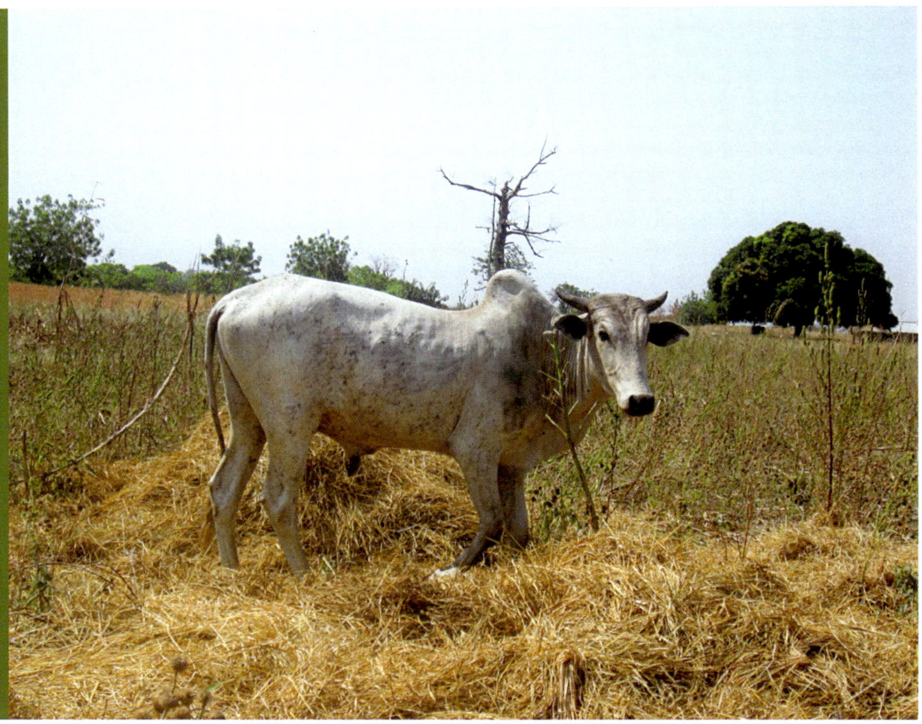

1 How long do cysticerci survive?

Cysticerci (*Cysticercus bovis*) are found in some muscle groups, mainly in the best vascularised muscle fascicles, where they develop better. Although preferably located in the tongue, masseter muscle and myocardium, they can also be found in the neck, intercostal muscles, diaphragm and other muscle groups. Similarly, they can be found in the oesophagus, liver and, less frequently, lung and kidney. Their survival depends on the animal's age at infection, but can range between one and three years.

Cysticerci withstand temperatures as low as -6 °C relatively well, surviving for about 150 hours, whereas at -19 °C and high relative humidity (86-90 %) they can survive for three or four days. At lower temperatures (-30 °C) they are destroyed within 30 minutes. In the liver, lung and heart they degrade after around 20 days, whereas they survive for 10-15 days in carcasses stored at 10 °C. Moreover, although putrefaction has no effect, they are particularly sensitive to heat, cold, radiation and chemicals.

Ingestion of these cysticerci by humans results in release of the scolex, its attachment to the intestinal mucosa and the formation of 10-16 segments/day. After 2-3 months, the strobilus contains around 900 proglottids, the last 100-150 of which contain eggs. The prepatency period is 4 months.

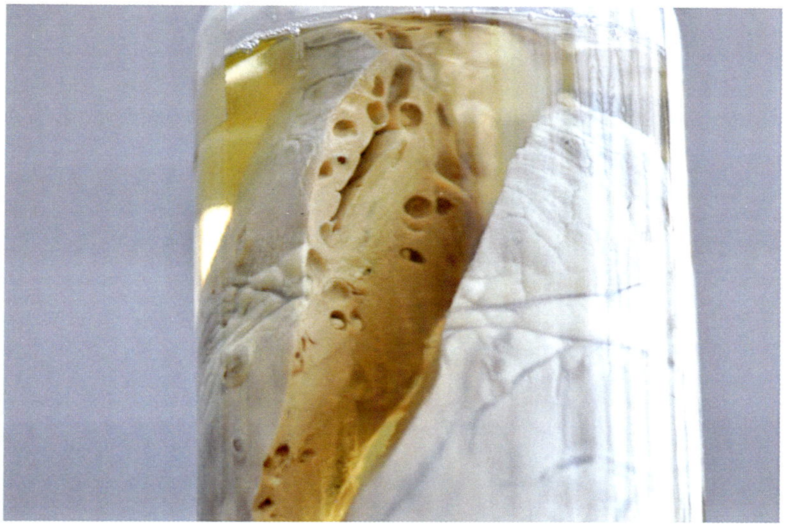

One of the human tapeworms, namely *Taenia saginata*, completes its biological cycle in bovines, in which cystic larvae known as cysticerci form. Specifically, the larval phase of *T. saginata* was named *Cysticercus bovis*, which is a small vesicle some 6-8 mm in length and 3-5 mm wide. The wall is thin and translucent and contains an amber-coloured liquid that allows a white punctiform formation (scolex) to be seen. Although they normally develop in striated muscle, they can also be found in cardiac muscle tissue.

2 ¿How can a *Taenia saginata* infection occur in a country with an adequate sanitation network?

Transmission to humans depends on several factors, including the tendency to eat insufficiently cooked meat and contamination of the environment (pastures, etc.) with faeces from people infected with *T. saginata*. The manner in which bovine cysticercosis was discovered in the mid-19th century after being completely unknown in ancient times deserves a mention. At that time, some European countries recommended the consumption of raw meat to combat childhood diarrhoea and to strengthen the weak. The frequent presence of tapeworms in these people became evident, and soon afterwards this was related to the "treatment" with raw meat.

Other factors, such as poor hygiene, also promote contagion. This is particularly common in underdeveloped countries, where animals live close to human dwellings and pastures become public places.

"Outbreaks" of cysticercosis have been reported in developed countries, such as Spain, as a result of epidemiological factors that favour establishment of the epidemiological chain for so-called "human taeniosis/bovine cysticercosis". Specifically, in some regions a bovine infection has occurred as a result of close contact between the animals and their caretakers, with the peculiarity that some caretakers were immigrants from countries in which *T. saginata* infection is quite prevalent. The poor sanitary conditions on these farms and the custom of using the cowsheds as "latrines" facilitated the cycle, thereby resulting in the infection of animals by infected humans. Furthermore, the acquisition of some of these animals by their caretakers and their subsequent slaughter according to certain religious rites, followed by consumption of the meat from these cattle, helped to complete the epidemiological circle, an event that would otherwise be practically impossible.

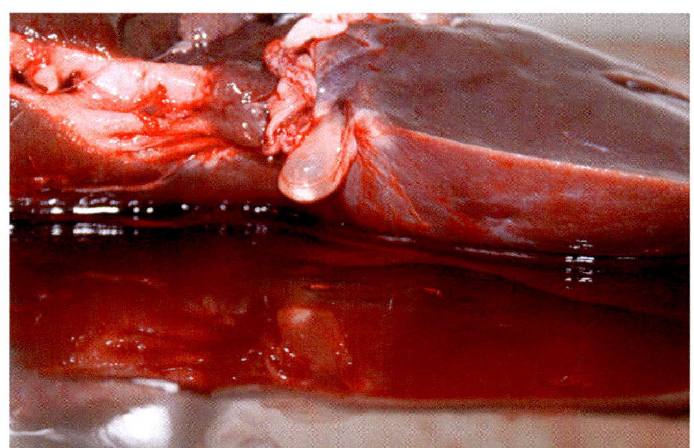

Cysticercus bovis can develop not only in some muscle groups parenchyma and the serous layers. It is found much less frequently in other organs such as the lung and kidney, where it can survive for several months, although survival appears to be related to the age of the host at infection.

3 How can degenerated cysticerci be identified in muscle?

Firstly, it should be noted that the number of cysticerci in cattle is generally very low, which is why cysticercosis passes essentially unnoticed during surface examination of the meat. As a result, a more careful examination, as well as incisions to detect cysticerci in muscle, is required. Cysticercosis is also observed in veal calves, with the heart being one of the most common infection sites.

The diagnosis of cysticercosis is usually relatively simple, with doubts only arising in those cases in which the "vesicles" have become completely infiltrated. Dead cysticerci undergo alterations comprising fibrous and caseous degradation and, finally, calcification. Cysticerci vary between 8 and 9 mm in length and 6 mm in width, and they present a small white mark the size of a grain of millet in the centre of the vesicle corresponding to the scolex. When observed under a microscope, the "unarmed" cysticercus has four suckers and a neck with numerous calcareous corpuscles. Once the degradation process is complete, remnants of these formations can be seen, although these are not always readily identifiable.

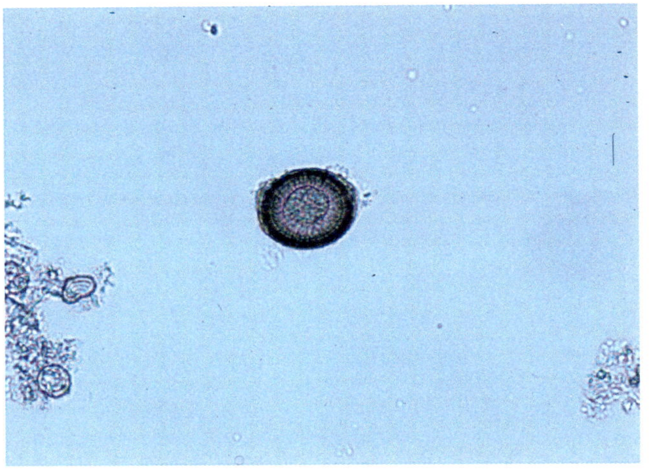

A large number of mature eggs, which are normally eliminated enclosed in each of the final proglottids, are found in the last proglottid of the cestode. They can also reach the exterior in the faeces of infected. Taenid eggs are very difficult to identify morphologically, and even experts have great difficulty in identifying them. Their most notable characteristics are the thick external cover that encloses the embryo, known as the oncosphere, which is globular and possesses six hooks (hexacanth embryo).

36 Can bovines have coenuri?

A two-year-old fighting bull was slaughtered due to continual undiagnosed neurological attacks. For over a year, the animals had presented muscle weakness, which was initially thought to be nutrition-related, but a change in diet did not result in any improvement. The breeder assumed that this was due to the animal's habit of hitting itself against other animals, which had already resulted in a fractured skull that caused a state of stupor from which the animal never fully recovered. Two coenuri, which were identified morphologically and characterised molecularly as being the larval phase of *Taenia multiceps (Multiceps multiceps)*, were removed from the animal's brain in the abattoir.

1. How did the bull become infected?
2. When was this process identified in bovines?
3. Is it very common?

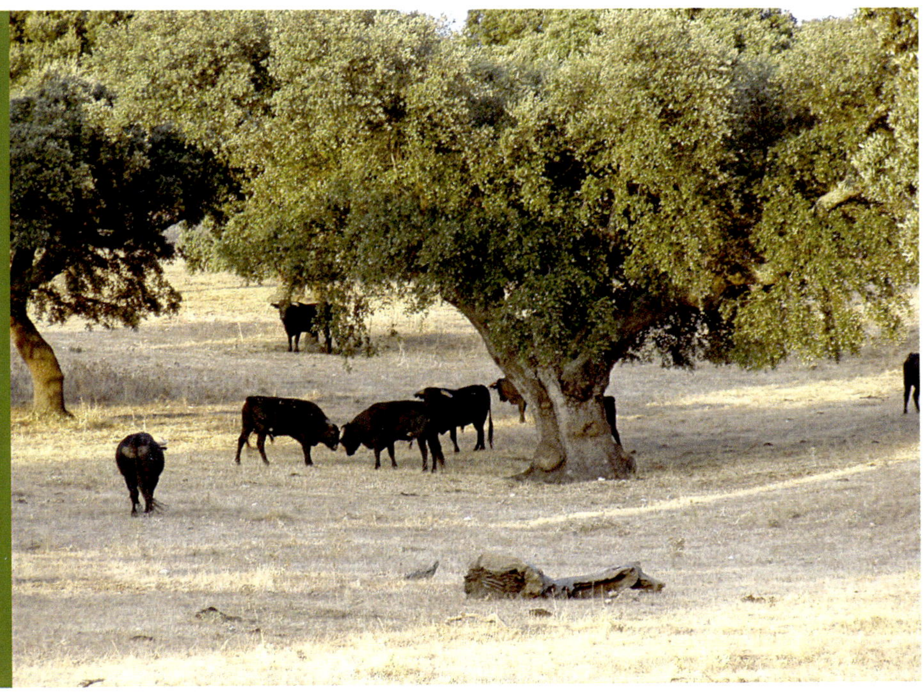

1 How did the bull become infected?

Coenurosis is a CNS disease of ruminants caused by the presence of the larval, cystic or vesicle stage (known as *Coenurus cerebralis*), of the cestode *Multiceps multiceps* in the brain or, less frequently, in the spinal cord.

Young sheep tend to be most commonly affected, although sporadic cases may appear in cattle.

The adult tapeworm *Multiceps multiceps* measures more than half a metre in length (40-70 cm) and lives in the intestine of dogs and other canids. Infected dogs excrete eggs in their faeces that are highly resistant to environmental conditions, especially in the event of sufficient humidity and if protected from sunlight. Contamination of the environment with eggs poses a risk to animals as they may ingest these eggs with contaminated grass, food or water and become infected. The embryos are released from the eggs in the intestine and transported to the CNS in the blood stream. Only those that get there continue to grow and transform into coenuri, although intrauterine infections are also possible. Development of the coenurus, which varies in size (up to a pigeon egg or a chicken egg), is complete within 7-8 months.

2 When was this process identified in bovines?

The agent responsible has been known since approximately 500 BC, when Hippocrates appears to have been the first to describe the coenurus as "thorns" in the brains of epileptic animals, especially sheep. Descriptions of the cysts from the 18th and 19th centuries are also available. Thus, in 1780 Leske recognised the coenurus as being the larval form of a tapeworm (*Taenia multiceps*), and in 1853 Kuchenmeister isolated cestodes from dogs fed with cysts taken from sheep (*Taenia hydatigena* from *Cysticercus tenuicollis* and *T. multiceps* from *Coenurus cerebralis*).

As bovine coenurosis is not a common process, identification of the disease may prove more complicated. Although more common in elderly cattle than elderly sheep, it is more frequent in young animals (1-2 years) than in adults.

The clinical manifestations coincide with a neurological presentation that onsets with relatively non-specific signs, such as difficulty in grabbing food, suddenly stopping eating, exhibiting drowsiness and slow movements and with the head typically raised and directed to one side due to continual convulsive contractions.

The forehead and base of the horns may also be hot, the pupils dilated and the pulse and respiration accelerated. Motor disorders are also observed. The animals walk forwards and stay close to the wall, and it is often difficult to make them move backwards. They may also follow circular movements or follow the same path. They occasionally fall violently to the ground in the stable, which may cause trauma, and suffer spasms.

3 Is it very common?

Bovine coenurosis is actually relatively rare. Despite this, "outbreaks" may occasionally appear in young animals, mainly on feedlots, with several individuals being affected. Such outbreaks are more common in wet years as the eggs remain viable for longer.

The rarity of coenurosis and the non-specific nature of its clinical signs may mean that this parasitosis is not diagnosed correctly as it may be confused with encephalitis, cerebrospinal meningitis, epilepsy, vertigo, cerebral neoplasms and other processes. Once coenurosis has been confirmed in a herd, the diagnosis in subsequent cases in much simpler.

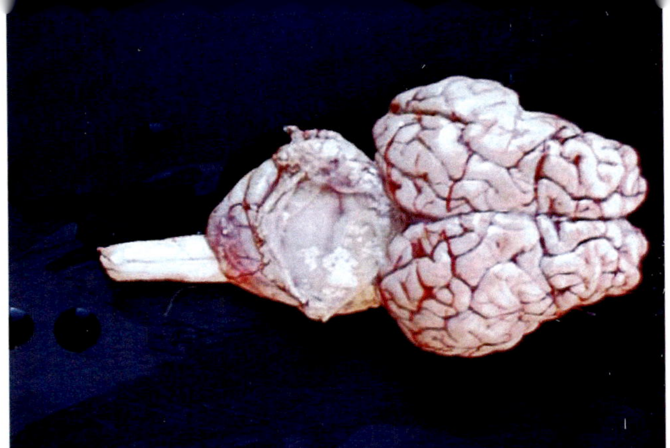

Although coenurosis is relatively common in small ruminants worldwide, mainly sheep, it has only occasionally been seen in the bovine nervous system, usually in young animals. The location of coenuri in bovines can vary, although they tend to be found in the cerebellum. They also develop in one of the hemispheres.

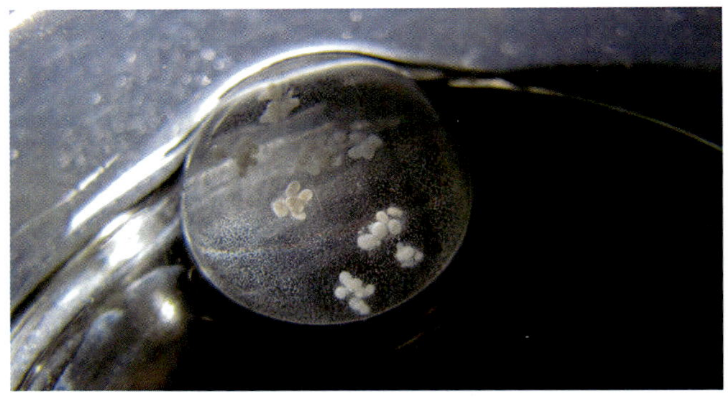

Coenuri are the larval stage of the canine tapeworm known as *Multiceps multiceps* or *Taenia multiceps.* This larval cyst is filled with an almost transparent fluid, and small formations (scolices) arranged in a branch-like manner can be seen in the cyst walls. Full development of the coenuri occurs at around 7 or 8 months post-infection. Their size varies from a few centimetres to that of a pigeon or chicken egg. When a definitive host (normally a dog) ingests these formations, each scolex will lead to an adult cestode.

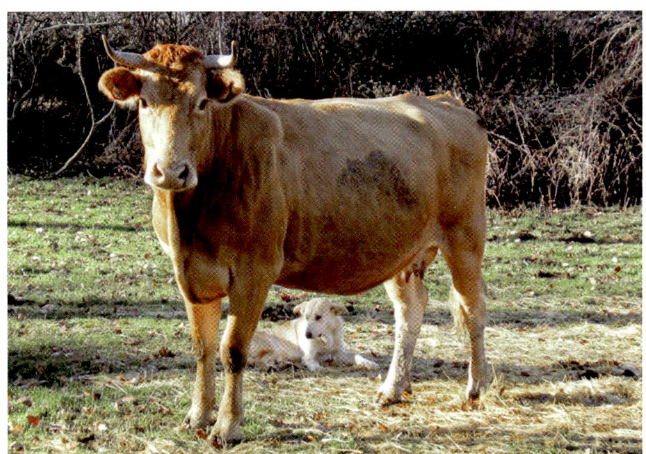

As dogs are traditionally associated with sheep herding, these two animals form a very important couple from a parasitosis viewpoint. Moreover, the presence of humans complicates the situation, especially as regards some parasitoses shared by these species. However, this pathogen "exchange""""""""""" relationship is also found in bovines, with some of them also being found in sheep, although the prevalence tends to be lower and human contagion much less common.

37 Are trypanosomes found in Europe?

During a blood test, a structure similar to that of a trypomastigote is seen and identified as *Trypanosoma theileri* on the basis of its characteristic morphology (undulating membrane and single flagelum) and large size. This unusual finding and the possibility of obtaining more blood from the animal allows a large number of parasites to be collected in a hematocrit microtube between the cell zones and the plasma. Directly under a microscope they are seen to be active and with undulating movements in this zone, and fracture of the microtube allows them to be deposited on a microscope slide. The animal presented with diarrhoea.

1. What clinical signs are related to this trypanosome species?
2. How are stercorarian trypanosomes transmitted?
3. What is the specific distribution of pathogenic species?
4. What clinical signs are closely related to these diseases?

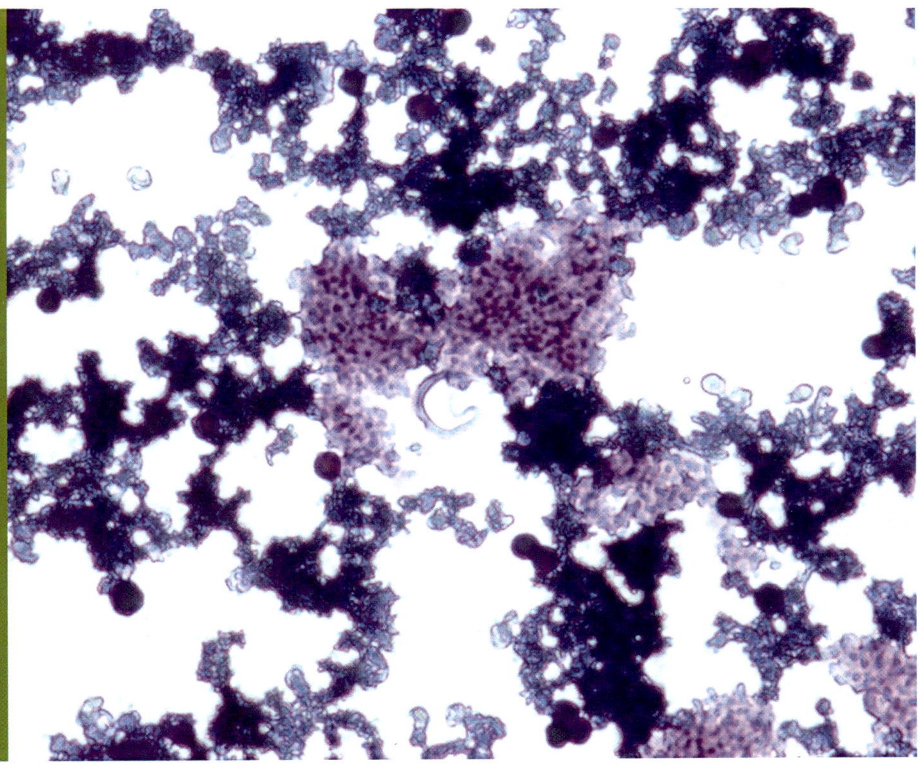

1 What clinical signs are related to this trypanosome species?

Trypanosoma theileri is a relatively large protozoan (60-70 µm or more). It is transmitted cyclically in posterior station development by tabanids. Both trypomastigote and epimastigote forms are found in cattle, and it mainly multiplies in the lymph nodes and internal organs.

Under normal conditions, *T. theileri* is a non-pathogenic trypanosome that is probably distributed worldwide, although there are no reports of its presence in some countries, including Spain.

A parasitaemic form may occasionally occur after splenectomy, in situations of stress or in the presence of concomitant infections with other pathogens. For example, it has been implicated as the cause of death in cattle after vaccination against cattle plague (rinderpest). Acute infections that produce symptoms similar to anthrax have been reported in some animals.

Although infection of both young animals (aged 7 months) and adults up to 15 years of age has been reported in animals naturally infected with *T. theileri*, this disease is rare in calves. Another peculiarity of this parasitosis is that not all infected animals test positive for trypanosomes in culture, and there is a wide variability between animals.

There is, however, a correlation between animals with trypanosomes and the presence of lymphocytosis. In any case, although not all findings agree, no clinical problems that can be ascribed to infection have been observed.

2 How are stercorarian trypanosomes transmitted?

Trypanosoma theileri belongs to the stercorarial group of trypanosomes. It has a heteroxenous cycle and normally requires an invertebrate to ensure transmission between hosts. In the case of *T. theileri*, and taking into account contagion of the parasitic form, transmission occurs by contamination: the infective form exits the invertebrate in faeces and penetrates the vertebrate via pre-existing breaks in the skin or those produced as a result of the intense pruritus caused by the bite.

Transmission of *T. theileri* occurs via tabanids. Some studies have shown that up to 14 % of tabanids in some regions contain trypanosomes. The vectors involved in some parts of Europe include *Haematopota pluvialis, Haematopota italica, Hybomitra micans* and *Tabanus bromius.*

Infected animals, asymptomatic carriers and natural reservoirs are important sources of infection for transmission between hosts. The last link in the epidemiological chain comprises ruminants, which can become infected by the parasite and develop the disease.

3 What is the specific distribution of pathogenic species?

In bovines, all trypanosomes use a vector to transmit themselves from one host to another. Irrespective of the type of transmission (cyclical or mechanical inoculation or by cyclical contamination), the species that act as vectors are arthropods, the distribution of which is restricted to specific regions (Africa, Asia, America).

No pathogenic trypanosome species are known in Europe. Indeed, as mentioned above, there have been no reports of trypanosomes in Spain, not even non-pathogenic species.

However, the possibility that favourable circumstances for the spread of some pathogens may appear means that the sporadic presentation of some trypanosomiases as a result of uncontrolled importation cannot be ruled out.

Species such as *Trypanosoma vivax*, *T. congolense* and *T. brucei*, which cause nagana, or Gambia fever, and *T. evansi*, which causes surra, "*mal de caderas*" and similar processes, are important at some latitudes. None of these species has been diagnosed in Spain.

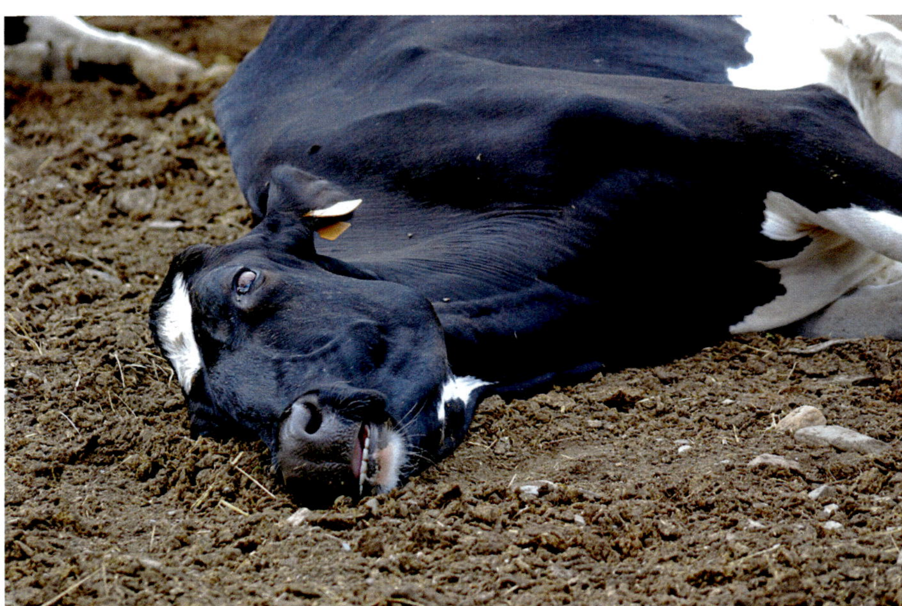

One of the trypanosome species commonly found in cattle herds is *Trypanosoma theileri*. This non pathogenic trypanosome can infect animals of all ages, as has been found for natural infections, without causing clinical alterations. Other trypanosome species present in bovines are responsible for similar processes to the so-called "sleeping sicknesses" in humans, which lead to symptoms of varying severity and are characterised by confusion, apathy and fever, with severe repercussions.

4 What clinical signs are closely related to these diseases?

From a clinical viewpoint, trypanosomiases have very variable prepatent periods that range from a few days to several months.

Similarly, the forms of presentation are also very widespread, ranging from acute or sub-acute to chronic processes.

The acute or sub-acute forms are more common in immunodeficient individuals or animals recently introduced into endemic regions that have had no prior contact with the parasite. In such cases the animals normally present a febrile syndrome with peak temperatures of up to 41 °C that repeats cyclically every 8-9 days. The lymph nodes close to the inoculation site are seen to be enlarged. If infection continues, a convulsive state that leads to flaccid or spastic paralysis presents.

Symptoms are more evident in the chronic form, with fever alternating with apyrexia or mild temperature increases, hypoglycaemia, hypogammaglobulinaemia (IgM), anaemia, haematuria, jaundice, oedema, hypokalaemia, various hepatic alterations (anisocytosis, etc.), progressive weight loss, including cachexia, and petechial haemorrhages in the mucosa.

Blood cells, haemoglobin, proteins, etc. can be found in the urine when there is renal involvement. As far as the nervous syndrome is concerned, locomotory ataxia, apathy, drowsiness, stupor, seizures, loss of vision, photophobia and general nervous attacks appear. Similarly, abortion, high perinatal mortality and very weak foetuses at birth may also present.

It may also present as a cryptic form essentially lacking parasitaemia and clinical signs due to an effective immune response. These asymptomatic carrier animals are very important from an epidemiological viewpoint.

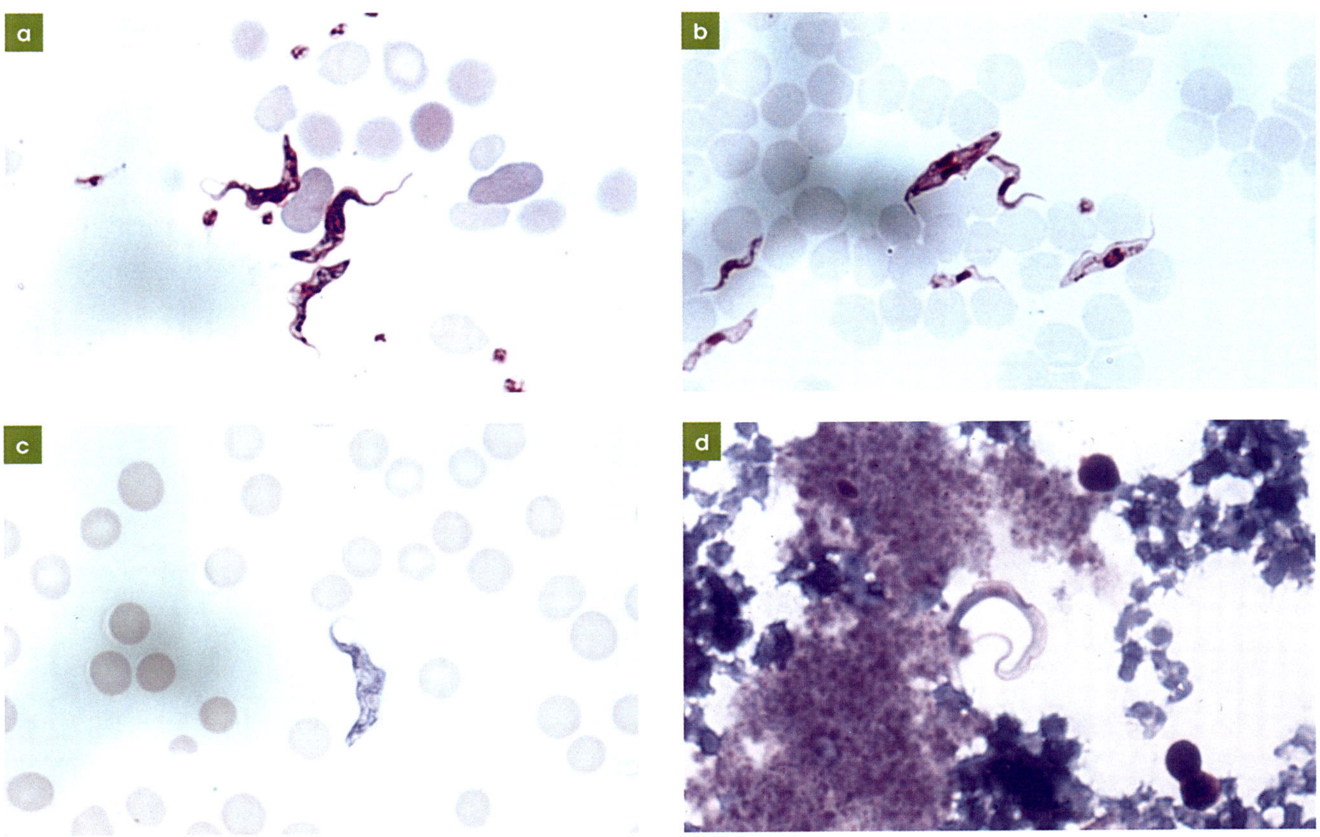

T. gambiense (a), *T. congolense* (b), *T. brucei* (c) and *T. theileri* (d). It is relatively common to find trypomastigote from the species *Trypasonoma theileri* in thin bovine blood smears. The smears are suitably fixed and stained with any of the Giemsa-derived or similar techniques. They are easily distinguished from other pathogenic trypanosomes under a microscope on the basis of their large size (up to 120 µm in length) and typical characteristics.

38 Can toxoplasmosis be transmitted to humans by eating beef?

During a gynaecological consultation, a pregnant woman requests information regarding the risk of toxoplasmosis infection as no antibodies have been detected in the blood test. She is aware of the risks of living with cats but, in light of her gastronomic preferences, she is keen to known whether she can continue to eat very undercooked meat or should avoid it completely.

1. How able are cows to transmit toxoplasmosis?
2. What is the biological cycle of *Toxoplasma gondii*?
3. What prophylactic measures should be recommended to pregnant women?

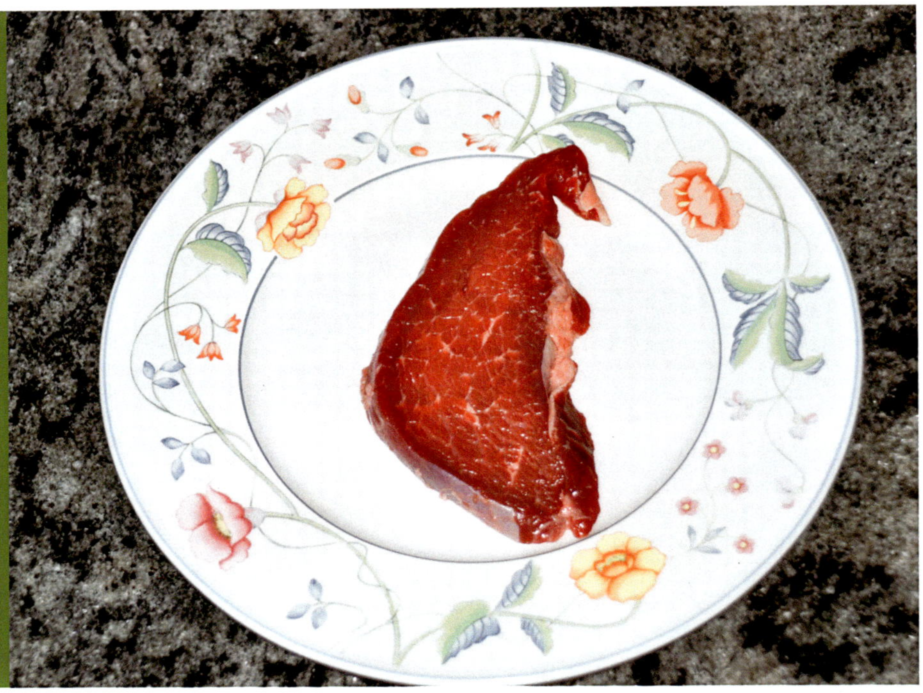

1 How able are cows to transmit toxoplasmosis?

Toxoplasma gondii is an infection that can be acquired via food of both plant and animal origin (meat and other organs).

The number of possible host species for this protozoan exceeds 300, including both mammals and birds.

In humans, the infection generally progresses asymptomatically, and in acquired forms infection is the norm and disease the exception. However, the real importance of toxoplasmosis in the public health field lies in the congenital forms, the severity and high frequency of which are particularly noteworthy.

Amongst definitive hosts, only representatives of the *Felidae* family, especially the cat, are considered here. Similarly, the most important intermediate hosts from an epidemiological viewpoint are herbivores and omnivores. In all these animals, oocyst ingestion represents the main or even only route of infection. In any case, domestic animals are an important infection source for humans.

Amongst ruminant livestock, toxoplasmosis is particularly important in sheep and is generally more serious in goats. Cattle appear to be less receptive and to play a less important role in its transmission, although this remains to be confirmed. Cattle are able to rapidly eliminate toxoplasma from tissue after the parasitaemia phase, or to greatly reduce their number. However, the parasite has been isolated from some tissues in experimentally infected calves after three years.

All indications suggest that the persistence of *T. gondii* in bovine tissue is probably of little relevance from a public health viewpoint.

2 What is the biological cycle of *Toxoplasma gondii*?

The biology of *Toxoplasma gondii* follows a host-prey model in which two types of host, namely intermediate and definitive, play a part. However, the epidemiological importance in this particular case lies in the fact that the definitive hosts are also intermediate hosts.

The most important definitive host is the cat. Not all intermediate host species play the same epidemiological role. Thus, from a practical point of view, three main groups can be defined on the basis of their receptivity (maximum, average and high), with the majority of domestic mammals falling into the second category.

Animals are mainly infected in two ways. One occurs upon ingestion of oocysts expelled in cat faeces and the other occurs as the result of ingesting cysts or pseudocysts that have developed in various tissues and organs.

In the first case the cycle is similar to that of classical coccidia. Asexual (schizogony) and then sexual multiplication (gametogony), which leads to the formation of oocysts that are subsequently expelled in faeces, occurs in the intestine of the cat.

In the second case, once sporozoites have been released in the intestine, they are distributed throughout the body via the blood, affecting cells from the mononuclear phagocyte system, brain and muscle in particular. They can pass into the embryo or foetus in pregnant females, thus leading to congenital toxoplasmosis.

In the environment, the oocysts sporulate and form two sporocysts inside which four sporozoites develop, leaving a residual body. These sporulated oocysts are infective.

Immediately upon penetration, the tachyzoites rapidly invade the host's cells and form pseudocysts, in which they begin to multiply so rapidly that the pseudocyst is filled with tachyzoites within only a few hours. The infected cell fractures and the invasion of new cells commences. The tachyzoites are distributed throughout the body, leading to a disseminated infection. Shortly after formation, the tachyzoites begin to develop tissue cysts of varying sizes (from a few to as many as 100 µm in diameter) containing several hundred thousand bradyzoites.

These cysts are mainly located in striated and cardiac muscle tissue, in the brain as well as in other parts of the nervous system, although they can invade any organ in the body. They tend to be found in the host cell with no direct exposure to the immune reaction, and can live for long periods of time like this. However, the latent infection reactivates if the walls of the cysts are broken.

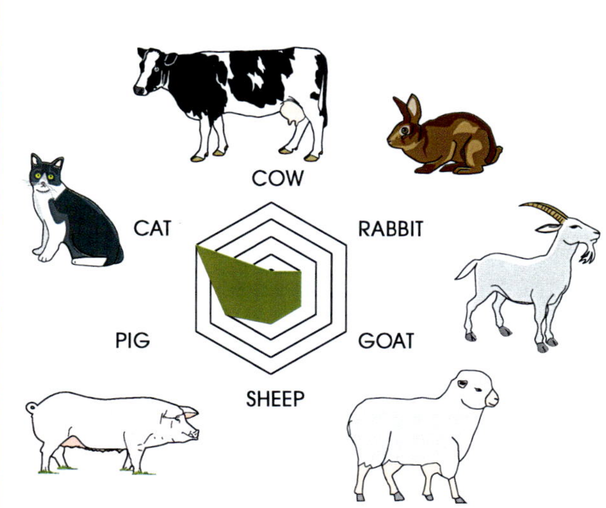

Cats play a key role in the dissemination of toxoplasmosis. The ingestion of tissue cysts from the meat of animals with a latent toxoplasmosis infection is also an important source of infection in humans. Pigs, goats, sheep and rabbits are important intermediate hosts in a domestic setting. In contrast, cows appear to be much more resistant and can rapidly eliminate the parasite. It is probably irrelevant from a public health viewpoint and mainly depends on gastronomic preferences.

3 What prophylactic measures should be recommended to pregnant women?

A large part of the success of toxoplasmosis infections is due to the ease with which they are transmitted from one host to another. The high prevalence of antibodies in humans and animals suggests that transmission by way of any of the three infective forms (oocysts, tachyzoites and tissue cysts) is relatively easy, although it also depends on parasite- and host-related factors.

The oocysts excreted in cat faeces contaminate the environment and can survive for more than a year under favourable conditions of humidity and temperature. Under favourable conditions, they can also survive for several months in water.

Cat faeces should therefore be considered to be a hazardous material and, as such, they should always be handled with great care as the risk of infection is high. For example, seroconversion has been observed in laboratory staff within 2-3 years of beginning to work with oocysts after having worked with tachyzoites and tissue cysts for 10 years without any problems.

Although tachyzoites survive for only short periods of time outside the host, they can survive for much longer in bodily fluids such as blood, milk, saliva, urine, tears and semen. Blood transfusions can cause infection if white blood cells are transfused. Unpasteurised or raw milk is also important in this respect.

Congenital transmission occurs when infection is produced during pregnancy, with toxoplasma passing into the foetus and causing a number of serious disorders, whose magnitude depends on the stage of pregnancy at which contagion occurs: the consequences are more severe in the case of early contagion.

The bradyzoites contained in tissue cysts can survive the action of digestive fluids for up to three hours. Moreover, although cooking destroys them, they can remain viable in large semi-raw or undercooked pieces of meat. The most common way of bradyzoite transmission is by ingestion of meat from other animals.

Some of the animal products that may be hazardous for humans, including muscle, various offals (liver, lungs), placenta, brain, etc., are the favourite implantation sites for toxoplasma, and they can remain viable at these sites for a long time.

As far as the prevention of human toxoplasmosis is concerned, a difference must be made between primary and secondary prevention, although any prevention proposed has a clear objective, namely preventing the congenital forms. The prevention of acquired toxoplasmosis is only considered in immunosuppressed patients.

Primary prevention of the congenital form aims to prevent pregnant seronegative women from acquiring toxoplasmosis during pregnancy and, if they become infected, establishes early diagnosis and treatment procedures to reduce the likelihood of transplacental transmission. Some countries perform serological controls of the female population of childbearing age, eliminating seropositive women from subsequent controls during pregnancy and the need to adopt specific measures due to the absence of risk of a new transmission in this population. Seronegative women are monitored during pregnancy to detect any possible seroconversion. If an acute phase (primary phase) diagnosis is reached in a pregnant woman, treatment to prevent foetal infection must be initiated.

The preventive measures that should be adopted in pregnant seronegative women are basically hygiene-related: washing hands after handling raw meat (or using gloves), washing fruit and vegetables, avoiding contact with cats or, if applicable, removing cat faeces and disinfecting bedding, administering cooked or canned food to cats and prolonged cooking of foods for human consumption.

The aim of **secondary prevention** is to diagnose congenital toxoplasmosis in a newborn (histological proof, isolation of the parasite from the placenta or a serological study) and treat it to prevent sequelae. Such a study should be performed in newborns whose mothers have been diagnosed with acute toxoplasmosis during pregnancy. If the child has not been monitored serologically during the pregnancy, this must be performed at birth.

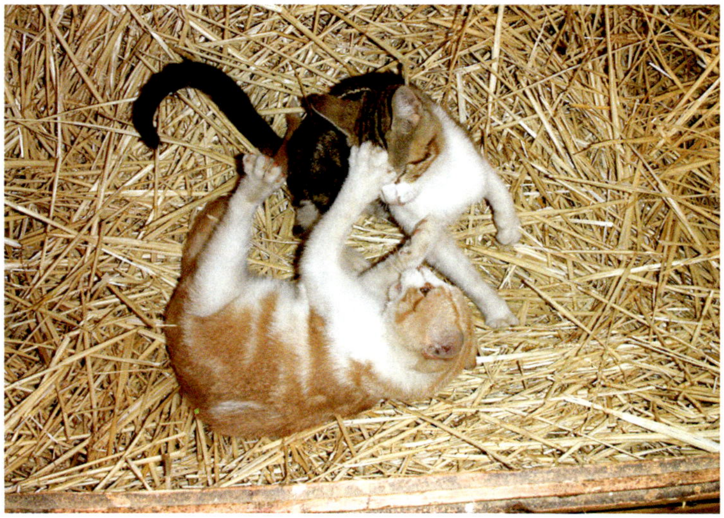

The presence of cats on farms is very common and they often defecate on stored straw or grain, going unnoticed due to their silent habits and tendency to hide their faeces. The contamination of feed with cat faeces is considered to be one of the main sources of infection for farm animals.

39 Which parasites cause abortion in cattle?

While preparing her new teaching activities, a young resident begins to prepare a series of lectures related to reproductive problems in cattle. She decided to concentrate on the diagnosis of abortions by undertaking a comparative study of the diagnostic methods available and the factors that affect the onset of parasitic diseases.

1. Which parasites can cause an abortion?
2. How does the abortion take place?
3. What other communicable diseases should be considered during the differential diagnosis?

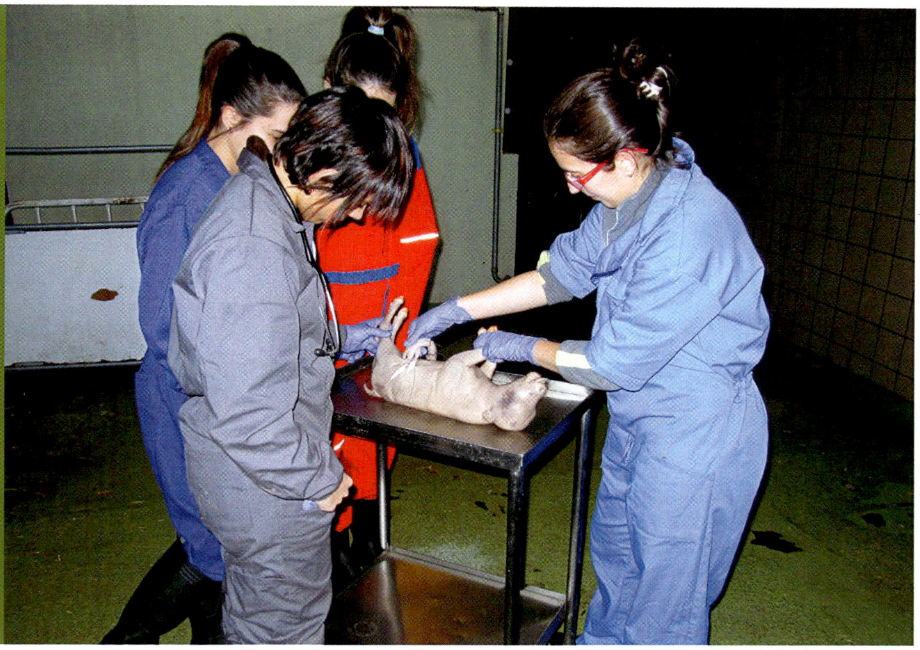

1 Which parasites can cause an abortion?

The fertility of a herd is one of the most important factors from a farming economics point of view. As such, disease processes that interfere with reproduction are of particular importance. From a parasitic infection viewpoint, reproductive diseases can be grouped into the following categories:

- Parasitoses specific to the genital region and foetus, including trichomonosis, toxoplasmosis and neosporosis.
- Non-specific parasitoses that can occasionally produce disorders similar to those in the previous group, such as sarcosporidiosis.
- Parasitoses of other systems and apparatuses that interfere with normal reproductive function, as is the case for helminths and some systemic parasites, such as piroplasmosis.

A brief mention should be made at this point of the nervous syndrome in trypanosomosis, which presents as locomotory ataxia, apathy, drowsiness, stupor, seizures, loss of vision, photophobia and general nervous attacks that can lead to abortion, high perinatal mortality and very weak foetuses at birth.

Any episode that causes stress, such as the stampedes that are sometimes seen to occur when cows attempt to flee from "fly attacks", is a potential risk that can lead to abortion in pregnant animals.

One of the parasitic diseases known to directly affect reproduction is **trichomonosis**, which had important effects on cattle breeding in the 1950s. Although the prevalence of this disease is currently nowhere near as high as previously, especially on intensive farms, it remains relatively common in regions of extensive beef farming and in herds that share stud bulls.

Problems almost always appear after the incorporation of new bull that carries trichomonas. The infection is mainly transmitted during mating, although mechanical transmission via insemination instrumentation, during vaginal palpation, etc.

is also possible, but less frequent. The parasite can survive in refrigerated and, on occasions, frozen semen.

It is not clear how the process develops. The cows are apparently covered, but shortly afterwards many of them come into heat again and exhibit vaginal secretions, with irregular but generally longer cycles.

Trichomonas is found in the reproductive apparatus. In bulls, it is found in high concentrations on the surface of penile secretions and mucosa in the preputial cavity without invading the epithelium. As the inflammatory response is limited, infection is difficult to detect macroscopically. Infected bulls are generally carriers throughout their life. In cows, the parasite can be found in the cervicovaginal mucous at around 1-2 weeks post-infection. The infection lasts around 90-95 days, although it can persist for one and a half and up to two years. In any case, it is self-limiting in most females.

Pregnancy is usually interrupted at around 18-20 days and 5 months post-mating. An initial mild inflammation of the uterine mucosa, with cellular infiltration, is followed by severe endometritis and foetal or embryonic death. This is followed by a uterine repair process. Pyometra occurs if the corpus luteum is retained.

Vaginitis, endometritis and a mucopurulent vaginal discharge occur. Although pregnancy is interrupted shortly after infection, this goes unnoticed and the majority of cows are classified as repeaters, infertile or not pregnant.

In extensive herds the periods between mating and calving, and between one calving and the next, become longer, thus meaning that the number of calves per season decreases. Abortions are more common in heifers that are pregnant for the first time. The process is usually more insidious in milk herds.

Bovine toxoplasmosis is much less important than in other species, such as sheep and goats. However, the parasite's cycle is identical and therefore comprises two phases: an asexual phase in a broad range of intermediate hosts, including cattle, and a second phase that only takes place in the intestine of the definitive host, in this case the cat.

The parasite initially multiplies rapidly in the intermediate host and then more slowly. In this initial phase, active multiplication in the host cells results in their fracture and the release of new tachyzoites, which move with the blood to invade new cells. This process continues until the host either dies or develops immunity, which leads to a chronic infection, forming cysts that remain in sheep and goats for their whole life. In contrast, the immune response in cows and other species leads to disappearance of the infection.

Bovine neosporosis mainly affects newborn calves and pregnant cows. In the former it is accompanied by symptoms such as ataxia and joint contractures in the limbs. In pregnant cows it is accompanied by foetal death together with retention or abortion, which occurs between the third and ninth month of pregnancy.

The presence of tachyzoites is more common in short-term abortions, whereas larger numbers of cysts are usually found in stillborn calves or in animals slaughtered within the first week of life. It has been found that *Neospora* can cause foetal death and retention or reabsorption and, under some circumstances, only the skeleton or mummified foetus is aborted or carried to term. Mummification is one of the clinical findings commonly observed in *Neospora*-related abortions.

The main manifestations in affected live-born calves are neuromuscular in nature. The first clinical signs are observed between 3 and 5 days after birth, although they can take up to two weeks to appear. Calves may be born underweight, weak and unable to stand due to limb stiffness.

An acute *Sarcocystis* infection during pregnancy can cause abortion, premature birth and stillbirths.

2 How does the abortion take place?

Bovine toxoplasmosis is accompanied by very vague symptoms, with pyrexia and central nervous system disorders, such as head and neck tremor, seizures and grinding of the teeth. Abortion or the birth of very weak calves that die shortly afterwards may occur if the cow is pregnant.

As discussed above, the biological cycle of *T. gondii* comprises two phases, an asexual phase with little host-specificity and a sexual phase that is confined to enteroepithelial cells on cats, which act as the definitive host.

The asexual cycle contains two stages, one in which rapid reproduction occurs (tachyzoite phase) and another in which reproduction is slower (bradyzoite phase). The tachyzoite, which is the first phase in the intermediate host, multiplies in the host cell by endodyogeny. This results in cell breaking and release of the new tachyzoites into the blood stream, from where they can parasite new cells. This process continues until the host dies or develops immunity, which occurs most often and coincides with the onset of a chronic infection. The extracellular stages disappear and intracellular

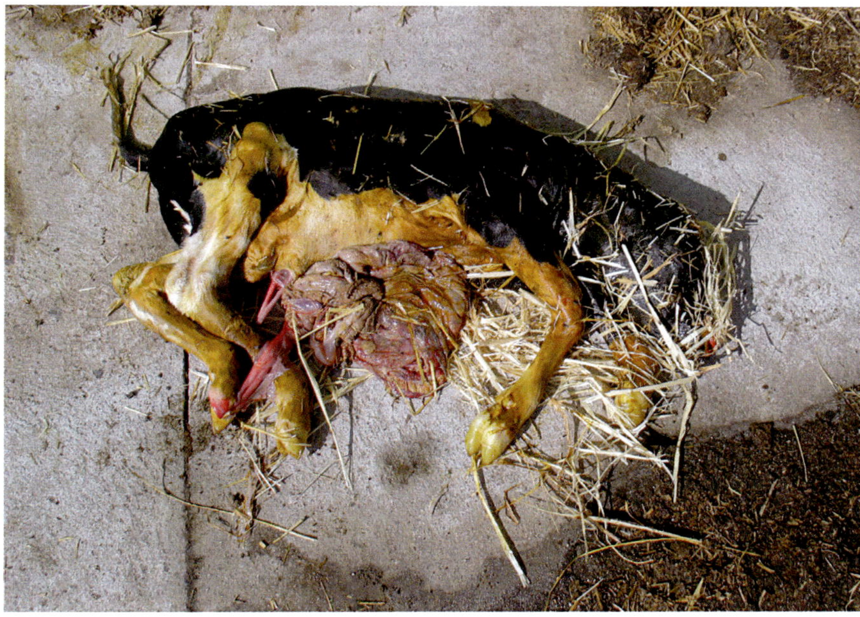

The best elements for sample submission are a whole foetus with placenta and paired serological samples. The placenta is important in some diseases, such as mycotic abortion and several bacterial diseases, where placentitis is the primary lesion. A complete necropsy examination of the foetus or placenta must be performed, searching for any visible lesions and estimating foetal age and degree of autolysis. Routine histopathological examinations of all organs, and bacteriological examinations of the lung, liver and abomasum, should also be performed. The contents of the abomasum can be examined by dark-field microscopy to detect *Campylobacter*. If lesions are present in the placenta, skin or other sites compatible with mycosis, a fungal culture should be performed. *Image courtesy of Dr. J. V. González.*

multiplication slows, leading to the formation of intracellular cysts and the second phase of the asexual cycle. These cysts are present in sheep and goats for their whole life, whereas in cattle and deer the host's immune response causes the infection to disappear.

The development of an effective immune response results in disappearance of the parasitaemia, which itself results in a change from fast to slow multiplication and bradyzoite production in the tissue cysts.

If cows are pregnant during the parasitaemia phase, the tachyzoites invade the caruncular septa, subsequently passing into the trophoblast cells and from there to the rest of the foetus. The onset of infection in the foetus depends on the phase of pregnancy.

In **trichomonosis**, inflammation of the endometrium leads to alteration of the intrauterine medium and embryo or foetal death. If the corpus luteum is maintained, which happens in some cases, and if there is foetal maceration, pyometra occurs and a chronic infection develops, which can cause permanent infertility if not treated.

Clinically, moderate vaginitis, cevicitis and endometritis lead to a mucous or mucopurulent vulvovaginal discharge, although no clear signs of infection are normally present. The embryo or foetus is almost always lost in the initial stages of pregnancy (6-16 weeks). Most abortions go unnoticed, and the cow comes into heat again 2-3 months after being covered and is considered to be a repeater, infertile or not pregnant. Pyometra is observed in less than 10 % of infected cows.

As far as **bovine neosporosis** is concerned, mother-to-foetus transmission and oocyst ingestion are the only demonstrated routes of transmission to date. In any case, *N. caninum* is one of the bovine pathogens for which transplacental transmission is most effective. This process may occur after infection resulting from the ingestion of oocysts after birth or by reactivation of a chronic infection.

Under natural conditions, the only means of transmission after birth is the ingestion of sporulated *N. caninum* oocysts that contaminate the environment.

3 What other communicable diseases should be considered during the differential diagnosis?

Diagnosis always involves bringing together the understanding of various factors that may lead to an initial suspicion regarding a specific problem.

All information referring to the recent history of a herd or herds in a specific region, starting with a consideration of what causes could have intervened in a clinical presentation that occurs during pregnancy, is of great value.

Clearly, the diagnosis of an abortion is relatively easy if it does not occur during the initial stages of pregnancy, although it is not always as easy to identify its cause(s). It is also easy to suspect problems in herds that come into heat again when they should be pregnant.

In the event of suspected reproductive disorders (abortions, infertility, etc.) of an infectious nature, it is always advisable to identify the agent responsible, although this is not always straightforward.

It is very important that samples are collected correctly. In this regard, it has been shown that a large proportion of abortions and reproductive failures are not diagnosed correctly because as the samples were collected incorrectly in terms of procedure (preputial massage, washes, aspirates, etc.), method used and storage conditions on site and during transport to a laboratory to confirm the diagnosis.

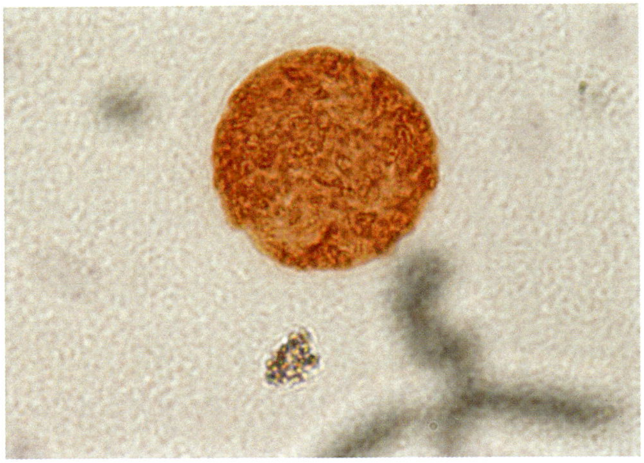

Neospora infection can be diagnosed by the presence of histological lesions and the positive staining of samples obtained from aborted foetuses using immunohistochemical techniques. The cysts are observed with bradyzoites as tachyzoites are difficult to identify in tissue from aborted foetuses. The most common lesions are multifocal, non-suppurative encephalitis, myocarditis, myositis and hepatitis. This is not a particularly sensitive technique due to the low number of parasites in affected tissue and the close relationship between false negatives, time spent and the number of sections performed. Moreover, the autolytic status of the foetus also affects diagnostic sensitivity.
Image courtesy of Dr. I. González.

The possibility that more than one pathogen is involved must always be taken into consideration and, if there is only one cause, the corresponding comparison should be performed to rule out possible aetiologies prior to requesting specific laboratory analyses.

The possible problems involved in reproductive disorders include nutrition-related infertility and strictly infectious processes. Possible bacterial infections include those caused by *Campylobacter* spp., brucellosis and listeriosis; viral infections include infectious bovine rhinotracheitis (IBR) and bovine viral diarrhoea (BVD); and mycosis and other parasitoses may also indirectly affect reproduction.

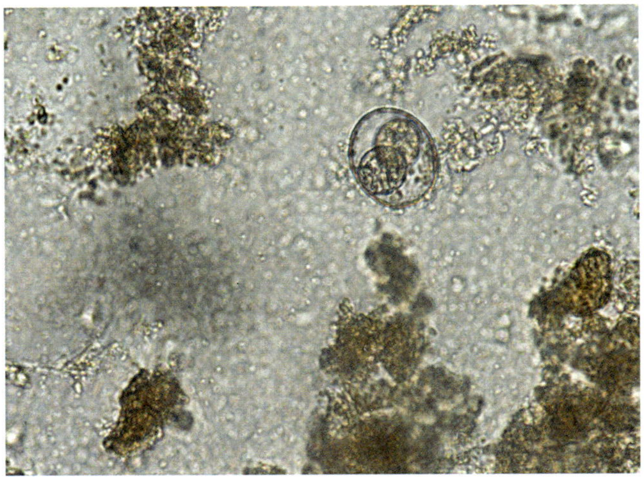

Unsporulated *Toxoplasma gondii* oocysts are excreted in feline faeces and remain infective for 1-5 days in the environment (soil). Sporulated oocysts are ovoid, measure 10-12 µm and contain two sporocysts, each of which has four sporozoites. Micronemes, rhoptries and dense granules are vitally important for adhesion, invasion, parasitophorous vacuole formation and nutrient acquisition in the infected cell. Parasite replication leads to cell lysis and dissemination of the tachyzoites to different tissues.

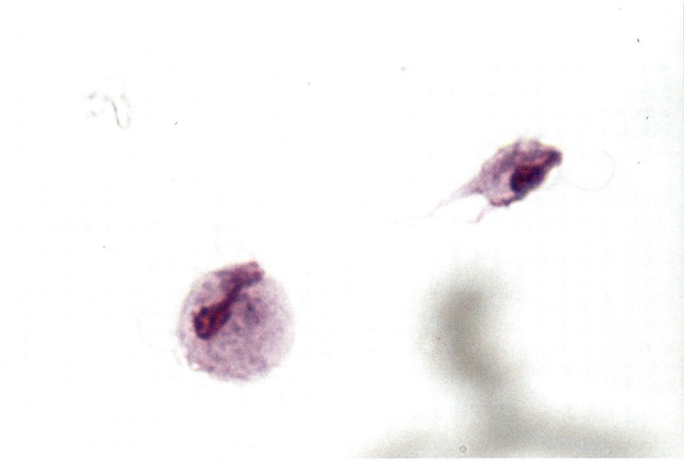

Tritrichomonas foetus infection causes embryo death, abortion and pyometra. The highest foetal loss occurs in the fifth month of pregnancy. Aborted foetuses are often autolytic and free from marked lesions. The placenta may be oedematous. Parasites are present in the placental or abomasal fluid. They are highly labile, therefore great care must be taken when collecting, storing and transporting samples.

Biological cycle of Apicomplexa, oral transmission (*Toxoplasma* and *Neospora*)

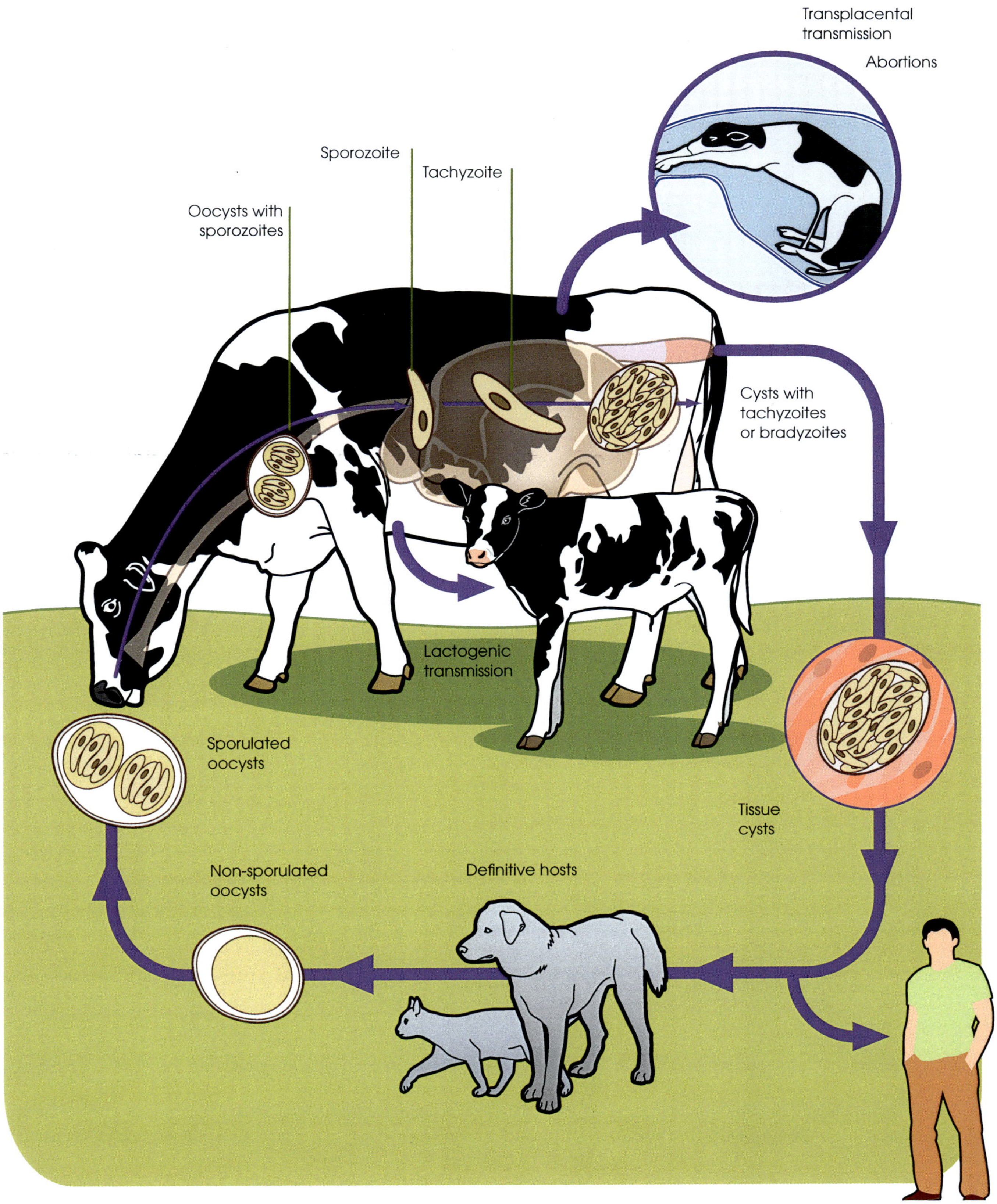

40 How is neosporosis diagnosed?

Over the past few years, five or six calves with neurological signs of unknown aetiology have appeared on a mixed dairy and beef farm from a total of around 150 calves per year. The two groups of animals are kept separate, only artificial insemination is used and, after ingesting colostrum from their own mothers, the calves from both groups are housed together and fed for four months prior to being separated for production. There is a history of abortion due to the vertical transmission of *Neospora caninum* in both groups of animals. In light of the possibility of congenital neosporosis, the vet sends three live animals to a university hospital for diagnosis. One of the animals is moribund, with marked neurological signs such as ataxia and ventromedial deviation of the eyes; another animal remains standing with help, with its forelegs bent since birth, although they can be straightened manually; finally, the third animal cannot remain upright as its hind legs are permanently extended and it has a spinal deformity that cannot be corrected manually.

1. What diagnostic methods are used in neosporosis?
2. How does the route of transmission affect abortion?
3. What losses does neosporosis cause?

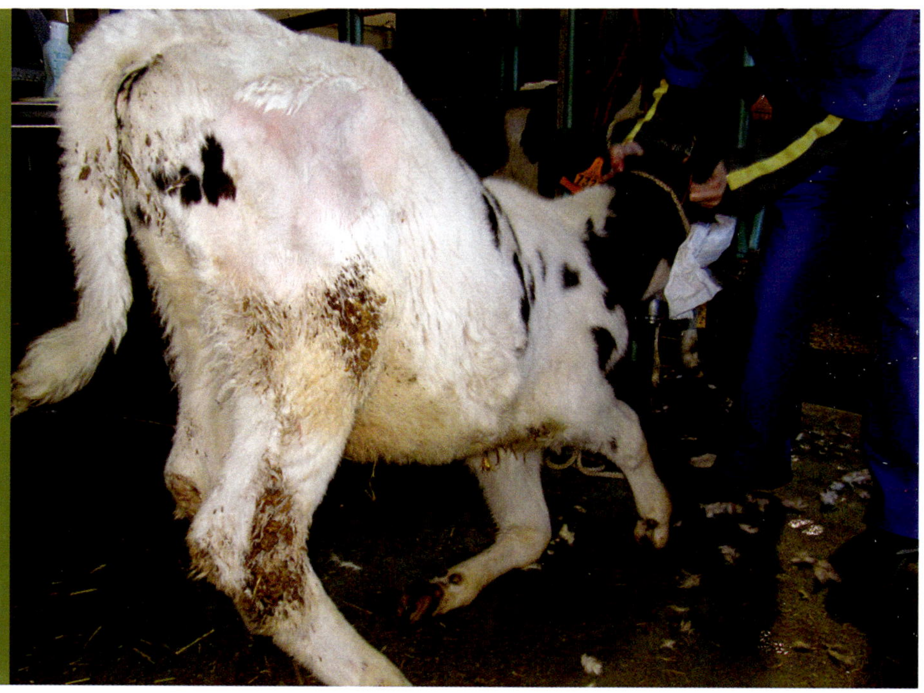

1 What diagnostic methods are used in neosporosis?

The diagnosis of congenital neosporosis in calves with neurological signs requires a comprehensive approach as currently available diagnostic methods are of limited value. Clinical cases of this type are very uncommon as the vast majority of congenitally infected calves are born normal.

It is not straightforward to establish a cause-effect relationship between abortions and *N. caninum* infection as asymptomatic congenital infections are common and determining the presence of the parasite or its DNA does not necessarily mean that *N. caninum* is responsible for the abortion.

A *post mortem* study and histological sections of the brain, heart and liver fixed in formalin and processed for routine histopathological and immunohistochemical tests are suitable diagnostic methods.

Indirect immunofluorescence can be used to detect serum antibodies. *N. caninum* tachyzoites obtained from cell cultures in an medium enriched with equine serum are used for this purpose. The serum is considered to be positive if the whole body of the tachyzoites body presents fluorescence.

Bulk tank milk serology can be used to estimate the prevalence of N. *caninum* infections in a herd. However, despite being relatively cheap, this method is not as suitable as detecting antibodies in serum.

From an epidemiological viewpoint, it is important to differentiate between acute and chronic infections, and various tests are available for this purpose.

Various techniques can be used to diagnose *N. caninum* infection. However, it should be remembered that antibody titres and white blood cell count can vary during pregnancy, even in animals that have not aborted, and some may be serologically negative. The type of antibody detected can vary with the clinical situation. Thus, IgG_2 tends to predominate in animals that abort, whereas either IgG_1 or IgG_2 can predominate in the remainder.

ELISA technique based on the protein NcGRA7 has been proven useful to differentiate cows that have aborted from those that have given birth normally.

Some studies have shown that the detection of certain substances in pregnant animals can help during the diagnosis of neosporosis. That is the case, for example, of the quantification of a pregnancy-related glycoprotein (PAG-1) which has been found to be of some utility. However, in some cases it appears to be more useful for determining the state of the foetus and placenta irrespective of *N. caninum* infection rather than being related to the chronic infection itself.

The use of various different yet complementary techniques is currently required to increase the possibility of detecting *N. caninum* infection in an aborted foetus. The diagnostic criteria should be based not only on demonstrating foetal infection and the severity of the lesions but also on the serological status of neosporosis in the herd.

2 How does the route of transmission affect abortion?

The key to the epidemiology of neosporosis lies in the oocysts excreted by the definitive hosts in their stools. Although the dog, Australian dingo and coyote are definitive hosts for *N. caninum*, viable oocysts have only been found in the dog under natural conditions (and also recently in the wolf). In any case, the number of oocysts eliminated in faeces is usually very low.

As is the case for other coccidia, the oocysts are highly resistant to environmental conditions. Furthermore, they are very similar to those of other species that infect dogs, such as *Hammondia heydorni*, therefore their identification is of great importance.

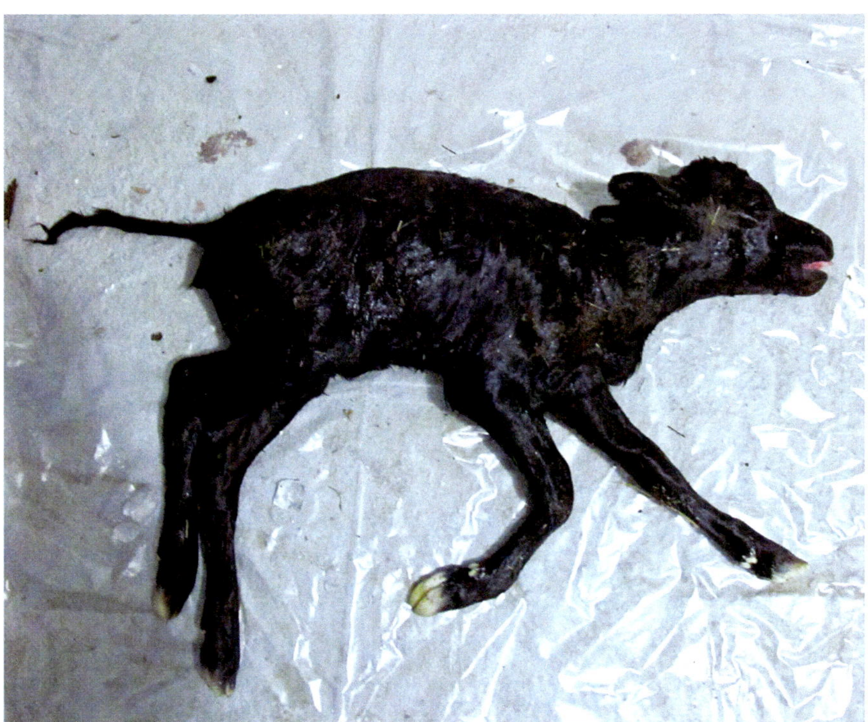

Abortion is the only symptom in cows infected with *N. caninum*. Cows of any age can abort sporadically or repeatedly from three months of pregnancy until term. In general, the diagnosis of bovine neosporosis is based on the detection of specific antibodies against the parasite in adult bovines and foetuses and the observation of compatible lesions in the brain, heart and liver of aborted foetuses, together with the immunohistochemical examination and molecular identification of *Neospora* in foetal tissue.
Image courtesy of Dr. J. V. González.

Although it is still not known exactly how dogs become infected, vertical transmission has traditionally been considered to be the most common route. However, in contrast to the situation found in cattle, this is unlikely to occur in the absence of horizontal transmission. It can also be transmitted from mother to foetus towards the end of pregnancy or to newborns via milk.

Faecal transmission does not appear to be important. Although seroconversion occurs in some animals post-infection, in many others this does not occur and neither is it possible to find parasitic forms or DNA in histological sections from seropositive animals. This suggests that faecal transmission may not be the most relevant route in the epidemiology of neosporosis.

Although most dogs are infected shortly after birth, prevalence is higher in older animals than in younger. The most common means of contagion is probably the ingestion of infected tissue, which theoretically is the most typical source of infection. This form of infection, which is related to the predator-prey coupling could explain why the seroprevalence in dogs from rural regions is higher than in urban areas.

Transmission can also occur when dogs have access to the corpses of infected cattle or wild animals. In all the above cases, the source of infection are various types of nerve tissue as well as other organs and tissues from infected cattle (masseter muscle, heart, liver).

As far as bovines are concerned, mother-to-foetus transmission and oocyst ingestion are the only demonstrated routes of transmission to date. In any case, *N. caninum* is one of the bovine pathogens for which transplacental transmission is most effective.

The vertical transmission rate varies from herd to herd, with values ranging from 37 % to 62 %. One of the means of measuring congenital infection is testing precolostral serum. In the absence of an active infection, the antibodies acquired via the colostrum decrease with time depending on their titre in the colostrum. Although it also depends on the technique used, it has been shown that the antibodies passively acquired via the colostrum can persist for up to five weeks.

Likewise, the seroprevalence values increase with age, ranging from 10 % in animals aged 1-2 years to 25 % in animals aged 3 years or more, irrespective of the competence of the herd.

Transmission can also occur via other routes, such as milk and semen.

3 What losses does neosporosis cause?

N. caninum infection causes severe disorders in cattle, dogs and other animal species. Infection tends to be common, but clinical manifestations are much rarer. However, this also depends on the *N. caninum* strain concerned. Moreover, the isolates obtained from various hosts are similar, although molecular studies have shown that many strains have unique characteristics. Indeed, as confirmed in serveral European countries, these characteristics are epidemiologically important.

Despite this, the relationship between strain variability and virulence remains unknown. It has been shown experimentally that the *in vitro* behaviour of some strains differs and that some are more virulent in mice than other, although it is still not known whether these differences are also repeated in other host species.

Cows have also been infected experimentally with strains from different sources. Some of these studies have shown that some isolates do not produce lesions in the foetus even though the cows were infected at the onset of pregnancy; however, infection of beef cattle at three and a half months of pregnancy can result in foetal death.

The most important repercussions of neosporosis are straightforward and due to reproductive failure. Another consecuences are: the costs of veterinary care and diagnosis;

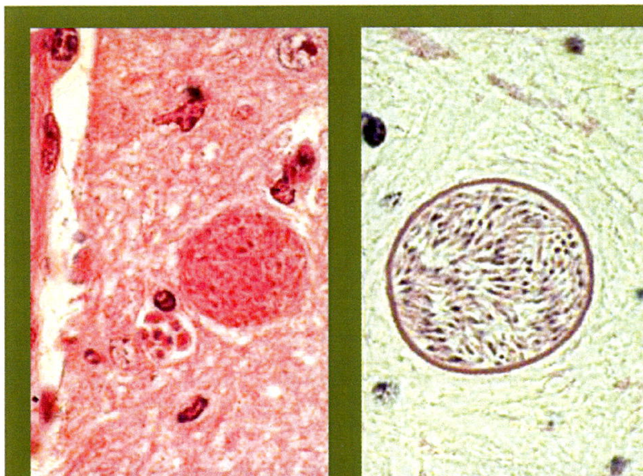

The most significant lesions are found in the brain and comprise a non-suppurative encephalomyelitis characterised by multifocal infiltrations in which the parasite must always be differentiated molecularly or antigenically from other protozoa, such as various species from the genus *Sarcocystis*, or even *Toxoplasma*, which can cause similar lesions.
Image courtesy of Dr. Dubey.

decreased milk production; and costs arising from replacement of those cows that aborted and were removed from the herd.

Neosporosis is difficult and expensive to diagnose. It is not easy to quantify postnatal neosporosis-related losses because, apart from foetal deaths, there are no other pathological effects. However, the removal of animals from dairy herds constitutes a major source of financial losses due to the difficulty in monitoring foetal expulsion in the first trimester of pregnancy.

Palliative measures aimed at reducing the consequences of *N. caninum* infection in cattle comprise:

- Embryo transfer.
- Artificial insemination of seropositive cows with semen from beef bulls.
- Elimination of infected animals.
- Chemotherapy and vaccination.

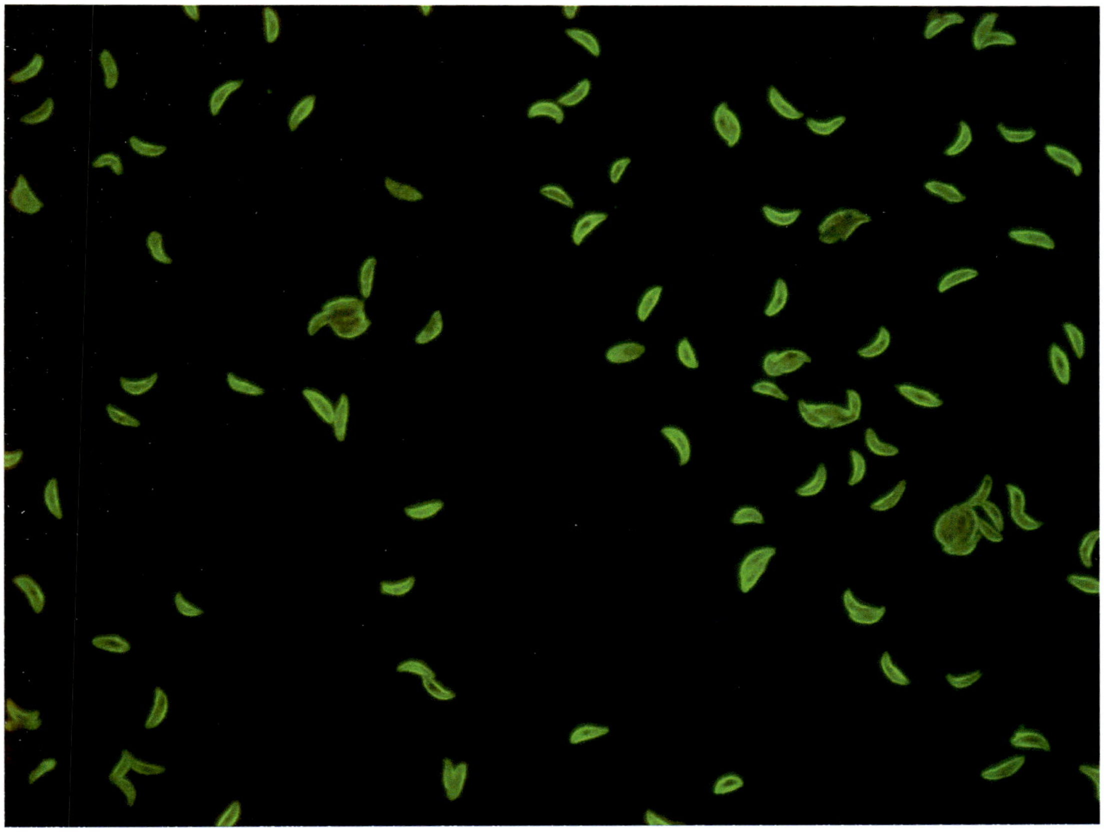

Immunological techniques, which detect specific antibodies against *N. caninum*, are normally performed with serum to confirm infection in adult cattle and in the herd, and to determine whether neosporosis is responsible for reproductive failure by comparing the infection prevalence in cows that have aborted and those that have not. The presence of antibodies in foetal serum or fluids is indicative of foetal infection as transplacental transmission of antibodies from mother to foetus does not take place in bovines.

41 Why are calves not diagnosed with trichomonosis?

In light of a suspected venereal disease on a fighting-bull farm on which the birth rate has been very low, the vet asks the farmer to round up adult male animals for sampling. The following day, the farmer has rounded up all females and young animals, explaining to the vet that the bulls are new and very healthy and that the problem is found in females, which abort, or calves, which are born very weak. The vet releases the animals and repeats his request to only round up adult males.

1. What is trichomoniasis?
2. How is trichomoniasis transmitted?
3. What factors are associated with the appearance of clinical signs of trichomoniasis?

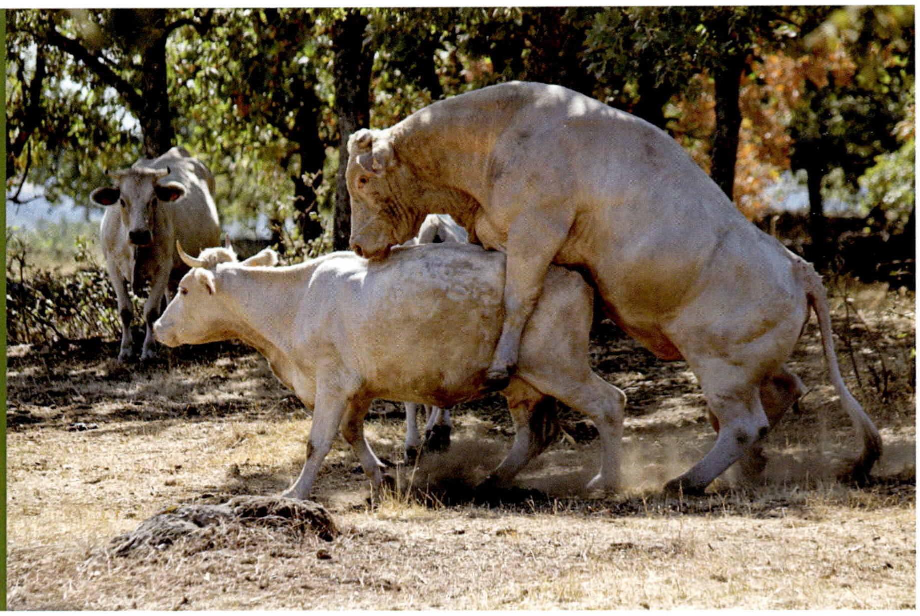

1 What is trichomonosis?

This parasitic disease is also known as bovine abortion caused by trichomonas and contagious vaginal catarrh, amongst others.

Bovine genital trichomonosis is a venereal disease caused by a parasitic protozoon known as *Tritrichomonas foetus* that courses with reproductive problems of various types. Thus, temporary fertility problems and embryo death occur on some occasions, whereas in others abortion and foetal mummification and retention occur. The most common signs are repeated oestrus and pyometra.

Tritrichomonas foetus is a highly pleomorphic flagellate, although ovoid and pyriform forms are common. It usually measures 10-18 µm × 4-10 µm and is characterised by possessing three anterior flagella and one posterior. The latter is associated with an undulating membrane and has a free end. There are numerous internal structures that are characteristic of this group with defined roles and a typical morphology. This flagellate reproduces by longitudinal binary fission and can easily be grown in artificial media.

It lives in the reproductive apparatus of males and females. In the bull it prefers the preputial cavity, where it is found in abundance in the penile mucosa and surrounding tissue. In cows, it is mainly found in the folds of the cervix, where it multiplies, although infection in females is self-limiting. The age of bulls is a risk factor as older animals tend to be carriers due to their greater exposure to the agent and anatomical changes, with a greater depth of the glandular crypts favouring the multiplication of trichomonas.

2 How is trichomonosis transmitted?

Transmission occurs almost exclusively during mating. However, mechanical transmission via the instruments used during artificial insemination or vaginal examination is also possible. Transmission of the infection from an infected cow to a receptive cow via a healthy bull is also possible if the time period between matings is sufficiently short. The possibility that the parasite could be transmitted mechanically via arthropods (flies, etc.) has also been reported, although this route lacks any practical importance.

Trichomonas survive in both fresh and refrigerated semen, and can even survive for short periods at very low temperatures (-80 °C) or in liquid nitrogen.

Although trichomonosis has been almost eradicated in regions where artificial insemination is performed, it is endemic in regions of extensive cattle farming where natural mating is performed.

As a result, the current prevalence of this infection is low or very low in many geographic regions. However, this disease was so important in many European countries until the mid-20th century that cattle breeding and farming was severely limited in some of them.

Spain was no exception to this. Although little information is available, very high prevalences have been reported. Nevertheless, such reports should be treated with care. Sporadic outbreaks of trichomonosis still occur in beef or mixed herds. The common denominator in this cases is almost always the acquisition of a new stud bull for reproduction by natural mating.

Although data regarding the economic repercussions of trichomonosis are somewhat lacking, it is easy to understand that once reproduction has been compromised, economic losses can be very high, especially in select herds. As a result, once the parasite has been introduced into the herd, the economic losses caused by it are considerable and mainly due to the lower number of calves/year and difficulties in controlling the infection.

3 What factors are associated with the appearance of clinical signs of trichomonosis?

The known pathogenic mechanisms include: direct mechanical action of trichomonas; the action of certain protozoon enzymes, for example cysteine proteases, which act on various host proteins (albumin, fibrinogen, lactoferrin and immunoglobulins G_1 and G_2); inflammation of the uterus and lymphokine-mediated cytotoxicity.

In males, the trichomonas present in secretions and the glandular lumen produces mild inflammation of the penile and preputial mucosa, although this is not normally accompanied by clinical signs. The absence of symptoms that

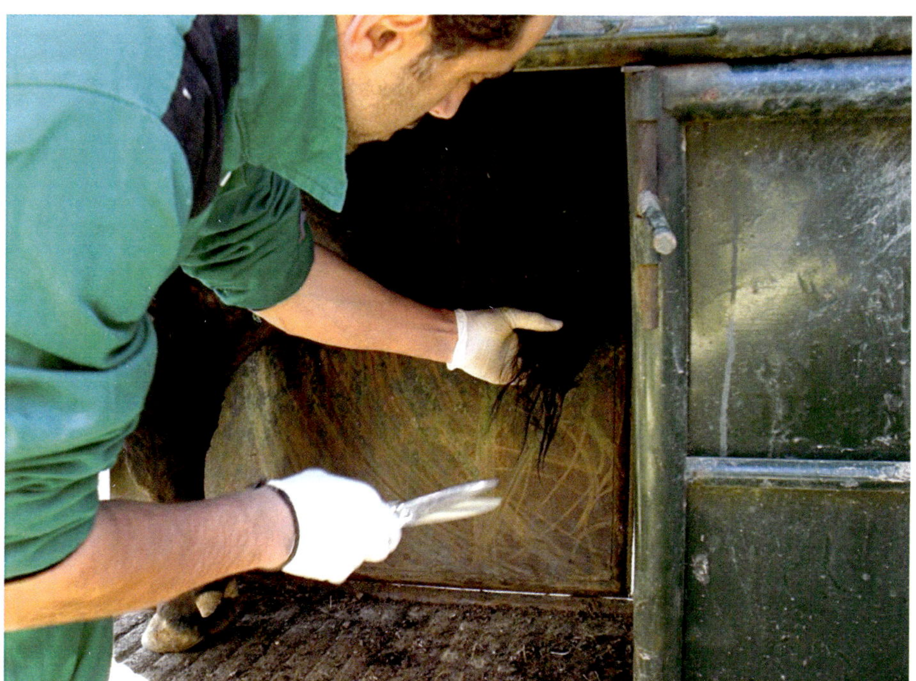

Appropriate samples for diagnosing trichomoniasis are a preputial sample from the male, vaginal discharge from the female and an aborted foetus. Preputial sampling can be performed by methods such as scraping, sampling using an insemination pipette or aspiration. Aborted foetuses are usually not found as they are very small and go unnoticed or disappear. The lesions caused by the parasite in bulls are minimal, and in the absence of natural immunity the male becomes a persistent carrier of this disease. *Image courtesy of Dr. J. C. Domínguez F. de Tejerina.*

indicate the presence of an infection means that animals can be carriers for long periods of time. As noted above, age is a key factor in an animal's role as a carrier.

In females, which can also be carriers, infection has an average duration of 2 to 5 months. Acute or moderate vaginitis and vestibulitis characterised by cellular infiltration (neutrophils, macrophages, lymphocytes and, occasionally, plasma cells) are observed at around 50 days post-contagion.

Inflammation of the endometrium leads to alteration of the intrauterine medium and embryo or foetal death. If the corpus luteum is maintained, which happens in some cases, and there is foetal maceration, pyometra and a chronic infection appear, which can cause permanent infertility if not treated.

Clinically, moderate vaginitis, cervicitis and endometritis lead to a mucous or mucopurulent vulvovaginal discharge, although no clear signs of infection are normally present. The embryo or foetus is almost always lost in the initial stages of pregnancy (6-16 weeks). Most abortions go unnoticed, and the cow comes into heat again 2-3 months after being covered and is considered to be a repeater, infertile or not pregnant. Pyometra is observed in less than 10 % of infected cows.

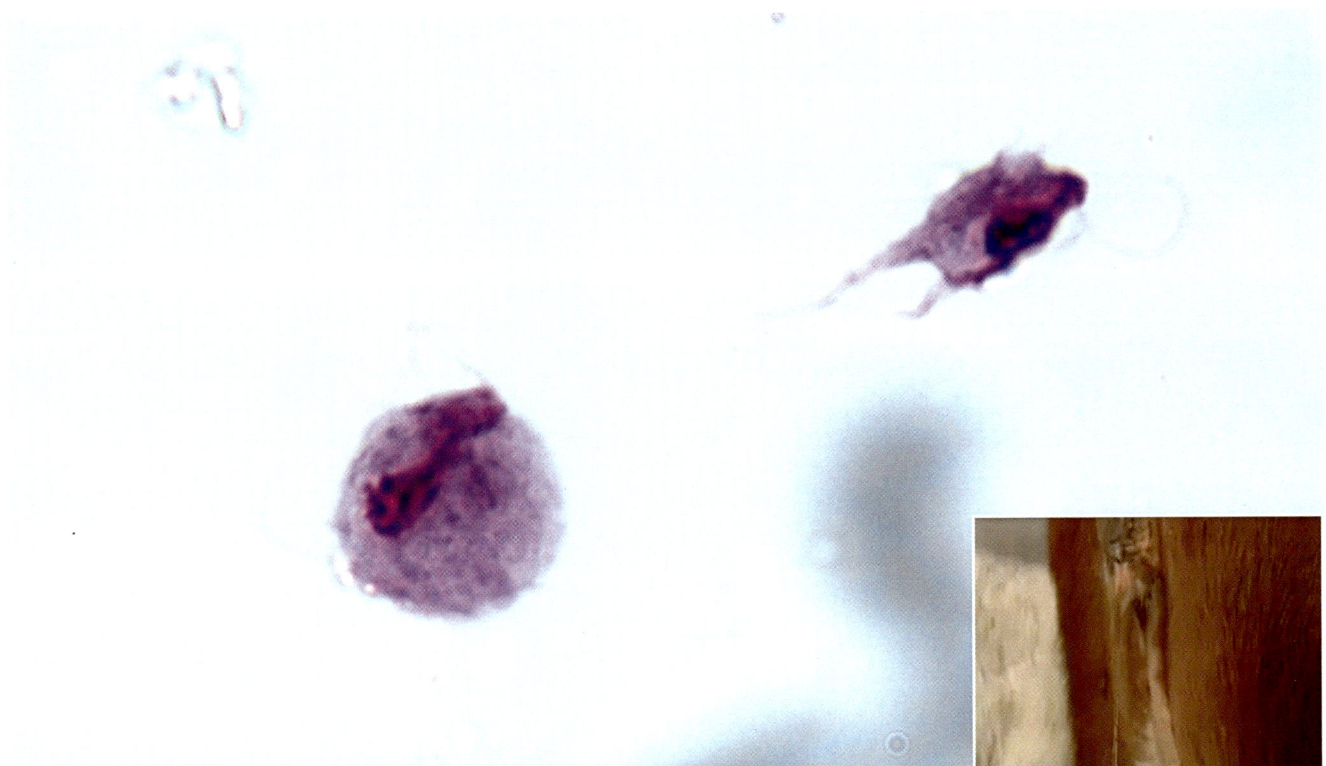

Trichomoniasis is characterised by females repeatedly coming into heat due to temporary infertility and embryonic death. Pyometra and abortion also occur. As pregnancy does not normally extend beyond the third month, these abortions often go unnoticed. Natural disease provokes an immunity that lasts for some time as damage to the female genital mucosa stimulates the production of immunoglobulins, which lyse the parasite in collaboration with the immune system, although reinfection is possible. *Image courtesy of Dr. J. C. Domínguez F. de Tejerina.*

42 How is trichomonosis diagnosed?

Two cases of trichomoniasis are confirmed on a farm in La Rioja during a diagnostic campaign, thus corroborating the entry of this sexually transmitted bovine disease into the region. However, this finding does not imply any risks for human consumption. These two cases were found amongst the samples collected by the Farming Health Defence Group (*Agrupación de Defensa Sanitaria Ganadera*, ADS), which covers various towns and villages and performed analysis on stud bulls from farms in at least four locations in the region. The farmer confirmed the recent acquisition of both bulls and a decrease in the reproductive success of his cows since their arrival. A more detailed clinical study showed that some of them presented a mucous vulvovaginal discharge ranging from vaginitis to moderate endometritis. The stud bulls did not present any visible signs of disease.

1. How is trichomoniasis diagnosed?
2. How are samples taken?
3. Why is it more common in extensive herds?

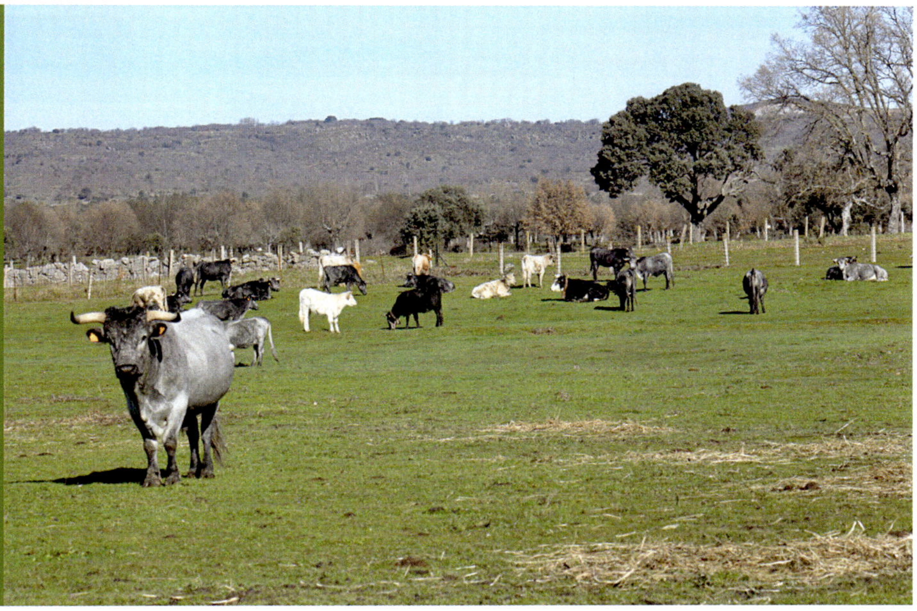

1 How is trichomonosis diagnosed?

The first warning that trichomonosis is present in the herd is a decrease in fertility. When taking the clinical history, the presence of some of the following should be taken into account: a decrease in the number of pregnancies, an increase in repeater cows, a longer time between births and lengthening of the birthing period. The presence of occasional abortions and the onset of pyometra in some animals is also indicative.

The clinical diagnosis is of little help as the infection goes unnoticed in males and is only moderate in females, with no pathognomonic clinical signs. Infection is confirmed by identifying trichomonas in the preputial secretions or cervicovaginal mucous. In the event of abortion, the parasite should be isolated from the placenta, placental fluid or contents of the abomasum. Laboratory diagnosis normally involves observation of the parasite in preputial or vaginal secretions from the suspected infected animal(s), or in foetal fluids or the foetal abomasum in the event of abortion. Male animals should be allowed one week after their last mating before a sample is collected. Preputial massage should be performed prior to collection in order to dislodge the trichomonas located in the epithelial crypts. Preputial smegma can be collected with a swab, an artificial insemination pipette or by lavage of the preputial cavity. In cows, vaginal mucous is

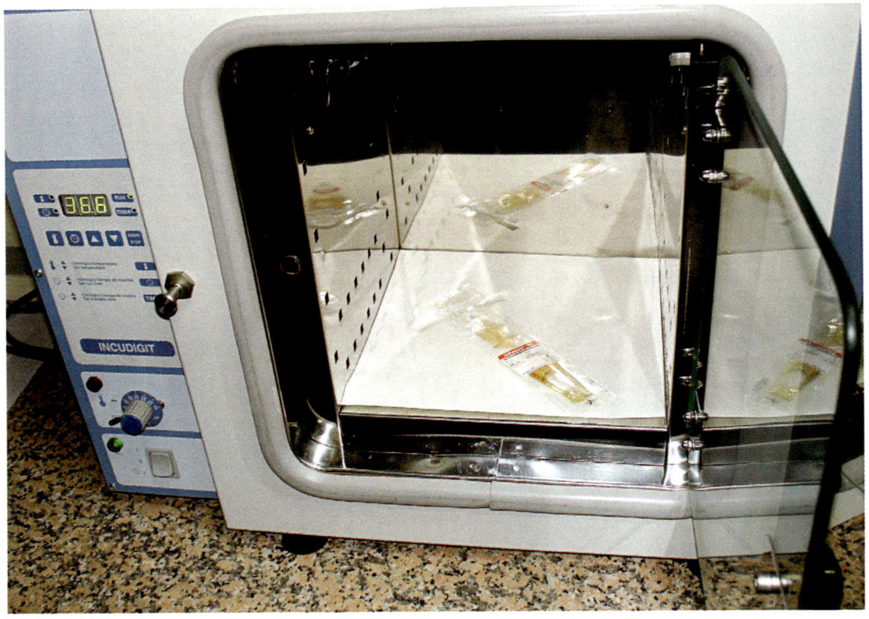

Genital samples should be placed in a transport medium suitable for direct culture in a trichomonas oven. They are then observed daily for 7-10 days, depending on the medium, to check for the presence of the parasite. All bulls should be sampled, including those that have not yet started to reproduce. The age of the bulls is a decisive factor as the risk increases with exposure to the parasite, with those older than 3 years more likely to be carriers. All animals added to the herd must also be checked despite having a clean health record.

collected from the cervix two days prior to, or two days after, coming into heat using an artificial insemination pipette or flexible catheter attached to a syringe. After collection, the sample should be observed directly or cultured, although direct examination is less sensitive. Other direct methods exist, but their sensitivity for some types of sample (vaginal mucous, etc.) is relatively low.

The number of trichomonas present depends on the location. They are abundant in aborted foetuses, remain in the uterus for several days and are also abundant in the vaginal mucous of recently infected cows up to 12-20 days post-infection. In males, *Tritrichomonas foetus* is present in the preputial mucosa but without apparently invading the submucosa. It is generally recommended to leave one week between the last revision and sampling of the preputial mucosa.

Indirect methods, such as agglutination of the vaginal mucous in females, intradermal reaction upon tricine inoculation, which can be used for herd diagnosis, and the detection of circulating antibodies, which has numerous drawbacks, also lack specificity and sensitivity.

It is also possible to detect the parasite in the embryo or foetus by studying the gastric contents and placental fluid. Immunohistochemistry is also diagnostically useful.

2 How are samples taken?

There are various possible techniques available for sampling the prepuce in bulls or the vagina in cows.

However, in all cases, it is important to avoid sample contamination in order to obtain valid results. One means of minimising contamination consists in eliminating external material and dirty hair from around the preputial orifice or vulva, although disinfectants should not be used as they may interfere with the diagnosis.

To collect samples from males, the preputial and penile mucosa can be scraped using an artificial insemination pipette or metal brush, a preputial lavage performed, or the artificial vagina washed after semen collection. This method is less advisable due to its low sensitivity.

Samples can be collected from cows by vaginal lavage or scraping the cervix with an artificial insemination pipette or metal brush.

If the time between sample collection and transport to the laboratory is less than 24 hours, a buffered saline solution at 4 °C to which foetal bovine serum has been added can be used during transport. For longer time periods, plastic recipients and an antibiotic-containing medium should be used if possible. The recipients should be protected from light and extreme temperatures, and should be maintained above 5 °C and below 38 °C.

Some classical (vaginal mucous agglutination, intradermal tests) and more recent tests (ELISA) used to diagnose bovine trichomonosis are not recommended for detection of the parasite in individual animals. Agglutination of mucous, which should preferably be obtained a few days post-oestrus, detects approximately 60 % of naturally infected cows. Antibodies appear at around six weeks post-infection and persist for several months.

Molecular techniques, such as PCR, have the advantage of being highly sensitive, fast and do not require viable parasites. This technique is able to detect very few parasites in laboratory cultures, although if preputial material is present a higher number of trichomonas are required to obtain positive results.

If only a small number of trichomonas are present and they cannot be detected directly, cell cultures using different compositions, which usually include meat extracts such as liver, are used. In any case, the addition of an antifungal agent to control fungal growth is particularly advisable.

Initial detection of the microorganisms can be performed by light microscopy on a wet mount slide prepared from the sample or culture directly, or via the plastic wall of a culture system designed for that purpose. Trichomonas can readily be seen to be actively moving under the microscope. Their characteristics (pyriform or pleomorphic forms, the flagella and undulating membrane) help identification.

Phase-contrast microscopy is very useful for revealing these traits, although they can also be stained to facilitate their observation.

3 Why is it more common in extensive herds?

As noted above, this infection has been essentially eliminated from regions and farms where artificial insemination is performed. In contrast, on extensive farms with natural mating it is still considered to be an enzootic infection whose prevalence varies widely.

There are even differences in extensive farms due to several factors. For example, some farmers incorporate animals from selective breeding farms into their beef herds, or purchase them from other producers, almost always with health guarantees. These animals can also be obtained from herds in which, as is becoming increasingly common, artificial insemination is performed.

In contrast, on some extensive and fighting bull breeding farms the bulls are obtained from the herd itself as a result of natural mating or from others, often without adequate health controls, especially as farmers often swap stud bulls.

Once this parasite has become established on a farm, the losses caused by it, and the difficulty in controlling the infection, can be considerable.

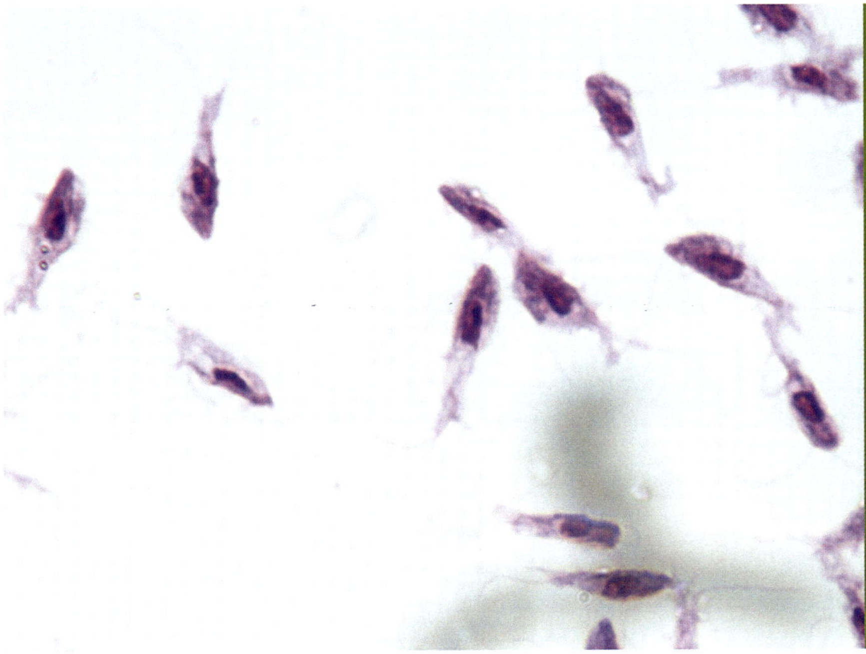

Trichomonas is a pyriform or ovoid flagellate protozoon with four flagella. Three of these are free at the anterior end and equally sized, whereas the fourth, which is directed towards the posterior part, is associated with an undulating membrane slightly smaller than that of the parasite and which binds to a support structure known as the costa at its internal edge. This recurrent flagellum remains free beyond the posterior end of the undulating membrane. Routine diagnosis involves identifying the agent in culture (stained or fresh samples) and subsequent confirmation by molecular identification.

43 How is besnoitiosis transmitted?

During a national study to locate emerging pockets of besnoitiosis, the existence of very few serologically *Besnoitia*-positive animals on two neighbouring farms was confirmed, whereas more than 50 % of animals on other farms in the same region were infected. It was decided to slaughter all positive animals on these two farms and to analyse all new animals purchased. On those farms with numerous infected animals, the repeated use of insecticides was recommended to control the vectors and thereby prevent transmission. Two years later, the two farms remained infection-free despite the presence of haematophagous insects.

1. How have the farms remained infection-free?
2. What are the clinical phases of besnoitiosis?
3. What measures are effective for controlling besnoitiosis?

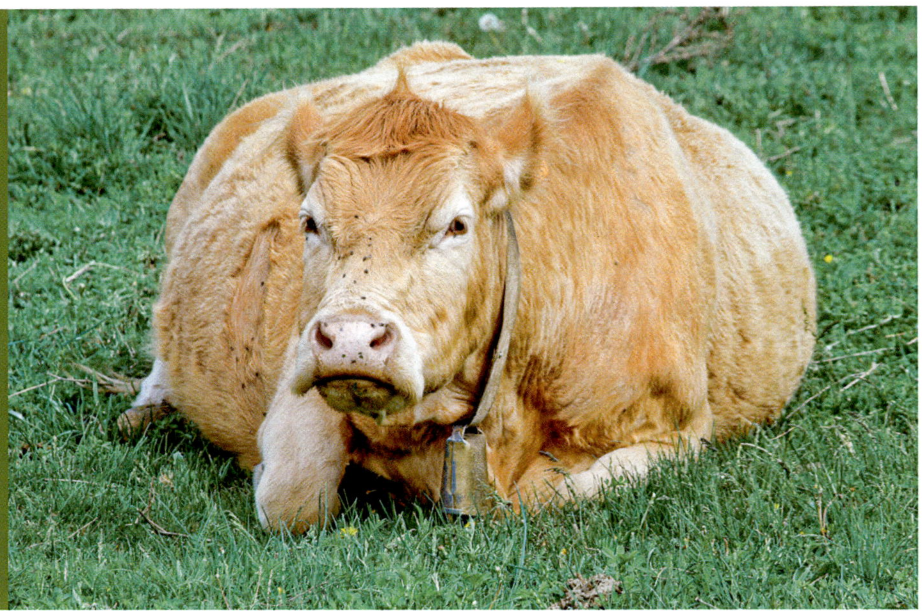

1 How have the farms remained infection-free?

As is the case with any disease process, the control of besnoitiosis is based on an understanding of the routes of transmission, risk, etc. Available epidemiological data suggest that various arthropods can act as vectors for *B. besnoiti*. The most likely route of transmission is transcutaneous.

Animals have been infected experimentally using blood tachyzoites or cutaneous bradyzoites.

Various haematophagous arthropod species act as vectors in transmission from one animal to another. Some seem to be better vectors than others. For example, tabanids are more effective than haematophagous flies as they can remain infective for 24 hours after taking blood whereas flies are only infective for around 3 hours. As a result, the number of animals infected on a farm increases markedly once the population of haematophagous insects reaches its peak. The house fly (*Musca domestica*) has also been considered to be responsible for mechanical transmission, although this route is yet to be confirmed. Biological transmission by biting arthropod species has not been observed.

Although infection is very widespread in sheep flocks in endemic regions and those where the problem is more sporadic, the proportion of infected animals that show clinical signs is very low. After infection, a small proportion of animals develop clinical signs and a large proportion of seropositive animals present scleroconjunctival cysts, whereas the majority of animals are seropositive but remain asymptomatic.

The prevalence of clinically affected animals in endemic regions is 1-10 % per year, whereas in regions in which the problem is emergent, up to 15-20 % of animals infected for the first time exhibit clinical signs.

There is currently no convincing treatment for this disease. Thus, although sulfamides (sulfadimerazine, sulfadimethoxine) are used to relieve the clinical signs, they are unable to cure the animals and relapses occur even when treatment is established correctly and in good time. Tetracyclines can also be used, although there is no evidence that they are really effective.

As chemoprophylaxis is also not possible and vaccination is not authorised in many European countries, control measures acquire particular importance. Serological analyses should be performed prior to the introduction of animals into herds previously considered to be free from *Besnoitia*. The state of the infection should also be evaluated if it appears in infection-free herds in order to eliminate it as soon as possible. The protection of animals against insect bites by regular use of pyrethroids is also effective.

It should be stressed that all these measures should be accompanied by correct "health education" for the farmers, especially in some regions, in order to achieve satisfactory results.

2 What are the clinical phases of besnoitiosis?

Normally only a small proportion of infected animals go on to develop clinical signs, probably due to both individual variations and difference differences in the virulence strains or the number of parasites transmitted by a single vector.

The incubation period for this disease is short (6-10 days) and the clinical manifestations can be grouped into three phases:

1. A febrile phase, which lasts between 2 and 10 days and is accompanied by an increase in body temperature up to 41-42 °C. Active multiplication of the tachyzoites in macrophages, fibroblasts and blood vessel endothelial cells occurs during this phase. The clinical manifestations include photophobia, epiphora, ocular or nasal discharge, cessation of rumination, anorexia and an increased heart and breathing rate; abortions may also occur. Diagnosis during this phase is not simple due to the lack of specificity of the symptoms, which are similar to those found for bluetongue and malignant catarrhal fever.
2. The following phase is characterised by a normal or slightly raised temperature, enlarged lymph nodes and oedema in the head, limbs and lower parts of the body. The animals remain immobile and their skin is hot, swollen and painful. Females exhibit congested udders and males orchitis with testicular pain and permanent or temporary infertility.
3. The chronic phase is characterised by the onset of numerous bradyzoite-containing cysts in the upper respiratory tract, connective tissue, conjunctiva, muscles, vulvar mucosa and, sometimes, in the spleen, liver and cardiac muscle tissue. The skin is very swollen, with hyperkeratosis and elephantiasis, and presents bald patches. The physical condition of affected animals deteriorates progressively. This does not remit even when the animals

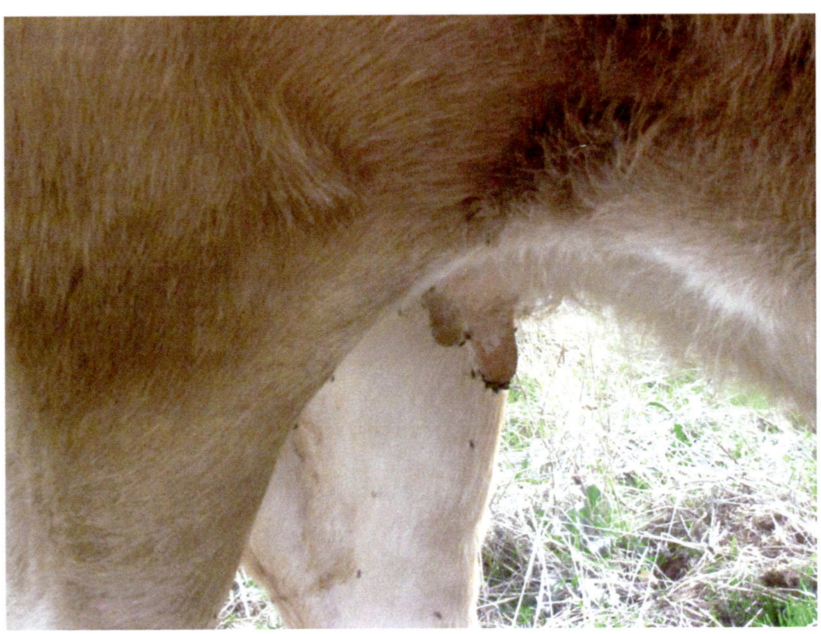

The role of felids in the biological cycle of *Besnoitia* and its transmission remains unclear. Haematophagous insects are considered to play an important role even though the introduction of animals from an endemic region remains the determining factor as regards spread of this parasite.

recover their appetite and can lead to cachexia. Some animals recover, at least partially, but in most cases the loss of value means that they must be sent for slaughter.

3 What measures are effective for controlling besnoitiosis?

Irrespective of the enzootic state or the sporadic appearance of *B. besnoiti* infection, there is some degree of seasonality in the onset of clinical outbreaks of the disease, with most cases occurring in summer. In other words, the dynamics of haematophagous insect populations could explain the seasonal incidence of the disease.

Although numerous studies have investigated antibody levels, the existence of different populations of vectors involved in transmission and the onset of besnoitiosis, very few conclusions can be extracted.

The direct relationship between positive animals and the presence of insects strongly suggests that the observed seasonality is related to vector activity, although this does not always appear to be the case. However, the decrease in antibody levels and vector populations suggests that continual transmission by bites from the corresponding vectors is required to maintain high antibody levels. Anyway, it has been shown that the presence of some vector species, such as *Stomoxys calcitrans*, in animal sheds during the winter could explain the seroconversion and high antibody levels observed prior to release of the animals to pasture in spring.

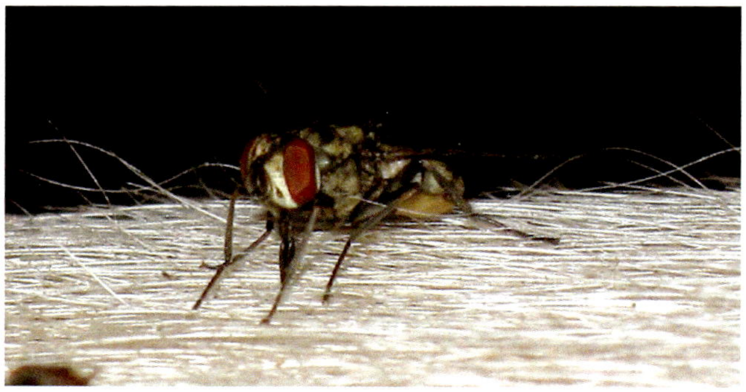

Some epidemiological findings support the hypothesis of transcutaneous transmission and the vectorial role of tabanids and haematophagous flies such as *Stomoxys calcitrans*. The parasites remain viable in tabanids for up to 24 hours after ingestion of blood, whereas in *Stomoxys* species they remain viable for only 3 hours. However, the larger population and ubiquity of the latter may compensate for its lower transmission capacity.

Three tabanids were able to cause a clear infection in comparison with more than 50,000 *Stomoxys* bites. *Image courtesy of Dr. P. Jacquiet.*

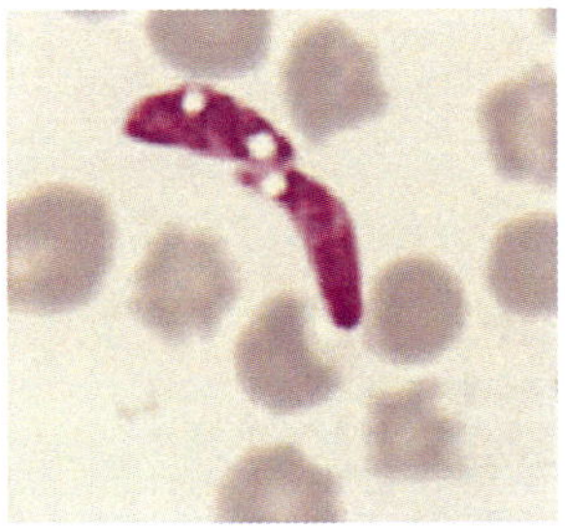

In a primary infection, the tachyzoites multiply rapidly in macrophages, fibroblasts and endothelial cells and the animals present fever with photophobia, epiphora and catarrh. Rumination stops, and anorexia coincides with a higher respiratory and heart rate. *Image courtesy of Dr. P. Jacquiet.*

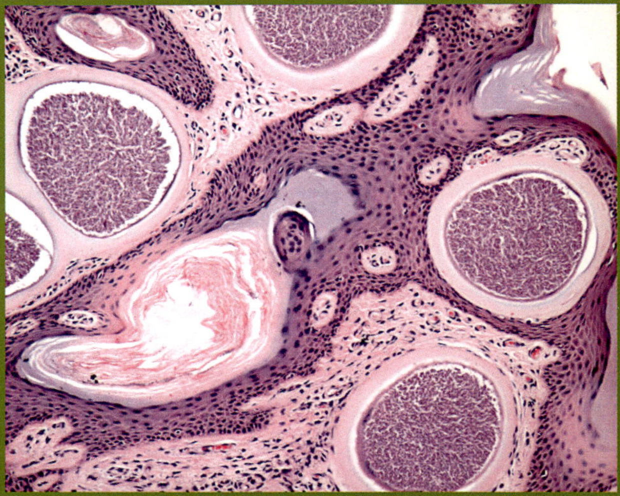

Fever is absent in the following phase, the lymph nodes become enlarged and generalised anasarca appears. The skin is hot, swollen and painful. Numerous bradyzoite-containing subcutaneous cysts can be seen. These cysts can be found in the skin, upper respiratory tract, connective tissue, ocular conjunctiva, muscles, vulvar mucosa and even in the liver, spleen and heart. The animal presents scleroderma with hyperkeratosis and more or less generalised alopecia. *Image courtesy of Dr. P. Jacquiet.*

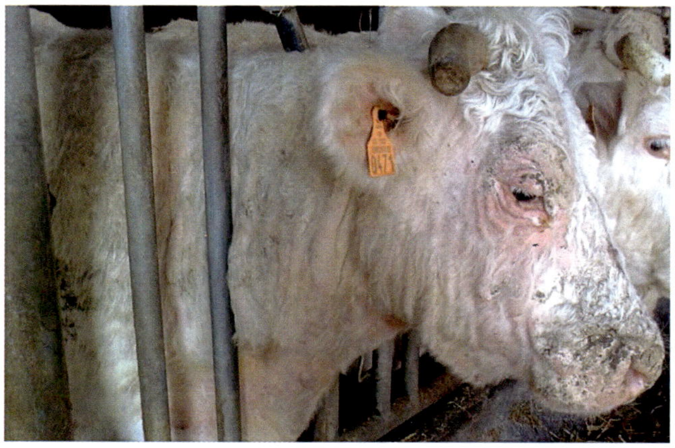

In a third phase, even though they have recovered their appetite, the physical condition is highly deteriorated and leads to cachexia. As the economic worth of the animals has decreased so much, they are sent for slaughter. In general, and for reasons that are still unknown, the proportion of animals that develop these symptoms is low. *Image courtesy of Dr. P. Jacquiet.*

Biological cycle of Apicomplexa (*Besnoitia*)

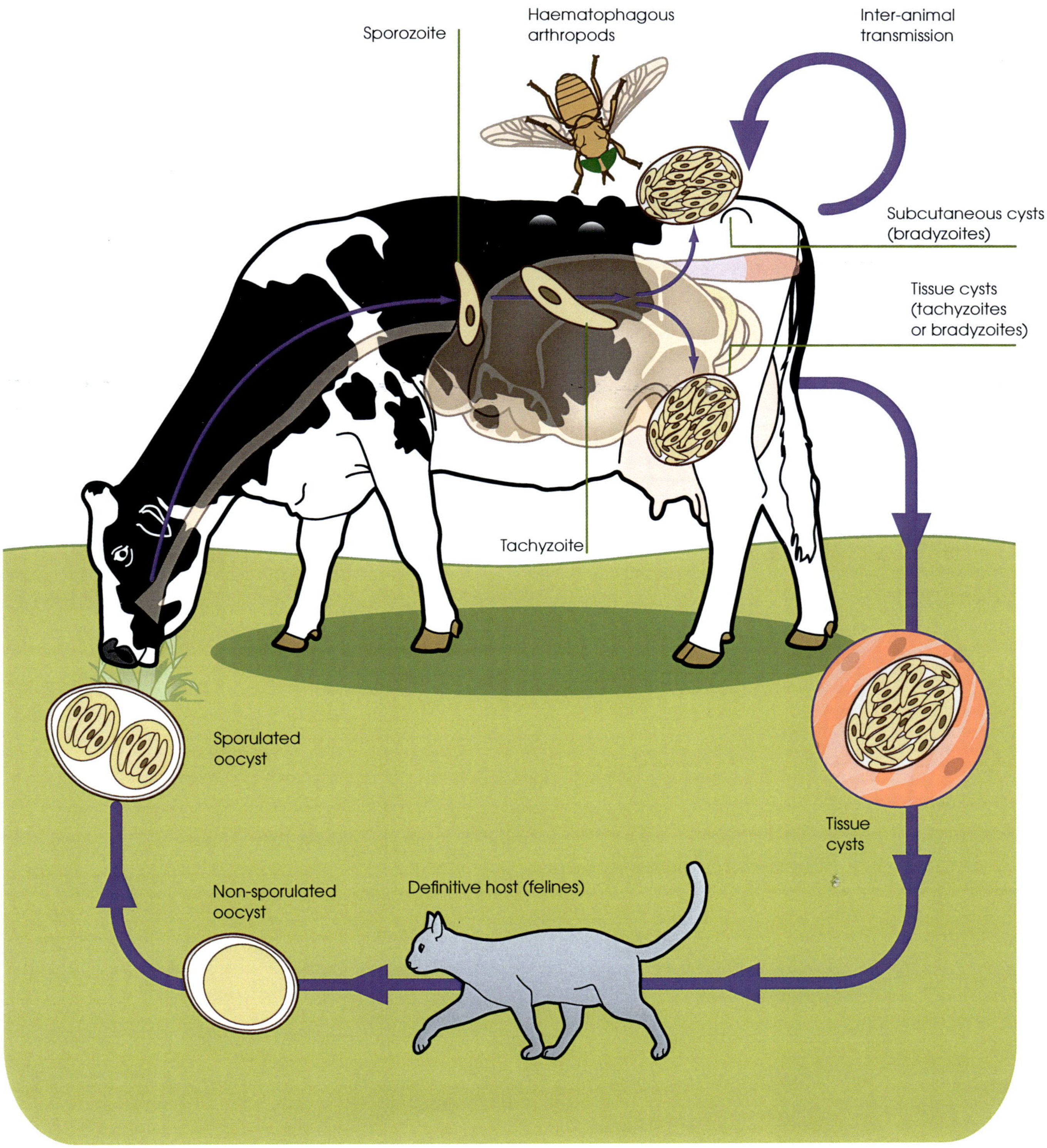

44 Are schistosomes present in European cattle?

Hepatitis with degenerative changes in the parenchyma, fibrosis and an unusual distortion of the lobes is observed during the necropsy of a one-year-old heifer from Salamanca province (Spain). A microscopic study shows the presence of abundant periportal granulomas in which ovoid structures corresponding to parasite eggs can be seen. The vascular alterations are characterised by hypertrophy of the middle layer and endothelial proliferation in all portal branches, with evident congestion and dilation of the sinusoids with stellate cells. Thick, robust, elongated parasites around 2 cm in length containing other, very fine and much thinner worms in a ventral canal are extracted from inside the venous, and some mesenteric, branches of the liver.

1. Which schistosomes can be found in cattle?
2. What is their biological cycle? How important are they?
3. Are they related to *Fasciola hepatica*?

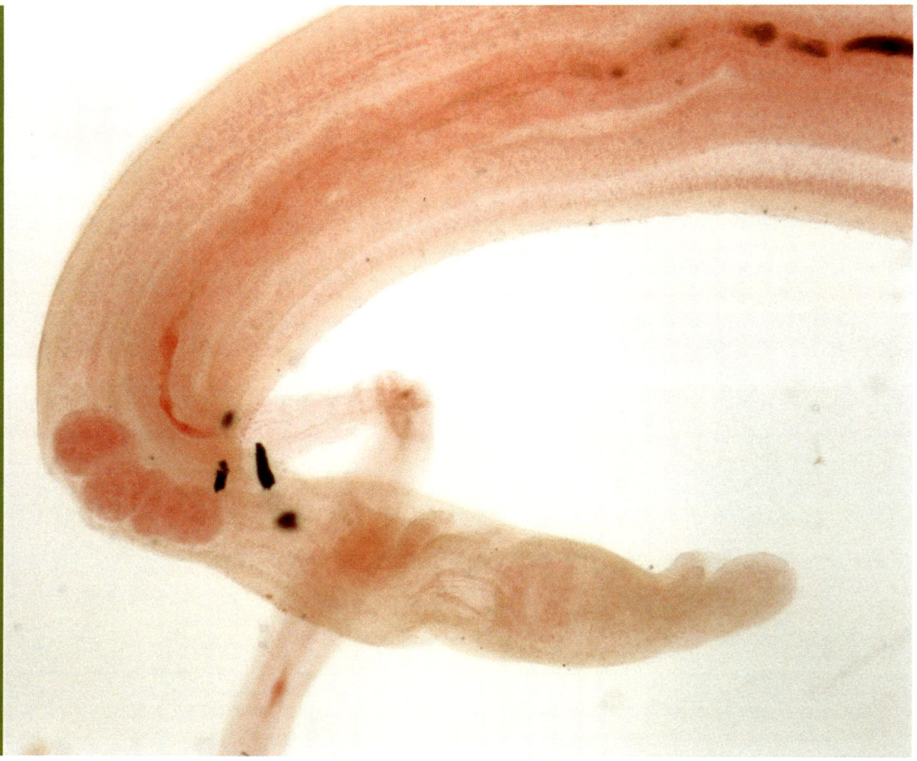

1 Which schistosomes can be found in cattle?

The geographical distribution of ruminant schistosomosis covers practically the whole of Africa, many parts of south-western and south-eastern Asia and some European Mediterranean regions such as Corsica, Sardinia, Sicily and Spain.

In Spain, schistosomosis was initially studied in sheep from Ávila province, and subsequently in cattle, goats and sheep from Salamanca and Zamora, more recently it has been found in Extremadura and Cordoba.

Schistosoma bovis is responsible for most infections in cattle, sheep and goats, whereas *S. mattheei*, which infects domestic ruminants, buffaloes and small wild ruminants, has not been found on the Iberian Peninsula. Horses, zebras, dogs, suids, camels, dromedaries, primates, rodents and, occasionally, humans, can also intervene in the cycle as secondary hosts.

Other wild ruminants, such as antelopes, tend to be infected by species with a much narrower distribution, such as *S. margrebowiei* and *S. leiperi*.

2 What is their biological cycle? How important are they?

The biological cycle of the species that infect cattle in Spain, namely *Schistosoma bovis,* has been known for over a hundred years. The external phase of the cycle bears some resemblance to that of *Fasciola hepatica* as it develops in an aqueous medium, although there are also some differences.

Adult schistosomes live in the venous branches of the portal system, in mesenteric veins, intestinal submucosal and subserous veins, pancreatic veins and, occasionally, in pulmonary venous branches. They are elongated worms with a size of between 5 and 30 mm, and the males are always much thicker than the females, which are thinner and finer. The latter are always found inside a medial canal of the male. The females lays large eggs with a size of 180-280 µm × 40-95 µm at this site. After passing through the blood vessels and intestinal wall, they reach the exterior in faeces. They need a minimum amount of water to remain viable. Under appropriate conditions, the embryo (miracidium) hatches and, actively searches for a snail in which to develop (from the sporocyst to the cercaria stage). Finally, the cercariae leave the mollusc. The climate conditions in the environment affect development, which can last for 17 days and 4 months.

Cercariae have great vitality and are very active for around 40 hours. If they "find" a suitable host they penetrate its skin, especially around its extremities and peribuccal region (lips), when the animals drink from pools.

After penetration, the worms emigrate via blood and lymphatic vessels to the lung, finally reaching the hepatic portal system and mesenteric veins via arterial circulation, where the endogenous cycle is completed.

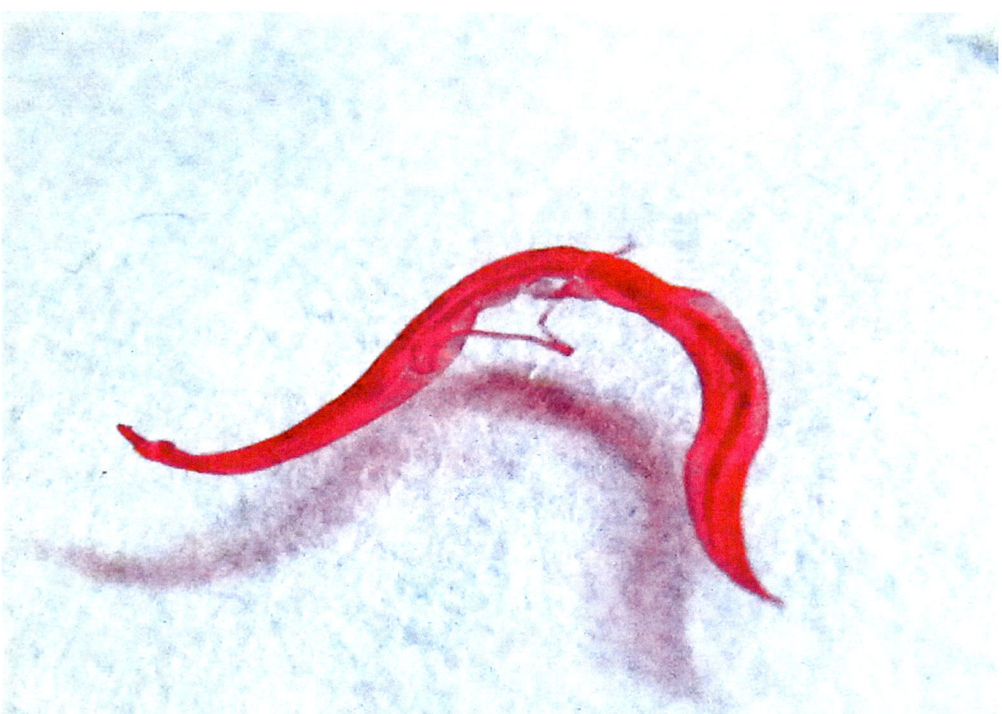

The peribuccal percutaneous (drinking) route gains importance as the most common entry for parasites in bovine infection. The pathogenic effects mainly arise due to passage of the eggs through the tissues. The liver presents degenerative changes in the parenchyma, telangiectasia, fibrosis and atrophy, with lobular distortion. Deposition of a large number of eggs may also cause catarrhal inflammation in the duodenum and rectum, with multiple petechiae and numerous granulomas.

3 Are they related to *Fasciola hepatica*?

From a phylogenetic point of view, there is no relationship between fasciola and schistosomes. However, the external phase of both parasites obeys a wholly aquatic biological model, although some phases of fasciola's cycle do not exist in schistosomes. The intermediate snail hosts are also different, even though aquatic molluscs or amphibious are involved in both cases. They also differ as regards their means of accessing the definitive hosts and the paths they follow inside the animal's body.

Despite this, the induction of resistance to *Schistosoma bovis* promoted by prior experimental infection with *Fasciola hepatica*, and vice versa, has been demonstrated. In this respect, the results of immunisation with native or recombinant antigenic molecules shared by both parasites are very promising in both directions.

It has also been shown experimentally that prior infection with heterologous species can significantly reduce the establishment of new parasites.

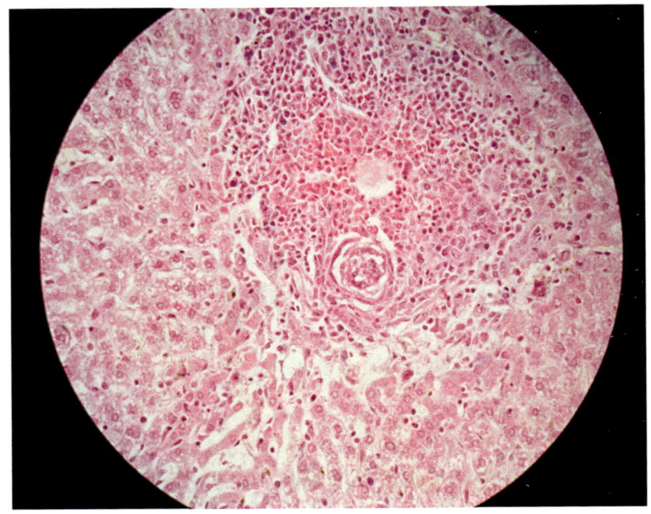

The parasites are mainly located in the portal and mesenteric venous system and, in some species, in vesicular plexi and nasal venules. They are dioecious, with the female being found in a ventral canal of the male. The somatic and sexual maturation of both requires coupling, which persists for most of their lives. The most common microscopic lesion is a granulomatous inflammatory process characterised by the presence of abundant nodules in different phases of evolution and at different sites, most commonly periportal, although they can also be found in other organs in response to the presence and action of eggs therein.

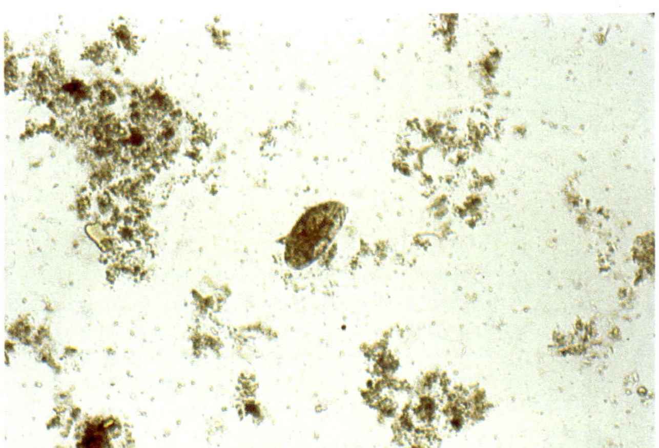

Schistosoma eggs are large and ellipsoidal with a smooth wall, although other structures such as a terminal spine may also be present. They are laid in veins in initial quantities of around a hundred per female and, after crossing the vascular and intestinal walls, reach the lumen. From there they exit the host in faeces, where they survive for a few days. Egg laying is reduced a few weeks post-infection as a result of the host's response.

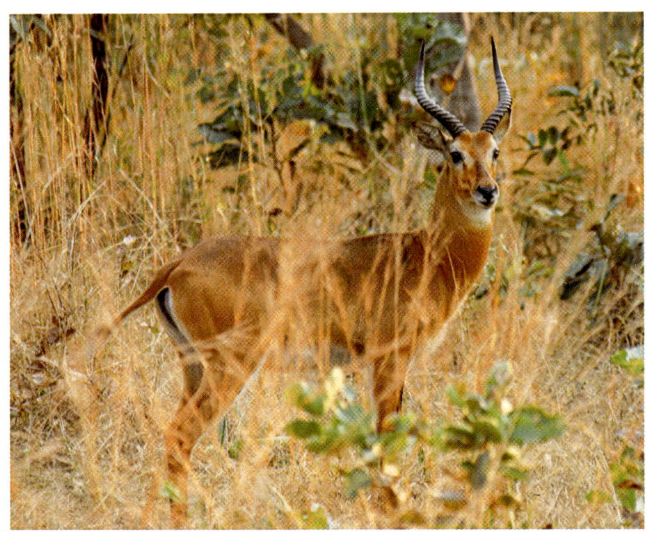

Ruminant schistosomosis is distributed throughout essentially the whole of Africa, Asia and part of Mediterranean Europe. In Africa, *S. margrebowiei and S. leiperi* are primarily hosted by antelopes and other small wild ruminants, and secondarily by domestic ruminants.

45 Which filariae affect cattle?

Various heads of zebu have been introduced from India into a village in Salamanca province (Spain) as a commercial alternative in the region. One of the animals presents heart failure with left ventricular hypertrophy, which manifests as a clear dyspnoea on exertion. The vet verifies that the animal has a slow-rising arterial pulse with a systolic murmur characteristic of ejection and fremitus. In the blood test, the laboratory reports the presence of a large quantity of microfilaria.

1. Which parasitosis is accompanied by heart failure and microfilaraemia in cattle?
2. What risk is there of transmission to other animals on the farm?
3. Why is it advisable to administer antibiotics to treat filariosis?

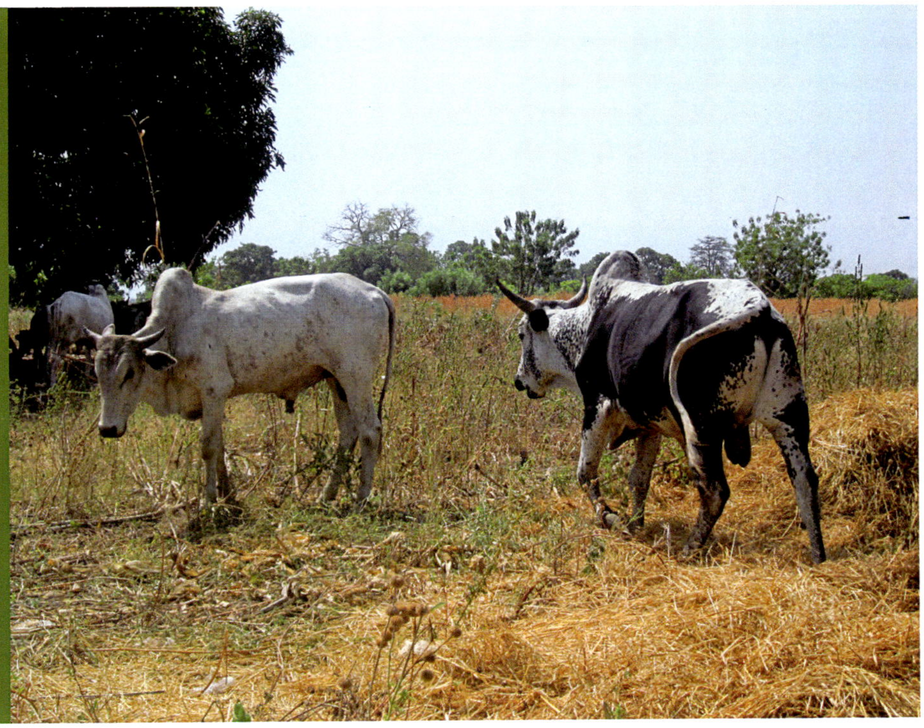

1 Which parasitosis is accompanied by heart failure and microfilaraemia in cattle?

A group of nematodes from the *Filarioidea* superfamily, the adults of which live in subcutaneous connective tissue, blood vessels, serous membrane or tendons, is known to infect animals and humans.

For transmission they use intermediates, namely haematophagous arthropods, in which the larvae, known as microfilariae (unsheathed or sheathed), develop. These microfilariae pass into circulation, from where they reach the intermediate host when it ingests blood.

They develop in these intermediates until they reach the infective phase (L3). The infection is transmitted when the vector feeds on the definitive host.

Some parasitic filaria in ruminants that are known to cause important disorders have been reported in the Iberian Peninsula, whereas others remain unknown. However, this situation can easily change in light of the movement and import of animals.

Some species responsible for onchocercosis are currently in this situation. Thus, although *Onchocerca linealis* has been found in Spain, other *Onchocerca* species, such as *O. armillata*, have not yet been reported here.

Of the known *Onchocerca* species, adult *O. armillata* are found in the aorta and, as such, can produce clinical alterations such as stenosis. In this case, exercise is accompanied by a normal decrease in arteriolar resistance without resulting in a marked decrease in resistance upon ventricular emptying. This phenomenon explains the drop in arterial pressure during exercise, which can lead to fainting.

2 What risk is there of transmission to other animals on the farm?

These processes are enzootic in nature and their presence is directly related to the existence of suitable intermediates. Various insect species, such as simulids (genus *Simulium*) and ceratopogonids (genus *Culicoides*), play a part in the transmission cycle.

Indeed, numerous culicoides species have been reported in both Spain and Portugal on the Iberian Peninsula. Reports in Spain tend to come from provinces bordering Portugal, such as Badajoz. A similar situation is found for the numerous species from the genus *Simulium*, which are much more widely distributed and have been reported in some provinces of Castilla y León.

Under appropriate environmental conditions, the parasites develop in the intermediate hosts within around three weeks, at the end of which transmission to a new animal is possible.

The intervention of simulids and ceratopogonids governs the time of year during which animals are at risk of infection, thus meaning that outbreaks tend to be seasonal, occurring more frequently in spring and summer.

Once the infection has been introduced into a specific region, and provided that the conditions required for the cycle to continue are present, "imported" animals may help to propagate the infection and new cases may arise at the most suitable times of year.

3 Why is it advisable to administer antibiotics to treat filariosis?

Onchocercosis control is based almost exclusively on "mass" treatment with the microfilaricidal drug ivermectin, which prevents pathological manifestations but does not destroy the adult worms.

Many parasitic filaria in humans and animals transport *Rickettsia*-like microorganisms of the genus *Wolbachia*, the recent discovery of which has stimulated research aimed at determining its possible role in the aetiology of filariosis, its functional relationship with filariae and possible treatments.

Four species of *Onchocerca* are known in African and Asian bovines: two of these are known to be "*Wolbachia*-positive" (*Onchocerca gutturosa* and *O. ochengi*), whereas the status of the other two is not currently known.

It has been shown that antibiotic treatment of bovines infected with *Wolbachia*-positive *Onchocerca ochengi* kills the adult filariae, thus indicating that their survival depends on the "bacteria". As a result, it has been shown that treatment of human onchocercosis with doxycycline has a significant effect on *O. volvulus* microfilariae, although daily treatment for 4-6 weeks is required.

The efficacy of antibiotic therapy in filariosis could be related to the action of these antibiotics against *Wolbachia*, the presence of which allows adult filariae to survive by preventing the action of eosinophils.

It has been shown in some *Onchocerca* species that the half-life of "*Wolbachia*-negative" strains is shorter than that of their "*Wolbachia*-positive" counterparts and that the environment of the former is dominated by eosinophils and giant cells. This hypothesis has been confirmed in some African onchocercia species that infect bovines.

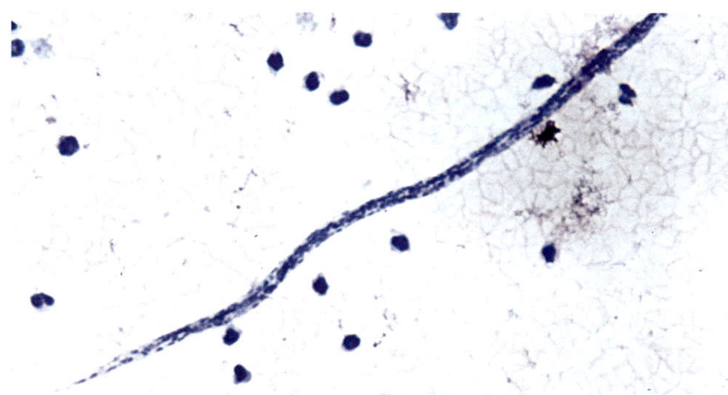

The unsheathed or sheathed microfilaria is ingested by the intermediate host directly from the skin or blood stream. It moults twice, reaching the infective L3 form in less than two weeks. If a large number of larvae are ingested, the vector can die as a result of intestinal perforation and destruction of its organs. Once the L3 larva has developed, it migrates to the proboscis and transmission occurs when the vector feeds on the definitive host.

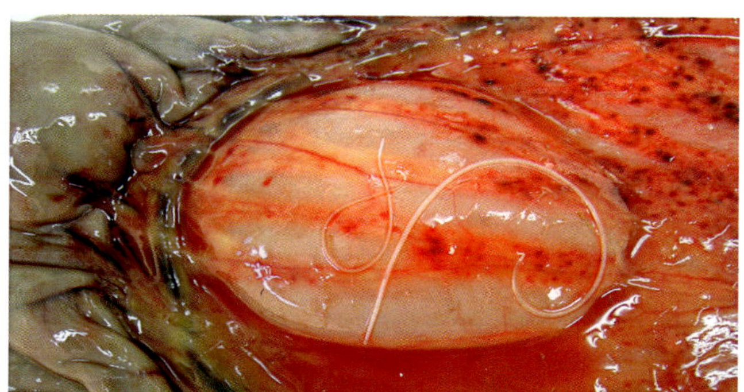

Filaria live in subcutaneous connective tissue, serous membranes and blood vessels or tendons. As these zones are difficult to access, they transmit themselves as larvae using intermediate hosts. During bovine necropsies, large apathogenic *Setaria* worms can be found in the peritoneum. If the larvae are passed from the intermediate hosts to an unsuitable host (sheep, goat, horse), they emigrate erratically via the nervous system. This "enzootic cerebrospinal nematodoses" is very serious and most common in summer and autumn, coinciding with the flying period of the intermediate hosts.

46 Which fly larvae can be found in the oesophagus?

Crystalline formations about 1 to 2 cm in length are detected in the oesophageal wall when slaughtering animals in an abattoir in January. After extraction with forceps, they are found to be cylindrical with rounded ends. Some are alive and moving. The majority are aligned longitudinally in the same direction as the muscle fibres. Numerous elongated structures are also present, some of which are clearly calcified, with larval remnants in their interior, as confirmed upon observing buccal hook remains under a microscope. A retrospective analysis in the same abattoir shows that these larvae tend to be found most often in winter.

1. What parasite are these oesophageal larvae from?
2. Why do they appear most often in winter?
3. Do they cause disease?

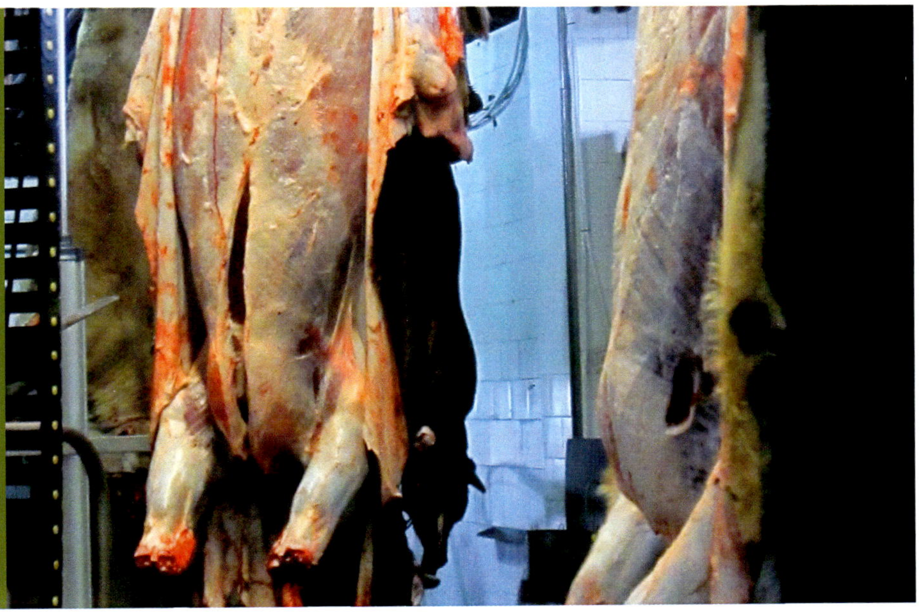

1 What parasite are these oesophageal larvae from?

The forms that appear in the oesophagus correspond to the first larval phase (L1) of *Hypoderma lineatum*, which is also known as the "heel fly" or "gadfly".

Although adult *H. lineatum* are very similar to those of *Hypoderma bovis*, they can be distinguished by the presence of white or yellowish hairs irregularly distributed over the abdomen without forming stripes. They are around 10-13 mm in size, with dark brown wings and legs covered with orangish-black hairs.

Adult flies lay their eggs from the base to the tip of the hair, in the form of a palisade, preferably on the legs and abdomen. Once the eggs have hatched, and after passing through the skin, the migratory route of the larvae includes the oesophageal submucosa. The L1 larva found at this site measure around 0.6-0.8 mm in length and are hyaline white in colour, with an almost circular cross-section. They present segments of very similar lengths covered with small denticles. The buccal hooks, which are curved in *H. lineatum*, are found in the cephalic skeleton. They grow to around 17 mm at this site.

2 Why do they appear most often in winter?

Firstly, one of the epidemiological factors that must be taken into account is the fact that hypodermosis is closely linked to extensive animal breeding systems, with large open spaces in which the animals are free to roam and can easily come into contact with flies.

The dynamics of *Hypoderma* spp. infestations are governed by various factors, especially the climate. During the exogenous phase, *Hypoderma* spp. requires moderate temperatures (20-25 °C), light and humidity for the fly to leave the puparium. Temperatures above 30 °C and the presence of cloudy and rainy days have a restrictive effect on the activity of adult flies.

These factors markedly affect the chronobiology of *Hypoderma*, thereby resulting in often significant variations from one region to another depending on the environmental conditions.

In southern Spain, where a temperate climate predominates, the cycle is 1-2 months in advance of that described in Central Europe, the same as in northern Spain. In southern Spain, *H. lineatum* flies from February to April/May, L1 larvae appear in the oesophagus between April and November/December, and L2 and L3 larvae can be found in the back between mid-November and late March.

This chronology is delayed somewhat in northern Spain, such that L1 larvae appear during the winter resting period in the majority of the provinces in this region.

3 Do they cause disease?

The clinical signs are limited and non-specific, with the appearance of "warbles" in winter or spring, depending on the region, being the most characteristic. However, during the flying period for hypoderma, the animals are seen to be restless as a result of the buzzing produced by the flies (similar to that of a bee) when they approach the animals to lay their eggs, although *H. lineatum* is less of a nuisance to cows than *H. bovis*. The lesions produced when the larvae penetrate the skin almost always go unnoticed.

Likewise, the negative repercussions for animal production (decreased milk yields, loss of appetite and growth retardation) are difficult to evaluate as they depend on various factors such as infective dose, age, health status, etc.

The most characteristic and significant lesions are dorsal subcutaneous nodules, which appear as well-defined semicircular lumps of varying size (as large as a walnut or larger), with regular borders and hard to the touch. These nodules present a clearly visible orifice some 2-6 mm in diameter, depending on the stage of development, in their apical part. Pressing this nodule with the fingers can release its serosanguineous or caseous contents, and a whitish, greyish or dark brown L3 larva may also be seen inside.

During the resting phase, *H. lineatum* L1 larvae appear in the oesophagus as cylindrical crystalline formations some 15 mm in length with rounded ends and enclosed in a translucent connective tissue. These formations cause deformations in the mucosa with a similar morphology to that of the larvae. These L1 larvae can be extracted by separating the keratinised mucosa from the underlying tissue and may be alive or dead, in which case they are more difficult to separate from surrounding tissue.

Although it may appear normal, the tissue surrounding the larva is often oedematous, with haemorrhagic trajectories.

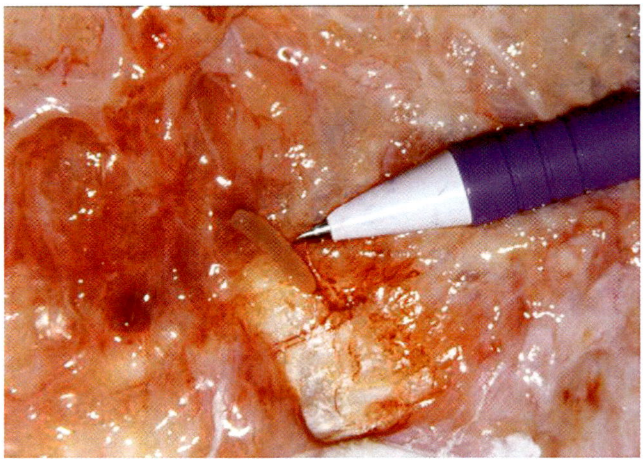

Hypoderma lineatum larvae tend to be detected in the oesophagus accidentally during carcass processing in an abattoir or during a highly systematic necropsy. They are readily identified as several are usually found in the same organ, with a size of more than one centimetre and with or without a surrounding reaction. Extraction is easy and allows the diagnosis to be confirmed due to the specific characteristics of the larvae. *Image courtesy of Dr. P. Morrondo.*

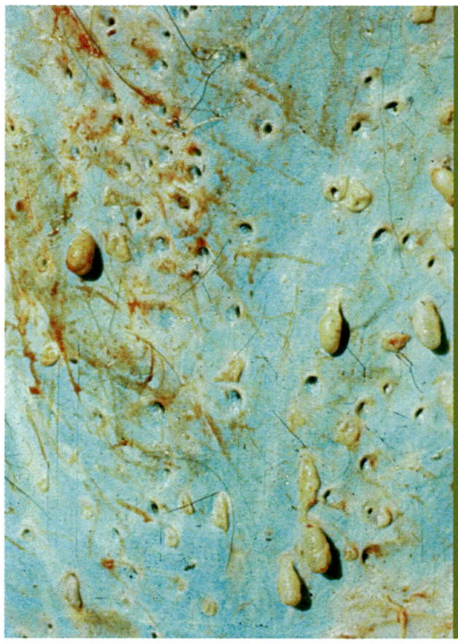

The presence of nodules in the skin is greater in young animals as individual resistance builds up as a result of successive reinfestation. Greater contact with the parasites leads to a stronger response, thus leading to isolation and death of the larvae and, consequently, a reduction in the number that become implanted in the back. *Image courtesy of Dr. C. Novoa.*

47 What are the risks of treating hypodermosis in winter?

After spraying of a group of cows and calves with an organophosphorus agent, the younger animals begin to exhibit ptyalism and some lie listless, with tremor and clear dyspnoea. They begin to suffer seizures within one hour and the youngest animals die. The vet confirms that the concentration of the product has not been calculated correctly and applies atropine and liver protectors to all animals treated. The following day some adult cows are prostrate with paralysis of their hind third and others are lame in their hind third. Corticosteroid treatment allows the majority to recover mobility after 2 to 3 days.

1. What causes the lameness in the older animals?
2. Why should hypodermosis not be treated in winter?
3. Are hypodermosis vaccines being developed?

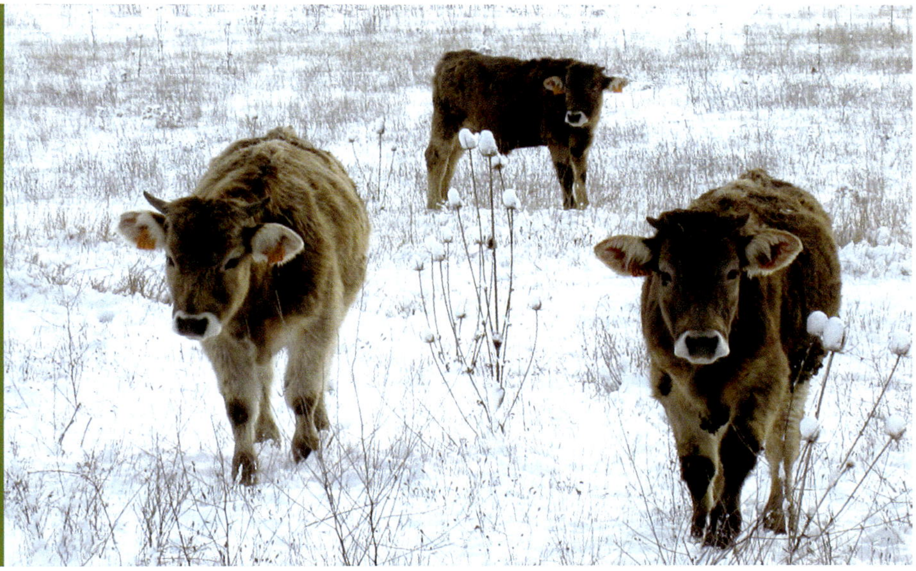

1 What causes the lameness in the older animals?

Undesirable reactions sometimes occur after treatment. The resulting problems represent a drawback, especially as farmers tend to withdraw their collaboration, thus interfering with the theoretical hypodermosis control measures.

Although the frequency of intolerance-type phenomena is low, their effects can be dramatic and serious, occasionally proving fatal. Although reactions can occur at any time of year, they appear to be more common between December and February as the L1 larvae accumulate higher quantities of antigenic and toxic substances during these months.

The onset of such incidents post-treatment is usually fast, more often than not on the same day the drug is administered and, although the most common manifestations are salivation, colic and diarrhoea, other signs such as oesophagitis, tympanites and locomotor alterations, which result in paresis and lameness, may also occur.

2 Why should hypodermosis not be treated in winter?

Although the path followed to reach the back is not known exactly, it appears that *H. lineatum* migrates via the diaphragm, caudal edge of the ribs, thoracic cavity and intercostal muscles before finally reaching the subcutaneous connective tissue in the dorsal region.

One of the keys to successful control, namely applying treatment at the most appropriate moment, is directly related to the chronobiology of the hypoderma flies in a specific region.

Although there are no "magistral formulations" and administration guidelines should be adapted to each specific region or zone, generally speaking treatment should be applied once the flying period of the flies has finished, thereby coinciding with the onset of the parasite's cycle inside the host. This prevents the animals from becoming reinfested with the eggs deposited after premature treatment, for example. Moreover, it acts against smaller larvae than those already present at the resting sites, thereby preventing the destruction and death of these larger larvae, which tend to release higher quantities of the antigens potentially responsible for undesired reactions.

The specific period varies by region. However, generally speaking, treatment should be applied around 2-3 months after the flying period of the flies has finished.

3 Are hypodermosis vaccines being developed?

Although chemoprophylaxis continues to be the most widespread method for controlling hypodermosis, other methods whose application could be a viable alternative in the future should be taken into consideration.

Thus, there is currently no "vaccine" against hypodermosis, but several promising studies may well pass from the purely experimental stage to field trials in the mid-term.

H. lineatum L1 antigens that stimulate resistance of the host to infestation are known to exist. This has encouraged work to develop protective vaccines based in the fractions obtained from the first larval phase of *Hypoderma*. Indeed, numerous protection studies have demonstrated the possibility of markedly reducing the number of hypoderma larvae in "vaccinated" animals. One of the most immunogenic such substances is hypodermin.

As a result, hypodermosis prevention in the most recent studies has aimed at achieving protection by immunisation. It has been shown that use of a raw antigen obtained from *H. lineatum* L1 larvae confers a degree of 95 % protection. However, despite this unquestionable protective efficacy, there are currently no authorised vaccines. It should also be noted that a protein known as hypodermin A has been obtained using recombination techniques and vaccine trials that may offer the possibility of immunoprophylaxis-based hypodermosis control are underway.

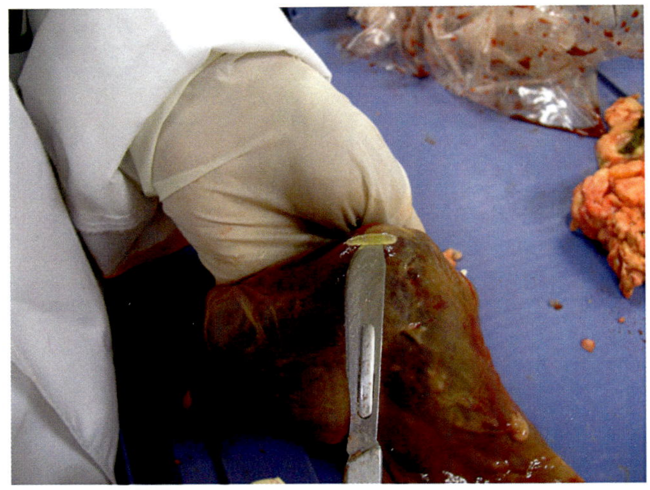

Continual and long-term contact with *Hypoderma* larvae during subcutaneous migration and maturation triggers an immune reaction from which various antigens with a promising future in immunoprophylaxis have been characterised.
Image courtesy of Dr. P. Morrondo.

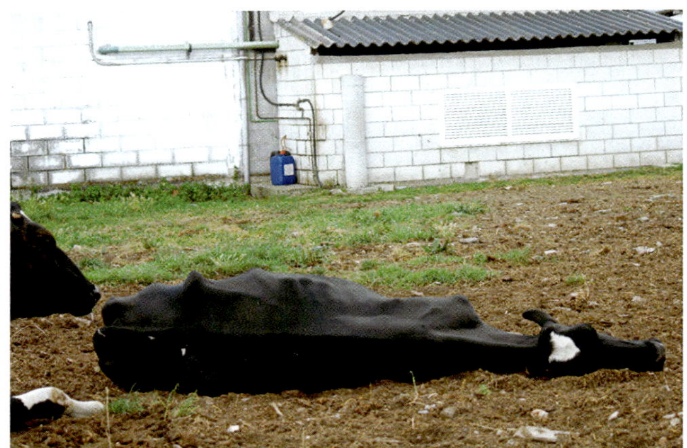

An anaphylactic reaction associated with the accidental or deliberate bursting of the hypodermic nodules may appear. Larval intestinal fluids and haemolymph produce a similar reaction in the body to phosphoric acid ester poisoning, namely tearing, dry cough, dyspnoea, muscle tremor and continual defecation/urination.

4

Q&A on cutaneous parasitoses

Chapter 4

Q&A on cutaneous parasitoses

Introduction

This chapter, which is dedicated to cutaneous parasitoses, describes various aspects of the most important processes in cattle. However, it should be noted that some of the diseases presented are not exclusive to this animal species and can also appear in other hosts, including humans.

The chapter comprises 13 clinical cases, three of which are dedicated to the different types of mange, two to hypodermosis, and five to the parasitoses produced by lice (true and false), ticks, adult diptera and myiasis, which are important in the majority of Latin American countries where it is called "*gusanera*". Moreover, three clinical cases describe processes whose aetiology involved nematodes and protozoa. These have become increasingly important in the past years even though pathology textbooks have described such processes since the late 19th and early 20th centuries.

The importance of many of the diseases described in this chapter 4 lies in the pathogenicity of the agents responsible for them, such as mange mites, "warbles" and other arthropods. Without underestimating the possible pathogenic role of ticks, flies, mosquitoes, etc., these parasites and insects are much more relevant at our latitude due to their ability to act as vectors for numerous pathogens of various types (viruses, bacteria, parasites). It should also be stressed that the more or less prominent climate changes, which have occurred recently have bestowed greater importance on those (animal or human) diseases whose transmission involves an arthropod.

Mange is specially important amongst cutaneous parasitoses. Despite being well known, it requires a much greater effort to ensure an efficient control that is not solely based in chemotherapy/chemoprophylaxis. Specifically, three clinical cases, which summarise the various types of mange, its aetiology, mode of transmission and detection, control and prevention methods, are dedicated specifically to this type of disease. These parasitoses continue to play a key role in animal diseases.

The vector role played by arthropods is undoubtedly highly important. Numerous viral or bacterial pathogens, etc. require the intervention of arthropods, mainly haematophages, to pass from one animal to another. The transmission role of mosquitoes, ticks and flies, amongst others, confers a marked protagonism on arthropods in various human and animal parasitoses. Moreover, the importance of arthropods in the transmission of certain diseases is increasing due to the modifications suffered by their habitats derived from climate change. It favours the geographical expansion of many of these processes which were, until recently, restricted to tropical and subtropical regions. However, it must not be forgotten that some arthropods also trigger clinical processes of some importance resulting from allergic and toxic reactions, etc.

Finally, there is a further group of parasites which must also be taken into consideration in this chapter on cutaneous parasitoses. It is the group of nematodes with a complex biological cycle (some of which are relatively unknown), which produce more or less evident cutaneous lesions that, *a priori*, are not initially assigned to nematodes. Similarly, this chapter also describes *Besnoitia besnoiti* infection, which appears to be emerging in some parts of Spain and presents highly characteristic clinical signs.

Agents for cutaneous parasitoses in cattle

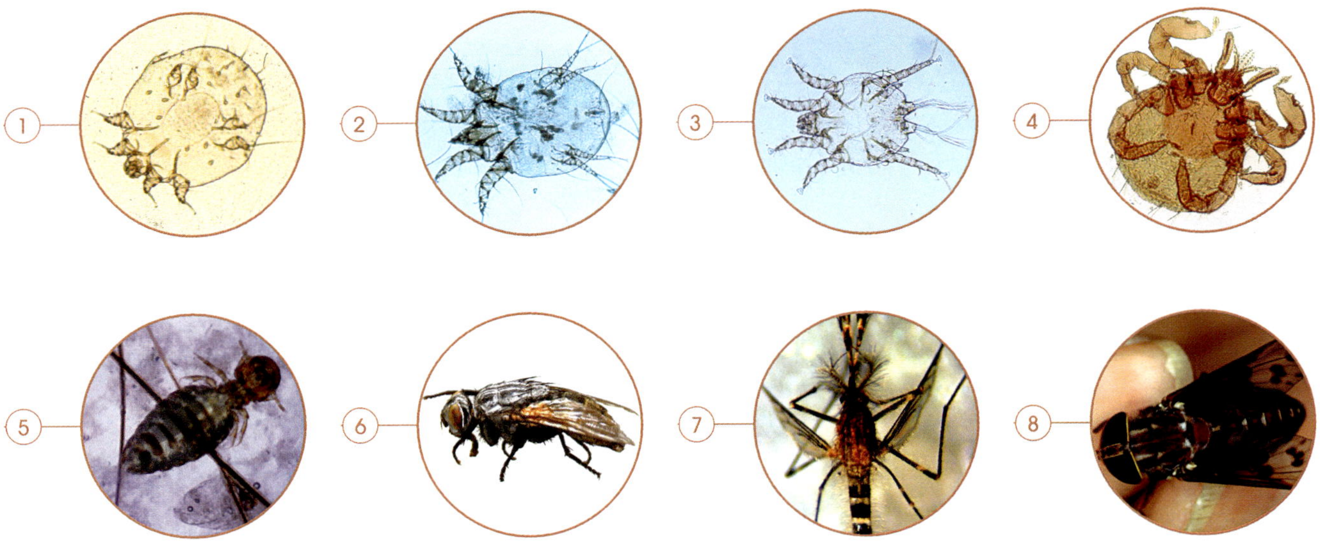

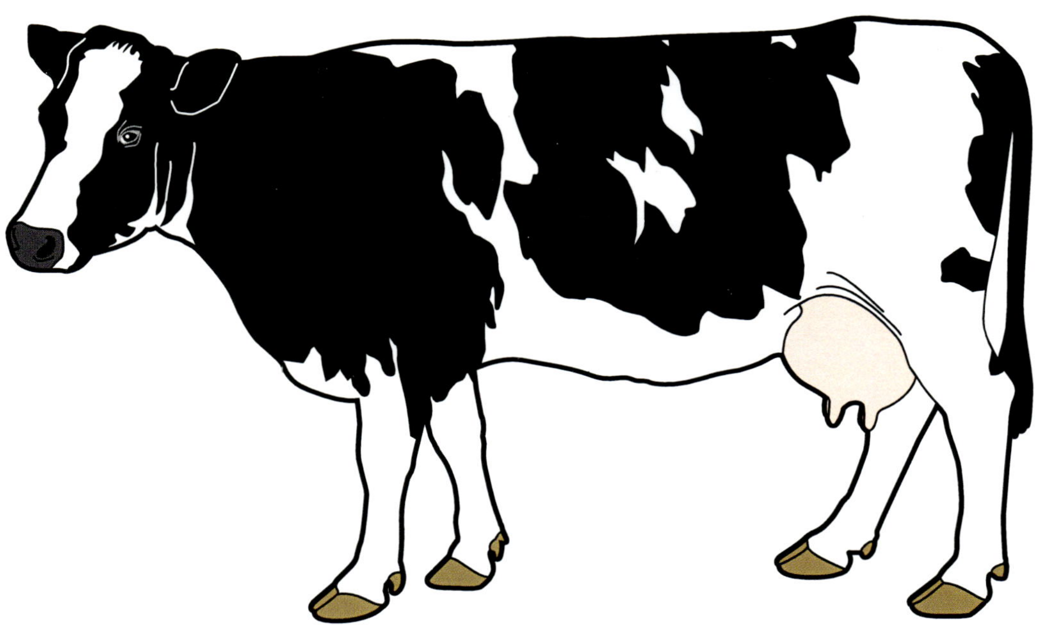

1. *Sarcoptes*
2. *Psoroptes*
3. *Chorioptes*
4. Tick
5. *Werneckiella*
6. *Wohlfahrtia*
7. Culicida
8. Horsefly

48 Which mange is found in cattle?

The owner of a beef farm decides to increase the number of animals after August. The new individuals are dewormed with an anthelmintic upon arrival but no additional quarantine measures are put into place. In autumn the farmer notes that many of the animals are restless and present lesions on both sides of the neck, the withers, the base of the neck and others even at the base of the tail. Some animals have lost weight. A visual examination of the affected regions of skin shows epidermal scaling, alopecia and dry brownish-grey scabs. Moreover, some animals have very swollen skin with a rough and warty appearance.

1. What parasitic process is consistent with this description?
2. How should the presumptive diagnosis be confirmed?
3. What are the characteristics of cattle mange?

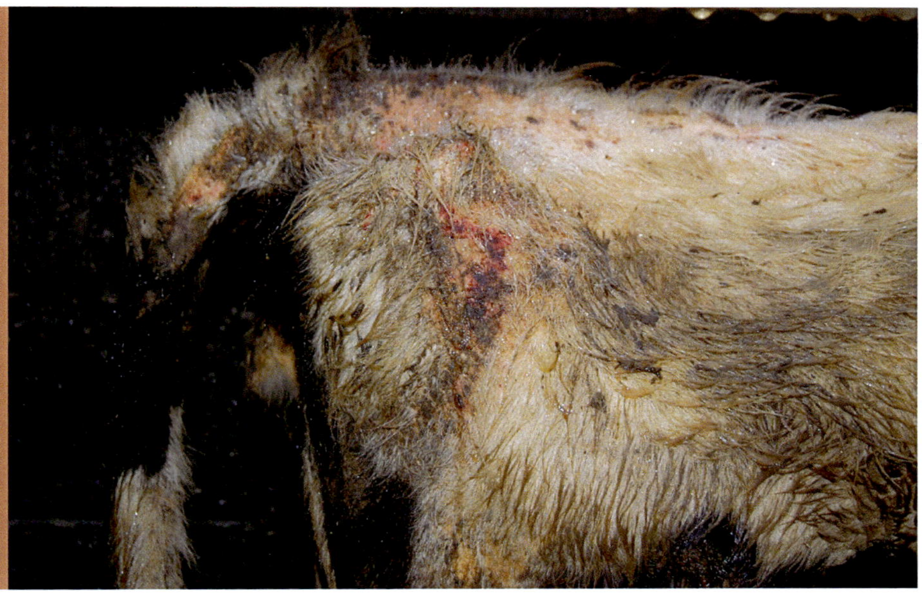

Image courtesy of Dr. S. Mitchel.

1 What parasitic process is consistent with this description?

The characteristics described in this case are almost certainly representative of an outbreak of mange.

Mange mites generally spread between animals very rapidly and easily. Once contagion has occurred, and under suitable conditions, various generations of mites can persist in the same host, thus leading to the characteristic manifestations of this disease. Considering that these parasites multiply actively under favourable circumstances, the infestation propagates rapidly. Thus, shortly after acquisition and incorporation of the new animals, and in the absence of health control measures, the first cases appear. The predisposing factors for mange include poor hygiene, low temperatures and humidity, as well as overcrowding, which favours contact between the animals.

Other diseases can also present similar clinical signs to mange. This must be taken into account when performing a differential diagnosis in the event of an outbreak with these characteristics. For example, surface pruritus and eczema caused by lice can be distinguished from mange as it is generally easy to detect these ectoparasites on the skin (adults, eggs, etc.). Some types of mycosis should also be considered. These are characterised by the appearance of rounded grey or yellowish scabs, with alopecia on some regions of the skin.

The most common mange found in cattle is psoroptic mange, which causes lesions in specific areas of the body. In this case, the characteristics of the outbreak described are compatible with bovine psoroptic mange.

2 How should the presumptive diagnosis be confirmed?

Irrespective of the information provided by the laboratory concerning the nature and causative agent of a disease, a methodical study of the clinical signs should provide sufficient evidence to help the vet reach a diagnosis. In other words, the symptoms that reveal a functional disorder or anatomical change in the animal should themselves define a presumptive diagnosis. As such, the clinical manifestations, such as the sudden onset, high contagiousness and rapid expansion of the initially affected regions allow mange to be suspected in cattle, even before the presence of mange mites is confirmed.

One of the most notable clinical signs is pruritus, which is usually much more intense than in other skin conditions. During the initial stages of the process, it is useful to note the location of skin lesions, which differ according to the type of mange concerned. Thus, sarcoptic mange lesions tend to start on the head, although they subsequently spread to nearby regions, whereas the lesions in chorioptic mange are found surrounding the limbs and anal region and in psoroptic mange they are found on protected parts of the body. In short, the three forms of mange can be distinguished by their clinical signs.

Psoroptic mange can also be diagnosed visually as the mites responsible are relatively large (up to 0.8 mm in length). In contrast, the other types of mange (including psoroptic mange, if necessary) need a microscopic study to identify the type of mite involved. To this end it is necessary to take skin samples, such as scabs and flakes, or to scrape a piece of skin off with a knife, scissors or scalpel.

For the microscopic study, the samples obtained should be placed on a Petri dish, heated in an oven at 30 °C for 5-6 hours and the presence of the parasites confirmed under a stereoscopic microscope. The mites can be seen as clear, round or moving dots. Each mite species is easily recognisable by its morphological differences.

If skin scabs are to be examined, they must be immersed in 10 % potassium hydroxide for at least 5 hours to soften and clarify them. In the event of an emergency, if an immediate examination is required, the scabs can be boiled for 10-20 minutes in a 10-fold greater volume of 0.5 % potassium hydroxide. Thin skin sections, which are examined on compression plates, can also be analysed.

3 What are the characteristics of cattle mange?

The most relevant types of mange in cattle are psoroptic, sarcoptic and chorioptic.

Psoroptic mange initially causes an intense pruritus in the animals and tends to be located on both sides of the neck, although regions around the withers, base of the neck and base of the tail may also be affected. It can spread from these sites to other parts of the body, such as the chest, base of the horns, back and even all over the body on occasions. The lesions observed on the skin are nodules, exudate secretions, increased epidermal scaling, alopecia and dry brown-grey scabs. The skin becomes coriaceous and swells, acquiring a rough and warty appearance. The clinical signs occasionally worsen in winter but improve in summer. If the process spreads all over the body the animals lose weight and can die.

Main distribution zones for bovine mange

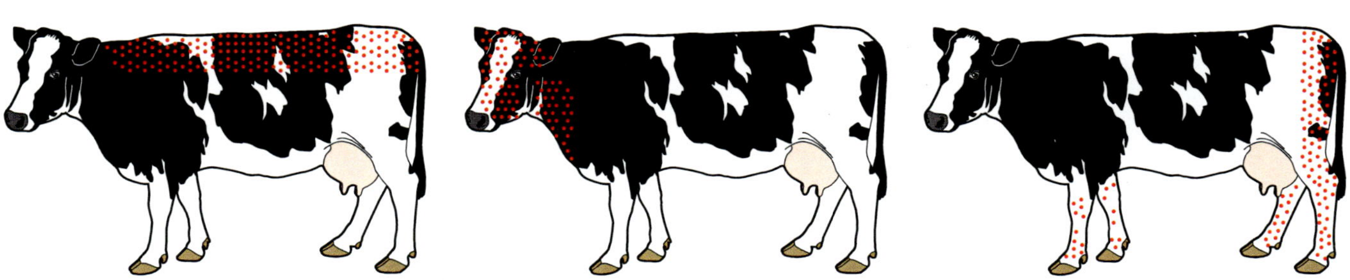

Psoroptic Sarcoptic Chorioptic

Sarcoptic mange provokes intense pruritus, especially on the face, neck, shoulders and hind third. This process is common in animals stabled over winter. It is characterised by the appearance of non-follicular papules and vesicles, followed by scabs, folds and alopecia. Serous or purulent exudates are occasionally seen due to secondary infections.

Chorioptic mange is also known as "tail mange". It is usually located in the hindquarters and close to the base of the tail, although in poorly kept animals it can affect almost the whole body (back, neck, loins) due to spreading of the primary foci. Cases characterised by coronitis, hoof and muzzle infections, anorexia and decreased milk production have also been described.

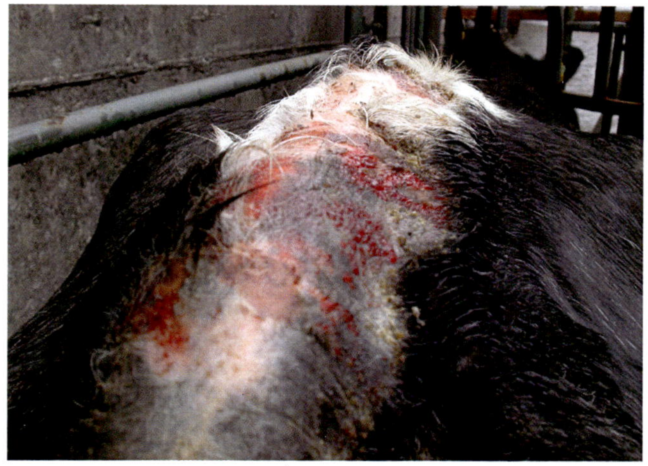

Psoroptes equi bovis causes psoroptic mange in cattle. The first symptom is pruritus. It preferentially presents on the sides of the neck, on its upper part, on the withers, on the base of the neck, in the fringe and at the base of the tail. Injuries caused by the animals themselves when they attempt to calm the pruritus by brushing or scratching themselves against any available surface are common.

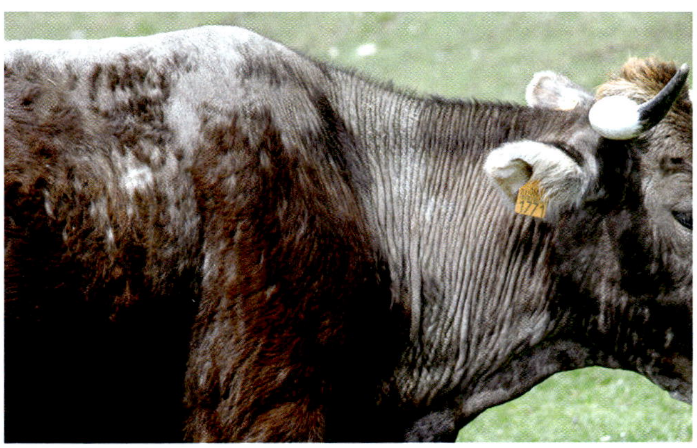

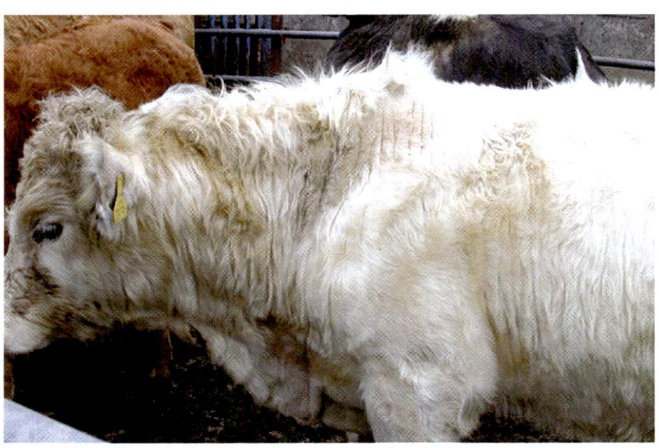

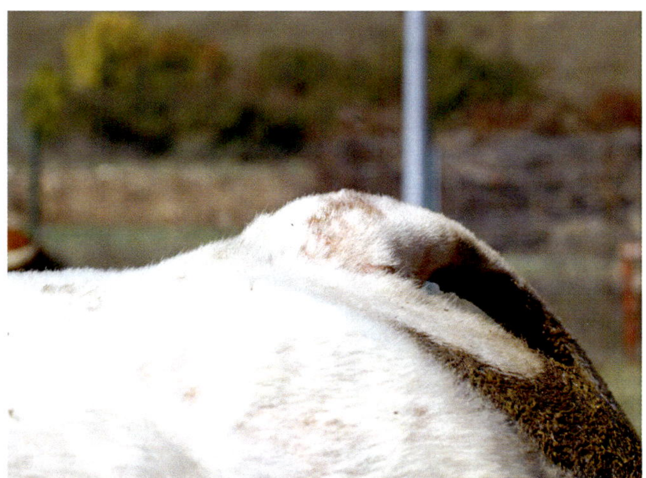

Chorioptes bovis bovis causes chorioptic mange. It is also known as "tail mange) and is common in cold stabling periods. This mange tends to be located in the hindquarters and close to the base of the tail, although it can spread all over the body (back, neck, loins) if the skin of the animal concerned is not cared for.

Sarcoptes scabiei bovis causes sarcoptic mange. It provokes intense pruritus, especially on the face, neck, shoulders and hind third. This mite is also known as "burrowing mite) as it forms tunnels in the dermis of its hosts.

49 How is mange transmitted?

An unusual case of chorioptic mange is detected in February on a dairy farm on which 82 % of new animals are affected. The cows present very extensive skin lesions with respect to the typical location, ranging from the tail to the back, loins and legs. The pruritus exhibited by the animals is more intense than would be normal for this type of mange. Some animals have lost weight and a marked decrease in milk production has been noted.

1. How were the animals infected?
2. What measures should be taken to prevent transmission of mange?
3. How do the biological cycles of the different mange mites differ?

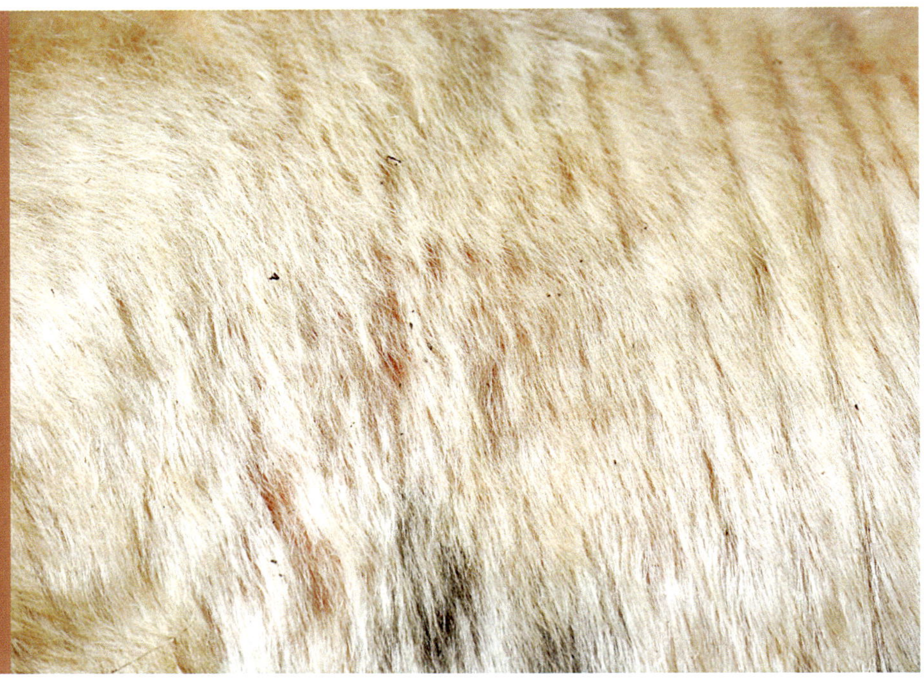

1 How were the animals infected?

Chorioptic mange is located in clearly demarcated regions of the body (base of the tail, ischiorectal fossa, pastern) and it only invades the hindquarters, back, perineum, loins and even the scrotum and udder if the process is ignored for a long period of time. This disease can persist for several months without major consequences at warmer times of year but worsens in the cold season. Under these circumstances it spreads from the initial regions to the hindquarters, back and shoulders. Practical experience has shown that mange is more common and spreads more rapidly when animals have less opportunity to graze.

Transmission usually occurs in cowsheds by direct contact between healthy and infected animals, although indirect contagion via cleaning or handling tools (examination gloves) may also occur. Chorioptic mange is poorly contagious.

The predisposing factors for mange include lack of hygiene, coexistence of other processes (mainly cutaneous, but also digestive, etc.), unsuitable nutrition and climate. Healthy and asymptomatic carrier animals are of great epidemiological importance as they are a constant source of contagion for the rest of the herd.

2 What measures should be taken to prevent transmission of mange?

Mange treatment should be accompanied by measures that facilitate mite control. The onset or reappearance of such processes can be prevented by following a few general guidelines.

Cleaning of the cowsheds and materials used is usually very effective in prophylaxis. It should also be remembered that some mite species cannot survive for very long outside

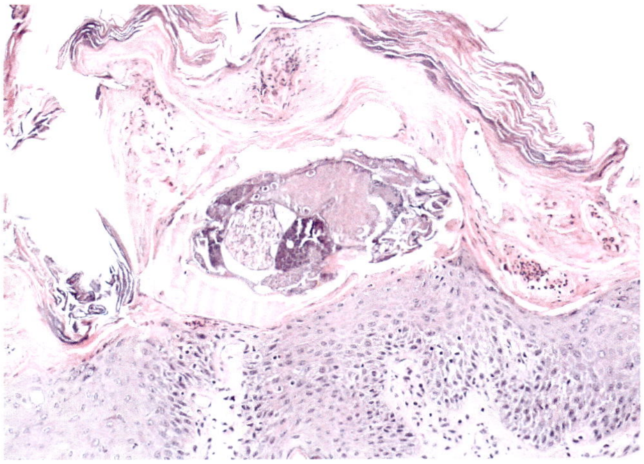

An impregnated *Sarcoptes* female excavates a single twisting gallery that increases in length by around 2-3 mm a day to a maximum of 35-50 mm. They dig tunnels in the skin, which produces a mechanical irritant action and releases metabolites and toxins that act on the nerve endings. This causes an intense pruritus.

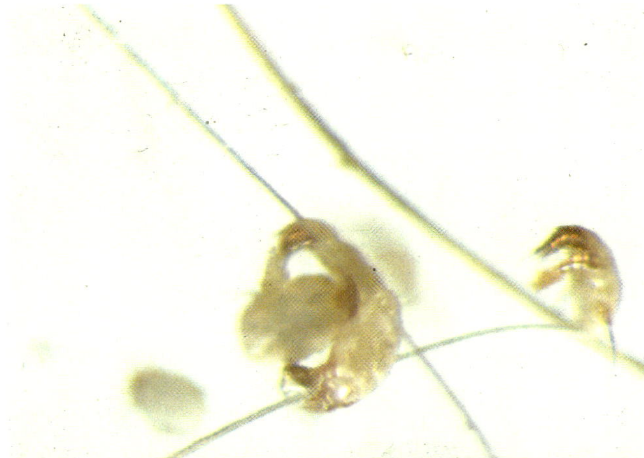

Mites only survive for a very short period of time outside the host. The most resistant is *Psoroptes*, which can survive for up to 48-70 days at low temperatures with a humidity of 75 %, although it only remains infective for 4 days.

the host, therefore cowsheds can be freed from mites by keeping them empty for around 4 weeks. There are, however, some exceptions, with *Psoroptes* spp., for example, being able to survive for more than two months outside the host. It is also advisable to avoid a high density of animals per surface unit. The main form of contagion is via direct contact. As both cold and humidity are also predisposing factors, it should theoretically be possible to prevent the problem with large installations and appropriate environmental conditions.

Any measures that facilitate direct contact of topical acaricide drugs with the parasites are highly advisable (removal of scabs, scales, etc.). Although systemic drugs are also used, their topical counterparts (spraying, sprinkling, etc.), which act directly on the most affected regions, should preferentially be used. An appropriate control of these diseases cannot be expected if the acaricide treatment is only applied once. As such, treatment should be repeated according to the biological cycle of the various types of mites and the activity of the drugs administered, as some also have ovicidal properties.

3 How do the biological cycles of the different mange mites differ?

The three most important genera of mange mites in cattle present very different morphological characteristics that aid their identification. From a biological viewpoint, each type of mite also evolves differently, although they share some characteristics.

Sarcoptes species are very small at around 0.25-0.6 mm in length. They penetrate the host's epidermis, creating galleries or tunnels. Females can lay 3-5 eggs per day for around 30 days. The larvae hatch within a week and transform into nymphs around 10-12 days later. They complete the cycle, which lasts for approximately 15-17 days, after sexual differentiation and fertilisation.

Psoroptes species are usually 0.4-0.8 mm in length. They are also known as scab mites. They do not penetrate the epidermis. Their cycle takes place on the tegumentary surface over a period of between 10 and 12 days, although it can last for up to 3 months.

Chorioptes species are morphologically very similar to *Psoroptes* but smaller, with a length of around 0.3-0.5 mm. They live on the skin and feed on detritus. In contrast to species from the other two genera, their biological cycle lasts for up to 2-3 weeks.

It should also be remembered that bovines can also be infested by *Demodex* (*D. bovis*), although such infestations normally pass unnoticed. Demodicosis results in the appearance of small nodules and pustules of varying sizes (ranging from the size of a pin head to that of a hazelnut) on the host's trunk, neck and back, with numerous mites in the centre of a purulent-caseous mass.

Comparative morphology of adult mange mites

	Psoroptes	*Sarcoptes*	*Chorioptes*	*Demodex*
	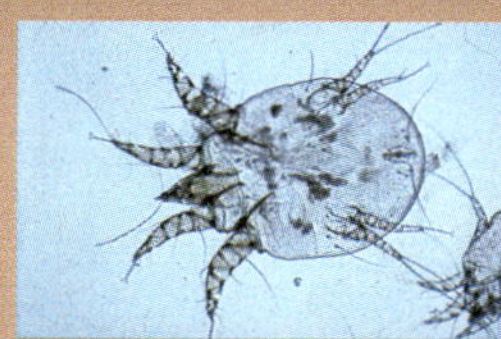	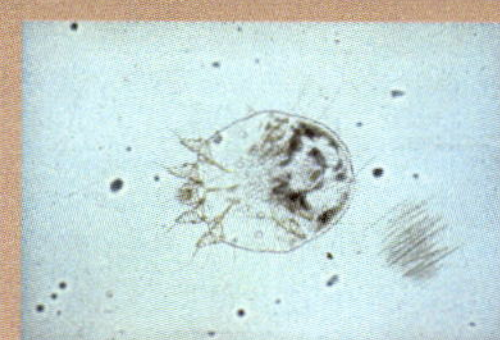	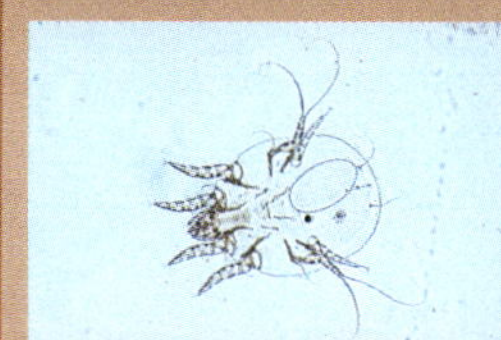	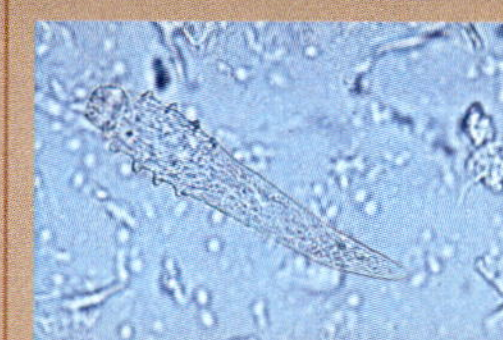
Morphology	• Oval body. • Elongated conical head.	• Rounded shape. • Small.	• Elongated body. • Slightly conical head.	• Vermiform. • With transversal striation.
Length	0.4-0.8 mm	0.25-0.6 mm	0.3-0.5 mm	0.3-0.4 mm
Morphological characteristics	Suckers on a triarticulate peduncle.	Cuticle with striations, triangular scales and spines.	Peduncles very short and unjointed on the legs.	Highly atrophied knuckles ending in spines.
	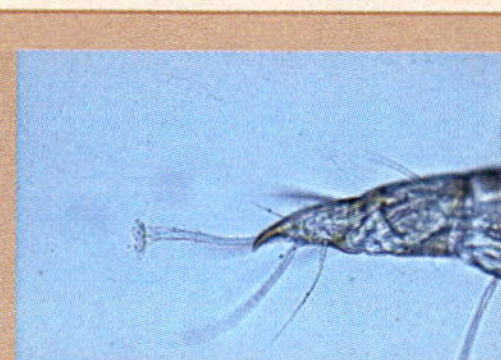	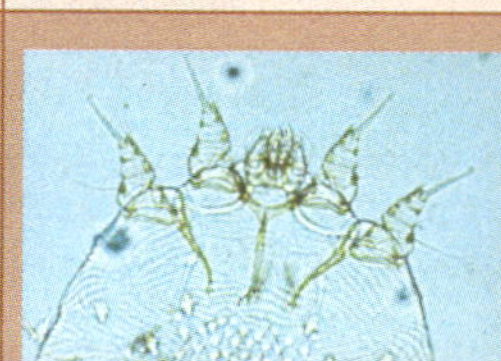	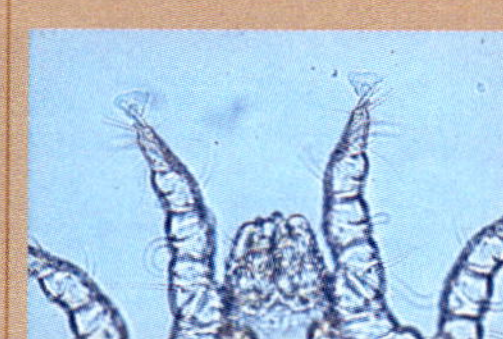	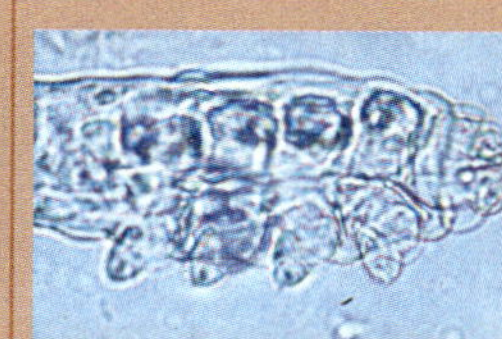
Biological cycle	10-12 days	15-17 days	21 days	18-24 days
Biological characteristics	• Lives on the tegumentary surface and is highly mobile. • Feeds on serosity and scales. • The female lays round 5 eggs per day for the 30-40 days of life. • The eggs hatch after an incubation period of 1-3 days to give hexapod larvae. The larvae mould after 2-3 days, passing through two nymphal stages. • The nymphs feed and produce the first females in 3-4 days and males in 6 days.	• Burrowing mite. • After incubating in the galleries for 7 days, hexapod larvae, which can also excavate small tunnels perpendicular to the maternal gallery or exit to the surface of the skin, hatch from the eggs. • Nine days after birth the larvae moult to nymphs and moult twice more in the next 3-6 days before becoming adults.	• Lives on the tegumentary surface. • Feeds on serosity and scales. • Lays its eggs in scabs on the surface of the skin. These eggs hatch to larvae after incubation for 3-5 days. • Larvae feed for a varying amount of time (3-12 days) and moult every 3-5 days, passing through two nymphal stages before becoming adults.	• Lives in the hair follicles. • Develops in four stages. • Feeds on cell detritus. • A hexapod larva that moults into an octapod nymph hatches from the eggs. Finally, the nymph transforms into an adult, which also has eight legs.

50 Can mange mites be eliminated?

The animals on a beef cattle feedlot are clearly affected by a fungal process. In some animals the pruritus is very intense and they also present lesions typical of sarcoptic mange on their face and neck. During the visit, the vet notes that the animal caretakers present highly pruriginous papules and twisting trajectories on their hands and forearms. The animals had been treated with subcutaneous ivermectin, although some calves continued to present lesions on the face, neck and shoulders.

1. What is the recommended treatment for mange?
2. Can mange mites survive outside the host?
3. Can animals infect the vet?

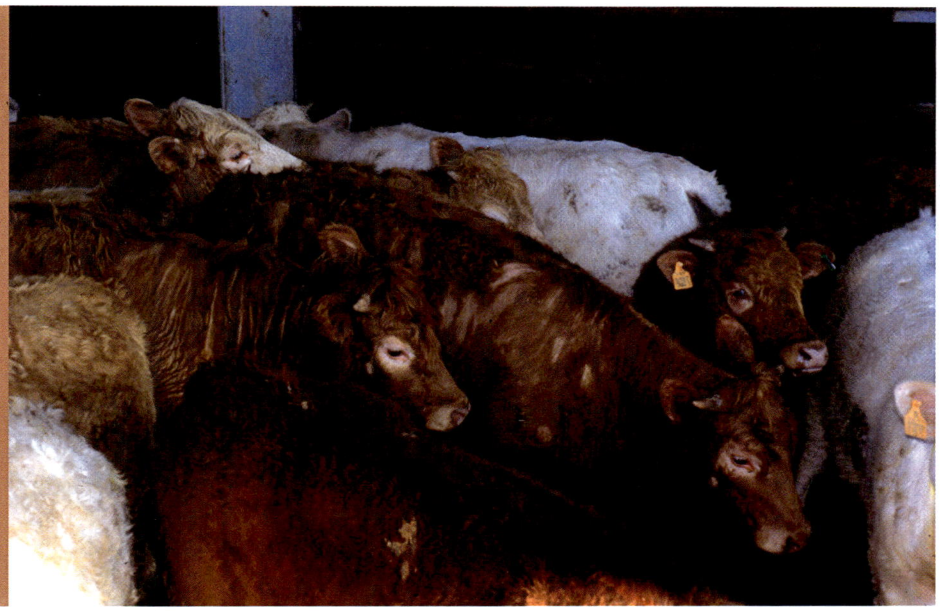

1 What is the recommended treatment for mange?

A series of general guidelines concerning the hygiene and disinfection of cowsheds, harnesses, various tools, etc. should be followed when treating mange.

In light of the survival capacity of the mites, a cowshed can be considered to be mite-free if it has been left empty for approximately one month. However, it should be remembered that *Psoroptes* spp. can survive for more than two months outside the host.

The efficacy of the topical drugs used is higher if the scales and scabs on the skin are softened and removed beforehand, and the hair in affected regions should also be removed if possible. Acaricides should be applied to both the lesions and the apparently healthy neighbouring regions. Obviously, if mange is very widespread the whole body surface area should be treated.

Numerous formulations of different products with acaricide activity are currently available, therefore it is advisable to use the simplest application, preferably one that is less stressful than a traditional anti-mange dip. Topical products (non-systemic acaricides), which are applied as a spray, those that are applied to specific regions (spot-on) or over the length of the back (pour-on), and those administered subcutaneously are perhaps the most important. Acaricides are considered to be systemic when administered orally, topically or by injection.

Mange can also be treated by spraying or by immersion of the animals in facilities suitable for such dips. Spray treatment tends to be tedious but can be applied to small groups. However, dips are more effective, although handling of the animals may be more complicated and the treatment more expensive (large volumes of water are required and

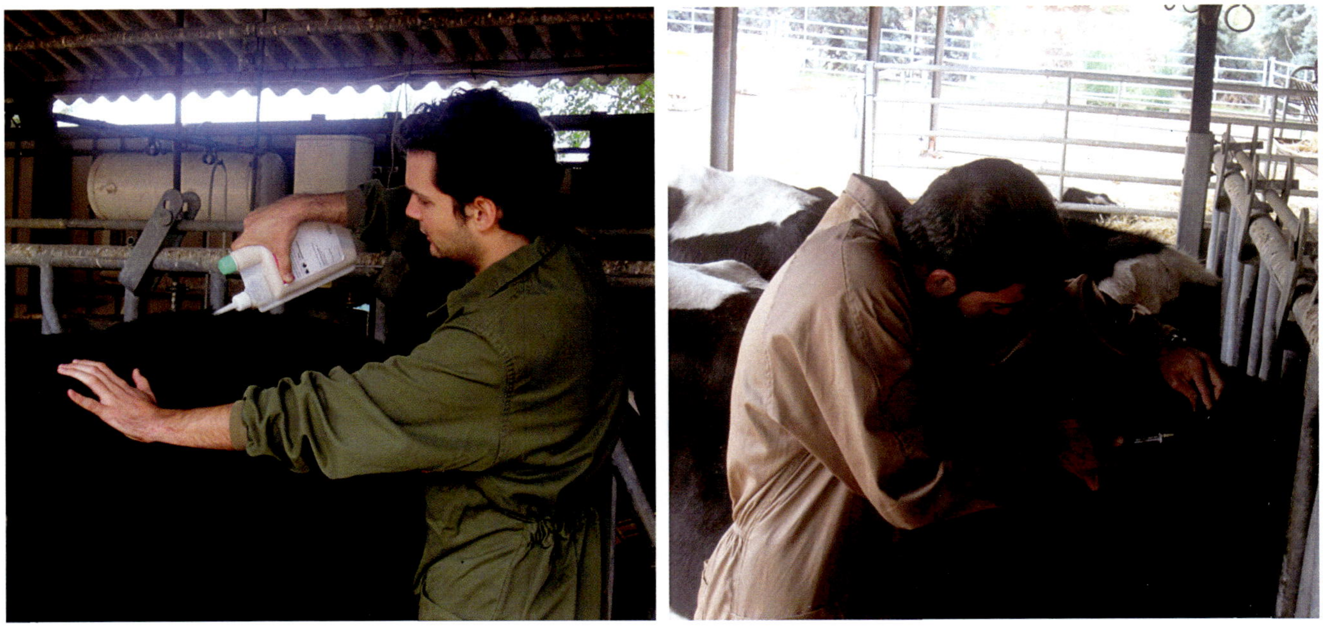

If clinical cases of mange appear in most of the herd, treatment must be applied to all animals to avoid the presence of carriers. If non-ovicidal injectable products are used, transcutaneous treatment should be repeated after 7-14 days.

residues must be disposed of following the safety guidelines). Although a single treatment may be sufficient, it is advisable to repeat treatment at 10-14 days and keep treated animals isolated from the others.

In severe cases, injectable treatment should be accompanied by the administration of pour-on acaricide drugs once the skin has recovered, as a single application of an injectable acaricide does not eliminate the parasites completely.

Treatment should be repeated according to the biological cycles of the various mite species involved, and the fact that most acaricides do not have ovicidal activity. Moreover, the milk or meat suppression period for each product must be taken into account, as should the possible drawbacks of treating lactating or gestating animals.

The time and frequency of anti-mange treatments depend on the circumstances of each individual animal. In most clinical cases, however, it is advisable to repeat the treatment a second time in order to control the problem for the stabling period. Although all animals should be treated at the same time, if they are treated in groups or batches each group must be kept isolated from the others, with no possibility of coming into contact with untreated animals.

The substances that can be applied topically include organophosphorus compounds (coumaphos, diazinon, trichlorfon, phoxim) and pyrethroids (cypermethrin or deltamethrin). Chlorphenvinphos, amitraz and even closantel also present acaricide activity. Although some of these drugs have no withdrawal period (coumaphos), the majority require a period of 21-28 days (toxaphene, phosmet).

Since their initial commercialisation, macrocyclic lactones have been widely used to treat animal mange, for both the psoroptic and sarcoptic varieties. Specifically, avermectins (ivermectin and doramectin) and milbemycins (moxidectin) are very effective when injected at a dose of 200 µg/kg, although they cannot be used in producing dairy cattle. Eprinomectin does not require a suppression period and can therefore be used to treat sarcoptic mange in lactating cows, with pour-on administration at a dose of 500 µg/kg. Transcutaneous administration to the back is also used, although injectable formulations are recommended for psoroptic mange. However, irrespective of the product chosen, the exact dose must be calculated to ensure that the animals are not underdosed, which can lead to the development of resistance to antiparasitic drugs in mange.

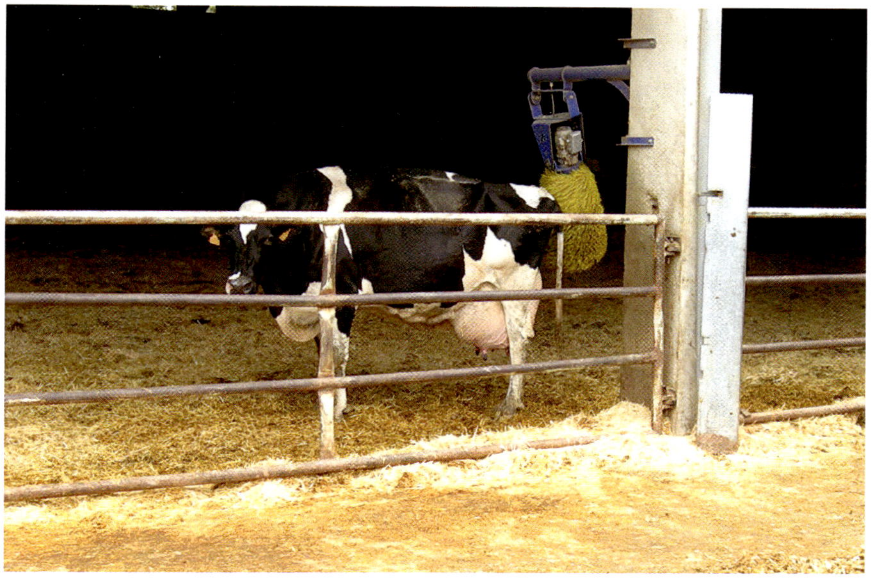

As contagion occurs upon direct contact between healthy and infected animals, or by mechanical transmission via scratchers, tools, etc., disinfestation of the facilities and zootechnical material is vital. Disinfestation must be performed regularly using authorised products.

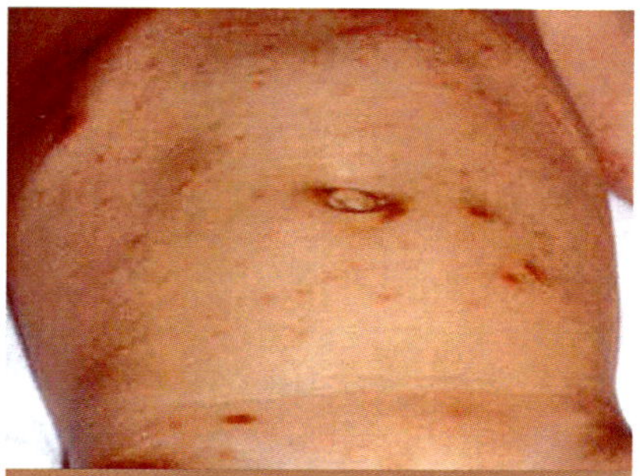

People can become infected upon contact with infested animals. This process normally remits spontaneously within a few days, although in the event of an inefficient immune response it can spread and lesions can appear on the arms and abdomen.

2 Can mange mites survive outside the host?

Mites can survive for some time outside the host depending on the temperature, humidity, sunlight and other environmental conditions. Low temperatures reduce the metabolic activity of the parasites, thus prolonging their survival. This characteristic is of some practical importance as it is not always possible to act against mites "hidden" in cracks in the cowshed walls. As a result, it is often necessary to maintain the cowshed free from animals for a specific time period in order to rid it of mites.

As all these factors affect the survival capacity of mites outside the host, the resistance of mites varies from one time to another. The least resistant species belong to the genus *Sarcoptes*, whereas *Psoroptes* spp., which can survive for more than two months (70 days) in the exterior, are the most resistant.

Various prophylactic measures should be followed to prevent contagion between animals. For example: the cowsheds should be cleaned, the bedding changed frequently, the tools and harnesses used with infected animals disinfected; infected/sick animals should be isolated, replacement animals examined and analysed before joining the herd, animals provided with appropriate amounts of feed, and a suitable number of animals per unit surface area should be established to prevent overcrowding.

3 Can animals infect the vet?

Sarcoptic mange can affect both domestic and farm animals, as well as some species of wild animals. The possible hosts for this type of mange include humans, with the variety *Sarcoptes scabiei* var. *hominis* being particularly relevant.

Animals infected with *Sarcoptes* can transmit their infection to humans, although the resulting infestation is usually transitory due to the host specificity of this mite. Consequently, anyone (such as a vet) who comes into contact with farm animals infected with *Sarcoptes*, either cattle or pigs, can also become infected. Sarcoptic mange of animal origin in humans can be distinguished from other types of mange by its rapid onset (around 48 hours) and other aspects, such as intense pruritus on the palms of the hands and forearms. Moreover, twisting and painful trajectories often present in the stomach region. The process is self-limiting and remits once exposure to the contagion source ceases.

Biological cycle of *Sarcoptes*

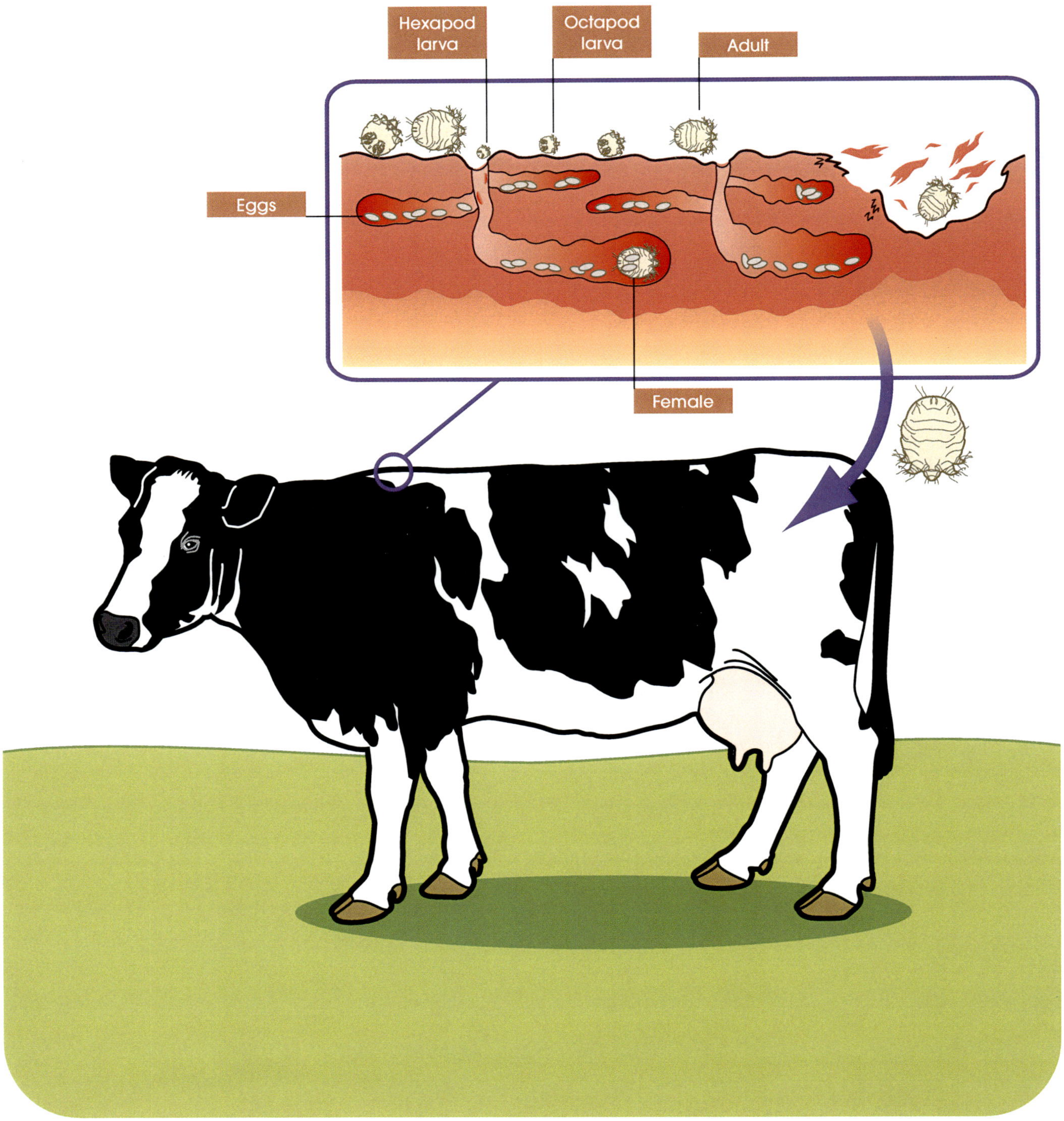

51 What clinical signs indicate the presence of lice in cattle?

The animals on a small farm in the north of Spain are overcrowded, dirty and have a poor coat. Some scratch and rub themselves vigorously. Easily identifiable nests of lice are commonly observed. The skin in those regions has been rubbed and scratched and is cracked; some animals even present secondary infections. The most affected animals are very thin. The owner states that the cows have been producing less milk since the process started and that even when lice cannot be seen directly they can easily be detected due to the presence of eggs in the hair.

1. What types of lice are found in cattle?
2. Are they a nuisance or can the animals live with them?
3. Do cattle and humans share the same lice species?
4. Can flies transmit lice between cows?

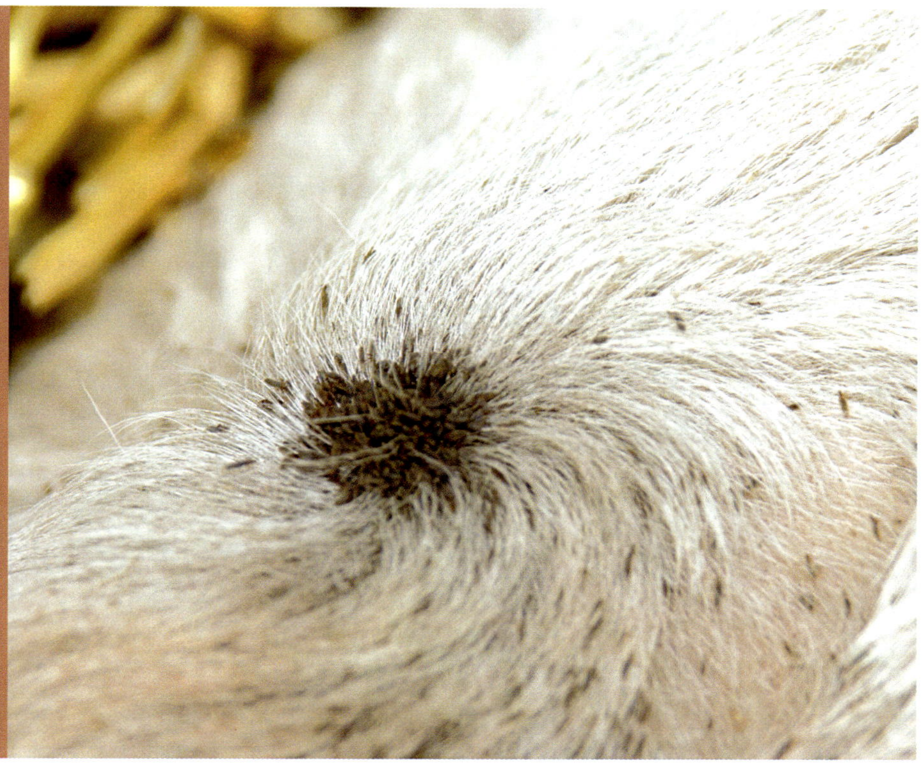

Image courtesy of the Clinic for Ruminants with Ambulatory and Herd Health Services, Ludwig Maximilians University.

1 What types of lice are found in cattle?

Cattle can be infested by various species of lice. These parasites can be mallophaga or false lice, which are chewing lice, or anoplura or true lice, which are sucking lice.

Amongst chewing lice, the most common and important is *Bovicola bovis*, the presence of which causes great discomfort in animals. *B. bovis* lives in colonies and can cause disorders of some importance. Females lay their eggs at the base of the hairs. After passing through three nymph stages adults complete the biological cycle in around 30 days, although this time period can vary with temperature and humidity. Adults measure between 1.2 and 1.4 mm in length, are whitish in colour and their head is almost as long as it is wide.

The most important anoplura, or true lice (sucking lice), in bovines are *Haematopinus eurysterunus*, *Linognathus vituli* and *Linognathus stenopsis*. They are slightly larger than mallophaga (measuring 2.5-2.7 mm in length), are yellow in colour and their head is narrow and elongated. Their cycle is complete in around 21 to 30 days.

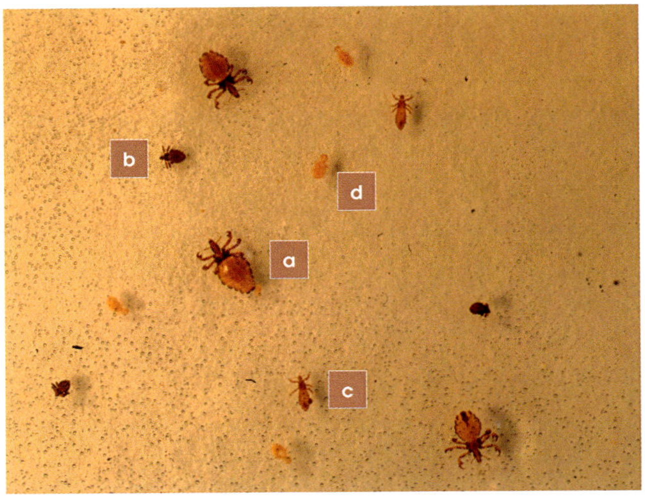

Lice exhibit high host specificity and are permanent ectoparasites. Although they vary in size and colour, they all have a dorsoventrally shortened body. They are known as large yellow louse (*Haematopinus*) (a), long-headed blue louse (*Linognathus*) (b), small yellow small-headed louse (*Solenopotes*) (c) and small yellow large-headed louse (*Bovicola*, the most common and harmful) (d).

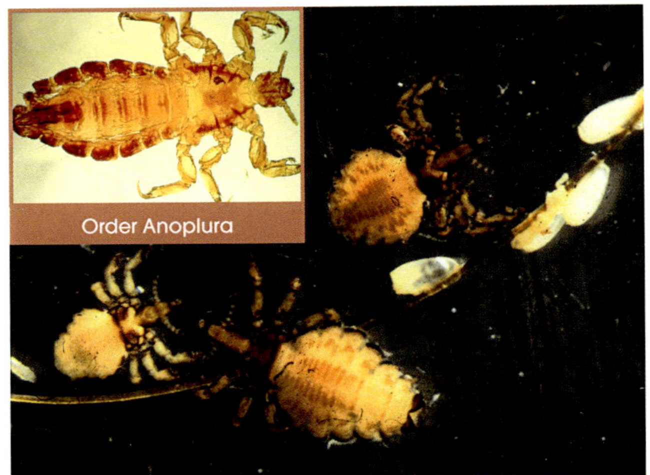

Anoplura (or sucking) lice are normally larger, measure more than 5 m in length, and have a small, pointed head with mouthparts in the apical part. Anoplura need to ingest blood in order for their eggs to mature.

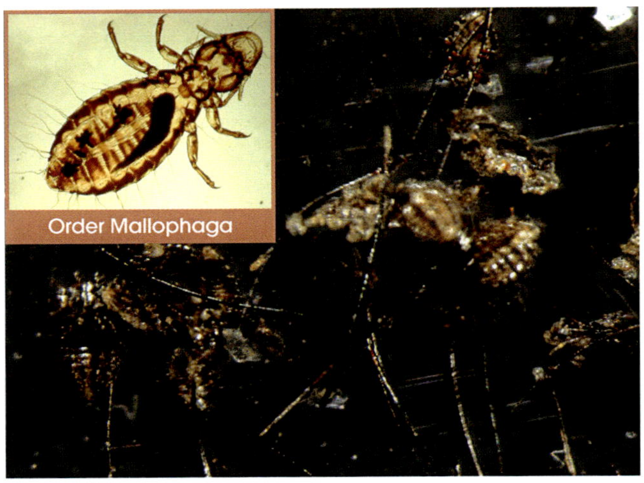

Chewing mites are generally small, not exceeding 3 mm in length, their head is relatively longer and often as wide as the body. Females lack a spermatheca, thus meaning that they need to copulate regularly in order for their eggs to be viable. The presence of large quantities of females suggests some degree of parthenogenetic reproduction.

The differences between these two types of lice (mallophaga and anoplura) are very important when it comes to controlling them. Thus, mallophaga (chewing lice) are best eliminated using topical products whereas anoplura (sucking lice) respond best to treatment with oral or parenteral drugs.

2 Are they a nuisance or can the animals live with them?

Sucking lice live in the animals' hairy coat, therefore thicker coats provide better conditions for their biological cycle. The anatomical characteristics of their legs allow them to grip their host's hair firmly. These lice feed on the animal's blood, for which they make a puncture in the skin that is easy to see. The constant movement of the lice results in restlessness and discomfort, as well as more or less intense pruritus, which forces the animals to rub and scratch themselves. This triggers inflammation, abscesses, hair damage, etc. A lice infestation results in marked unrest, which itself causes lower yields, weight loss, poor coat and restlessness in the animals.

Due to their mode of feeding, mallophaga do not provide so many alterations in the animals. However, their continual movement and small bites also induce pruritus and discomfort, thus meaning that the animals suffer similar consequences in both cases.

3 Do cattle and humans share the same lice species?

Both true and false lice have a marked host specificity. Although lice are highly ubiquitous, they do not infect humans, even those people who have come into contact with infested animals (cows). It is possible that humans may accidentally and temporarily become "contaminated" if they live

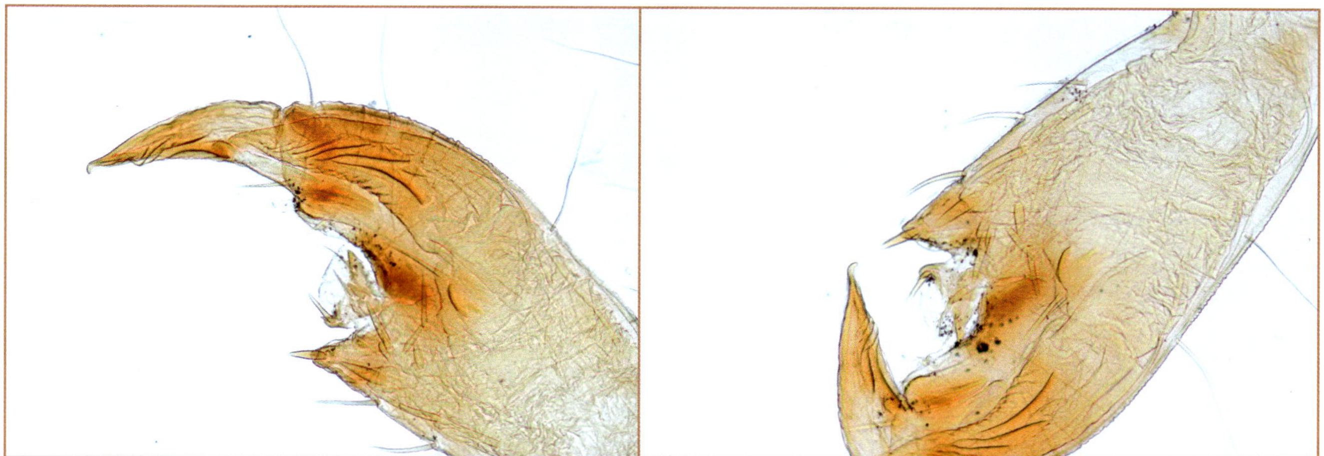

The high specificity of lice is directly related to the adaptation of their legs. The louse's leg forms a prensile ring between a protuberance on the tibia and an opposable nail that matches the diameter of the host's hairs. They are generally sedentary and tend not to move from the region of the body in which they live.

(even for a short time) in a region with poor hygiene conditions. However, each host has its "own lice", which it does not share with other animals species or humans. There are no studies to indicate the possibility that humans and animals share anoplura or mallophaga lice species.

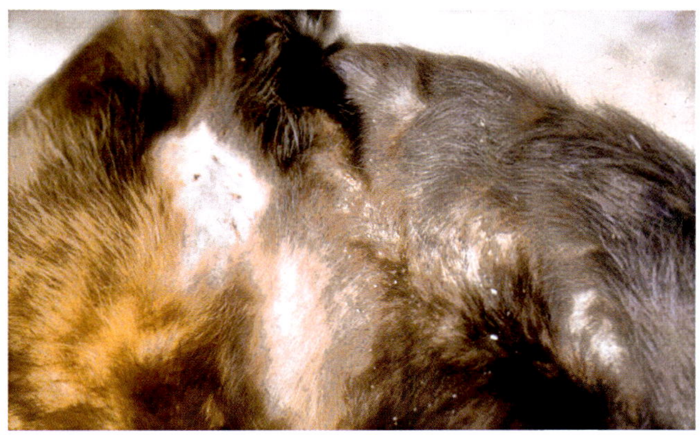

The presence of lice is very uncomfortable; the animals scratch and rub themselves vigorously, which results in alopecia and skin wounds. This activity leads to weight loss, a decrease in milk production of up to 10 % and a higher susceptibility to other diseases.

4 Can flies transmit lice between cows?

The most common means of lice transmission is direct, when healthy and infested animals come into contact, thus allowing the parasites to pass from one animal to another. From an epidemiological viewpoint, this is the most important and significant form of propagation. In practical terms, it can be considered to be the contagion pathway that should be taken into account when establishing control and prevention measures against lice.

However, the survival capacity of lice in the external environment (outside the host) may favour indirect contagion as tools, installations, etc. may "vehiculise" lice after some time and become a potential, although normally not significant, source of contagion.

In addition to the above, it is possible that some lice (mainly mallophaga) attach themselves to certain living creatures, including insects, which allows them to be transported to suitable hosts. This occurs when flies feed on the secretions from skin damaged by lice nests, although such cases are few and far between.

52 Are ticks present in the cold season?

During a visit to South America, numerous ticks were detected in permanently grazing animals on a series of extensive farms in Argentina. The quantity of ticks hosted by each animal was very high in comparison with prior experience in European countries. Local experts noted that tick species in Argentina differ from those found in Europe and that the latter have become adapted to the cold climate, and they can even multiply in winter.

1. What tick species can be found in a European winter?
2. How do ticks attach themselves to their host?
3. What is Haller's organ?
4. How can they harm their host?

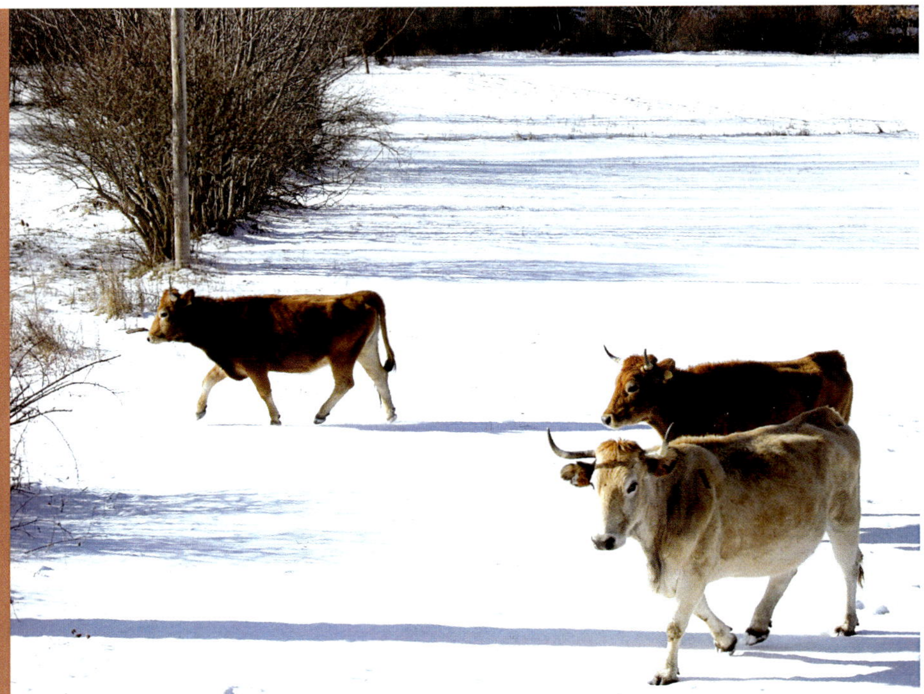

1 What tick species can be found in a European winter?

Ticks generally prefer the warmth. Indeed, the majority of species are found in warm and humid regions. As they are fairly sensitive to drying, they tend to inhabit regions of dense vegetation with high levels of groundwater, such as wet woodland, shaded valleys, etc.

During their "non-parasitic" period ticks are especially sensitive to environmental conditions, which therefore govern their activity or inhibition over several weeks or even months. Ticks pass through three stages of development, not including the egg, namely larva, nymph and adult (male and female). These forms of the parasite must survive adverse environmental conditions. The mechanisms by which these parasites can survive for long periods of time are complex and determine the activity periods of each species.

In the wetter northern regions of the Iberian Peninsula, the most abundant cattle ticks are *Ixodes ricinus,* which is active throughout the year; *Haemaphysalis punctata*, in autumn; *Rhipicephalus bursa,* in summer; and *Dermacentor reticulatus,* in autumn and winter. In contrast, ticks from the genera *Hyalomma* and *Dermacentor marginatus* are most abundant in drier regions, especially in spring and summer (first generations) and autumn and winter (second generations); *R. bursa* is also common in summer.

Ixodes ricinus is a three-host tick found in temperate or cold and wet climates. The main limiting factor for this species in Spain is the humidity —it only survives for a few days at less than 80 % relative humidity. This therefore limits its distribution to the northern part of the peninsula, and it only appears in residual populations and specific habitats in Spain. *Ixodes ricinus* can remain active throughout the year in wetter regions of Spain. In the rest of the country, although individual adult ticks can be found throughout the year, their period of maximum activity is autumn and winter. Nymphs appear in spring and larvae approximately one month later, depending on the climate conditions each season.

Haemaphysalis punctata occupies wet habitats in the north of the country and, like *I. ricinus*, sporadically in the rest of the peninsula as well. This three-host tick, which has low specificity, is most active between autumn and spring at our latitudes.

Rhipicephalus bursa is a medium-sized tick typically found in extensively farmed ruminants, although it can also be found in other animal species, mainly equidae. It has been identified essentially throughout the Iberian Peninsula. During its biological cycle *R. bursa* alternates between two hosts: one on which the immature forms feed and the other on which the adults feed, although both hosts tend to be ruminants. This tick is active between autumn and winter (larvae and nymphs) and spring and autumn (adults).

The two tick species from the genus *Dermacentor* found in our country are highly characteristic. However, their distribution varies, with one species being most abundant precisely where the other is lacking. Thus, *D. reticulatus* is widely spread throughout the north of the country, whereas *D. marginatus* is abundant in the centre and south. Their appetite for hosts is the same: the larvae and nymphs tend to infest small mammals whereas adults infest larger mammals. It should be noted that *D. reticulatus* is commonly found in the dog in regions where *R. sanguineus* is uncommon. Although adults from both species are active in autumn and winter, the activity of their immature forms differs, with *D. marginatus* being active in spring and *D. reticulatus* in autumn.

Tick species from the genus *Hyalomma* (*H. lusitanicum* and *H. marginatum*) are adapted to warm dry climates, therefore they are most abundant in central and southern Spain from spring to autumn, depending on the specific conditions in each region.

The species *Boophilus annulatus* is a single-host tick that lives in open spaces. Its distribution in Spain is limited to the Balearics and the Guadalquivir estuary in warm wet months.

2 How do ticks attach themselves to their host?

In light of their status as obligate haematophagous ectoparasites, ticks have adapted their morphology over thousands of years while conserving the general characteristics of the Acari subclass to which they belong. They have a typical morphology divided into a buccal apparatus, or gnathostome, and body, or idiosome. The buccal apparatus contains the structures required to cut the skin (chelicerae) and anchor itself (hypostome). All these elements are protected by the pedipalps, which remain closed when the tick is in the environment and open on the host.

During all stages of development, ticks head for grass or shrubs and climb to a height sufficient to allow passing animals to brush against them. At this point they attach themselves using the first pair of legs and then grip with the

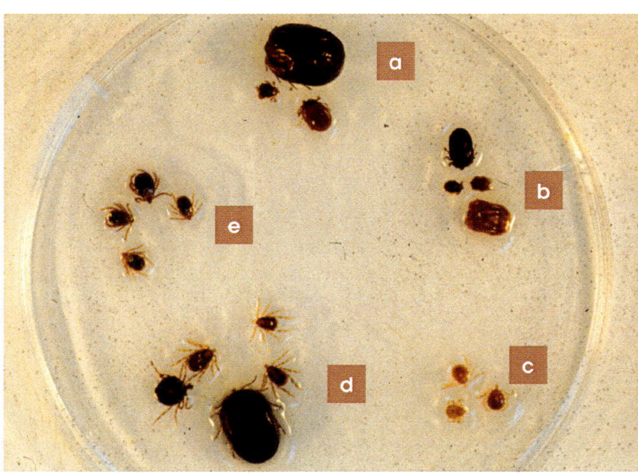

Rhipicephalus (a); *Hyalomma* (b); *Ixodes* (c); *Haemaphysalis* (d) and *Dermacentor* (e). In the wetter regions of Spain *Rhipicephalus* is abundant in summer and *Haemaphysalis* and *Dermacentor reticulatus* in autumn and winter. *R. bursa* is also found in the drier regions of Spain in summer, *Hyalomma* in spring and summer and *Dermacentor marginatus* in autumn and winter.

remaining legs. Although they can use Haller's organ to distinguish animals by their smell, they do not in fact select their host in this way: it is actually the sensation of movement and touch that stimulates them to launch themselves onto their prey. After coming into contact with their host, each species (and evolutionary phase) tends to attach to a specific region of the body, generally the head, neck, back or inguinal region.

Ticks perforate the host's skin using the toothed distal segment of the chelicerae; enzymes secreted by the salivary glands may also play a role in this process. As the chelicerae scrape the skin, the hypostome gets inserted. In some ixodida the hypostome and chelicerae come into direct contact with the tissue, whereas in others the salivary glands begin to secrete a whitish liquid mainly containing lipoproteins, which hardens to form a tube around the appendages.

3 What is Haller's organ?

Ixodidae are species which have become ecologically and biologically adapted to "exploit" hosts in open habitats. For example, these ticks lack antennae (organs that are difficult to conserve). Their visual organ comprises one or more pairs of simple eyes. Their legs are jointed and finish at the tarsus and metatarsus. The tarsi on the first pair of legs possess a dorsal depression, the centre of which contains an orifice with numerous sensory hairs known as Haller's organ.

The various types of hairs (setae) in Haller's organ are able to perceive temperature, humidity, smell and vibrations, amongst other stimuli. During all developmental phases of ticks, but especially in the immature phases, the morphology of these setae and their distribution are the most important characteristic as regards species classification.

4 How can they harm their host?

Even in the absence of an infection, the mere presence of ticks and the way they feed can cause disorders of some importance in animals.

The local action of the tick bite depends above all on the secretions from the salivary glands. The tissue surrounding the bite is digested, which results in small haemorrhages and oedemas, and the region becomes surrounded by connective tissue. The consequences of the inflammation resulting from a bite depend on the region of skin affected. In the most extreme cases, bites can trigger pain, lameness, visual and auditory disorders and paralysis of the face or eyelids, amongst other signs in ruminants. Clinically, the toxic action leads to skin reactions with pruritus or erythema, fever, paralysis and spasms. The half-life of these salivary components is rather short, given that paralysis disappears a few hours after elimination of the parasites.

The acute anaemia often observed in heavily infested animals can be explained by the fact that hard ticks

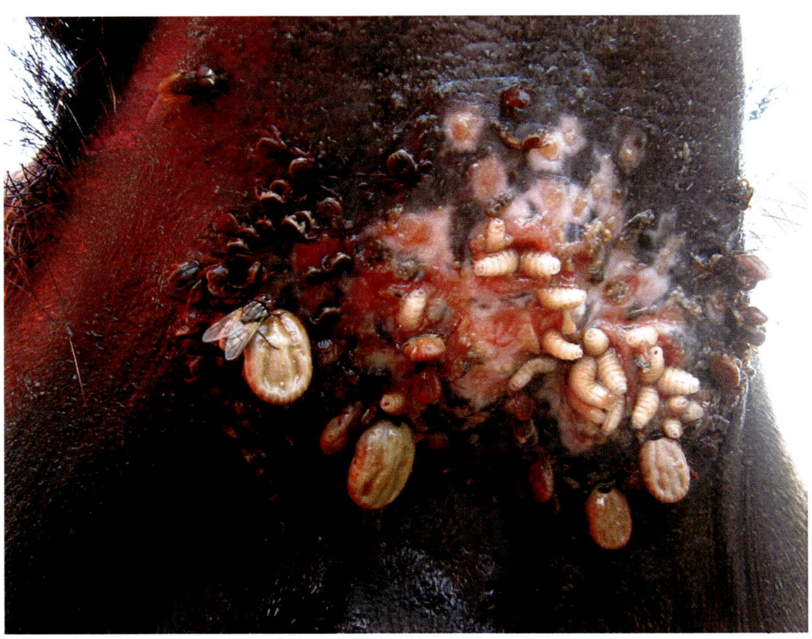

Tick infestations are important as they feed on blood, act as vectors for very serious processes and cause skin wounds, which themselves predispose the animal to secondary infections or myiases.
Image courtesy of Dr. A. S. Olmeda.

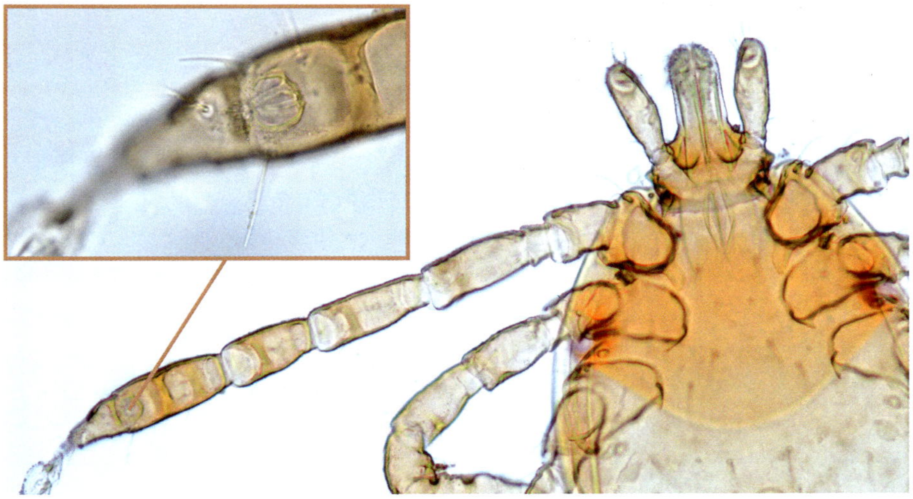

Haller's organ is present in the dorsal surface of the tarsus of the first pair of legs in all stages of the tick. It contains up to six types of setae inside a capsule, one of which is trifurcated and of major taxonomic, functional and phylogenetic significance as its presence indicates a higher evolutionary speciation.

re-concentrate the blood they ingest in their body, removing the water from it and returning it to the host. As a result of this process, it has been calculated that each female tick from the larger species can extract up to 2-4 grammes of blood.

All tick species are relevant to a greater or lesser extent in veterinary medicine due to their ability both to transmit diseases to animals and from animals to humans. This fact broadens their clinical/veterinary repercussions. The importance of ticks on cattle farms results from the direct pathogenic action of their feeding (bites) and the reactions they cause as well as their ability to transmit numerous pathogens. Their efficacy as vectors is due to their status as obligate haematophagous parasite, their complex life cycle, in which they can alternate between up to three hosts, their high degree of adaptation to the various ecosystems in which they are found and the close relationship they maintain with the pathogens they transmit. Indeed, the vector/agent association is so strong that identification of the ticks that infest farm animals in a specific region throughout the year allows the pathogens that could be transmitted to the farm to be predicted.

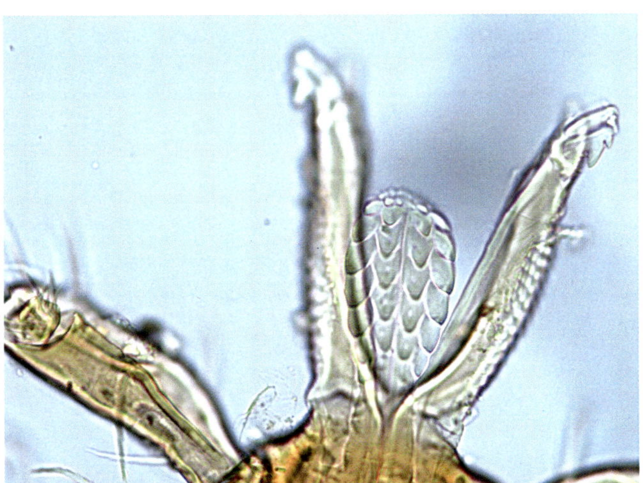

The buccal apparatus of ticks comprises a basal structure, or base of the capitulum, two segmented and two protective palps, two chelicerae that act like knives and a hypostome, which contains diagonal teeth, as an anchoring organ.

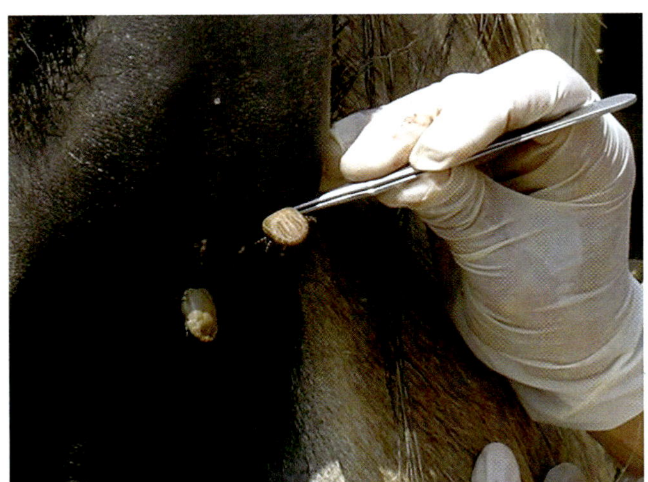

The method for extracting a tick directly involves its removal using fine tweezers. These tweezers should be placed as close to the skin as possible, holding the parts of the buccal apparatus. The body of the tick should not be squeezed. Always pull in a direction perpendicular to the skin, using a smooth yet firm motion, without making sharp movements.

53 What are "warbles"?

In Galicia, as well as in other northern and north-eastern parts of Spain, it is relatively common to observe subcutaneous nodules on the back of animals in late winter or early spring. In Spain they are also known as "*engordaderas*) or "*crecederas*) by farmers and locals, clearly referring to the nodules that appear in children when maternal milk is rich in fats and other nutrients. In cattle they appear as well-defined bulges the size of a walnut (or bigger) with a regular outline and hard to the touch. A vet new to the region inspects these nodules and notes the presence of an orifice several millimetres in diameter in their upper part, which is easily detectable upon moving the fingers against the grain of the hair. Some of these openings are covered with a whitish or yellowish exudate, and upon localised pressure the nodule releases a serosanguineous fluid. In one case, increasing the pressure triggers a spectacular collapse of the animal and its sudden fall to the floor in a state of shock.

1. What are these nodules?
2. What repercussions do they have in animals?
3. What caused the state of shock in the cow?
4. How are they diagnosed *in vivo*?

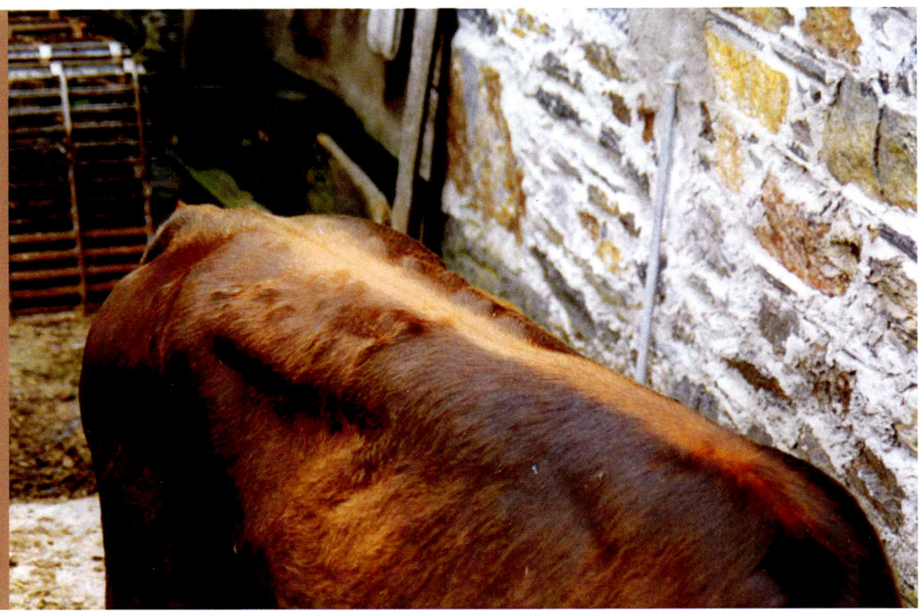

Image courtesy of Dr. P. Morrondo.

1 What are these nodules?

Warbles are nodules that appear in the dorsolumbar region of animals, mainly bovines. However, their correct name is hypodermosis. This disease is characterised by the presence of small abscesses under the skin on the back and loins on both sides of the dorsolumbar line. The larva of a fly wrapped in a purulent cream-coloured secretion with a doughy consistency is found inside each nodule.

Hypodermosis is actually an obligatory myiasis caused by larvae of flies from the genus *Hypoderma*. This seasonal parasitosis is closely linked to climate conditions, the characteristics of the land and, above all, to extensive farming systems, although it may very occasionally present in animals farmed intensively. Hypodermosis appears due to contact with the environment during the flying phase of the fly.

This parasitosis is also known to affect equids. As well as presenting in the same form as in cows, an atypical form due to the aberrant migration of L1 larvae exists in this host.

Since humans can also suffer from hypodermosis, it is considered a zoonosis. Human hypodermosis presents in people who come into close contact with infested cattle, although the larvae do not mature in the majority of cases.

2 What repercussions do they have in animals?

Except for the most typical sign, namely the appearance of warbles on the animal's back, hypodermosis is normally accompanied by few and non-specific clinical manifestations. These nodules represent the final developmental stage of the parasite in the host. Depending on the geographical region concerned, warbles may appear from late autumn, during winter, until late spring. The intraorgan migration of hypoderma larvae results in a series of alterations that negatively affect yields, such as decreased milk yields, loss of appetite and growth retardation.

During the flying phase of *Hypoderma* flies, the animals become restless due to the buzzing sound produced by nearby flies and when they approach the animals to lay their eggs. This can even cause stampedes with serious repercussions (trauma, etc.).

The most significant lesions correspond to the subcutaneous dorsal nodules. They contain an opening around 2-6 mm in diameter at their apex, depending on the degree of evolution of the warble, which is easily visible upon removing the hairs surrounding it. This opening has a regular border that is usually covered by a whitish or yellowish exudate.

Organisations such as the FAO have traditionally claimed that hypodermosis-related repercussions and losses, such as decreased bodily defences, greater ease of contracting other infectious/contagious diseases, low fertility and even sterility in heavily infected cows, poor vaccine efficacy and less efficient feed use, amongst others, are difficult to calculate. However, the main losses related to this disease can be grouped as follows: deterioration of the skin, cachexia-related loss of meat, and decreased milk production.

The holes in the top of the nodules can reach up to 2-6 mm in diameter. Moreover, as the number of larvae can be very high (more than 200 in a single animal), it is easy to understand the enormous damage they cause to the skin and its subsequent loss of value. This varies with the number of larvae or holes present in the skin. As far as cachexia-related meat loss is concerned, farmers commonly state that the general appearance of dewormed cows improves and their weight gain is obvious. Some data aimed at quantifying the weight gain in such animals suggest an increase of up to 30 kg in the 2-3 months post-treatment with respect to untreated control animals. Finally, the continual disturbance to which animals with hypodermosis are subjected explains why milk production suffers and decreases markedly.

3 What caused the state of shock in the cow?

The content of the warbles, which is usually serosanguineous or occasionally purulent/caseous, is forced out upon pressuring them. As the pressure increases, the opening and the whitish, greyish or brownish L3 larva, depending on its degree of development, can be seen inside the nodule.

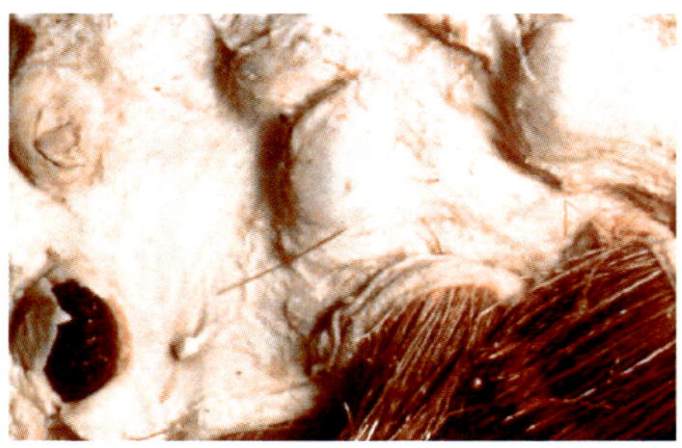

The L3 larvae exert their pathogenic action in the subcutaneous tissue on the back. They cause prominent nodules various centimetres in size known as warbles, in which the larvae remain for between 5 and 11 weeks. These parasites secrete bacteriostatic substances that prevent secondary infections while they are present in the nodule. Once the larvae have matured and left the cavity, abscesses that affect the deepest layers of the skin, and even the subcutaneous muscle, often appear.

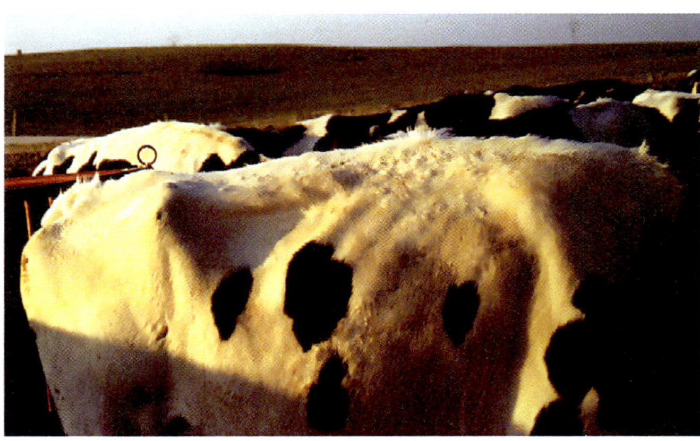

Hypodermosis is a typical disease in extensively farmed cattle left on large open spaces where the animals are free to move around and flies can readily come into contact with the animals. During the exogenous cycle of *Hypoderma*, warm but not excessively hot temperatures in the range 20-25 °C, with significant sunlight and humidity, are required for the puparium to hatch, thus meaning that this cycle varies in each region or ecological zone depending on the environmental conditions.
Image courtesy of Dr. S. Hernández.

It is not recommended to remove warbles mechanically by pressing with the fingers to remove the almost mature larvae, even in mildly affected animals. This procedure is uncomfortable, tiring and painful for the animal and accidents may occur due to the toxic and antigenic action of the secretions released after lysis of the larvae. Indeed, undesired reactions such as that which occurred in the animal in this specific case may occasionally occur after such treatment.

Once inside the body, *Hypoderma* larvae begin to migrate internally due to the release of proteolytic substances (hypodermins). These also play a key role in the phenomena which allow the parasite to evade the immune response and resist reinfections. As no local inflammatory response is observed upon passage of the larvae through the animal in primary infections, the parasite is free to circulate through tissue until it reaches the subcutaneous tissue in the back. In contrast, in the event of a reinfection the host presents an increasingly intense inflammatory response that restricts or inhibits larval migration. Large-scale larval death results in the release of large quantities of larval antigens, which can provoke type I hypersensitivity phenomena similar to those caused by larvicidal treatments administered during the migration phase due to their sensitizing properties.

4 How are they diagnosed *in vivo*?

A presumptive diagnosis can be established by observing the flies during their flying period or confirming the presence of eggs attached to the animal's hair, although these methods are very unreliable.

Hypodermosis is easy to diagnose once warbles appear on the backs of infested animals. Indeed, it can be seen with the naked eye or checked by palpation that the nodules are distributed irregularly on both sides of the dorsolumbar midline. However, a diagnosis at this point has one major drawback, namely that the damage caused by migratory larvae and, in many cases, perforation of the skin, has already occurred. It should also be added this larval migration is not synchronous, therefore regular examinations must be performed for at least three months. This increases costs and therefore the losses caused by this parasitosis.

If the different phases of the intraorganic cycle of *Hypoderma* can be detected and identified in the regions where the parasite rests, or in subcutaneous tissue, during examination of the animal, the diagnosis of hypodermosis can be confirmed.

Methods that confirm the reaction of the host to the parasite are also of great utility as regards clinical diagnosis. Although the first such method used was passive haemagglutination, immunoenzymatic methods (ELISA) are currently considered to be most suitable for epidemiological studies irrespective of the species of *Hypoderma* responsible for the infection. Moreover, such methods are easy to use and only present around 5-7 % of false negatives. The best time to perform the analysis is when antibody levels are high and easy to detect, in other words during the first larval migration before they reach their overwintering zones. An early diagnosis of hypodermosis allows appropriate treatment to be initiated at an early stage.

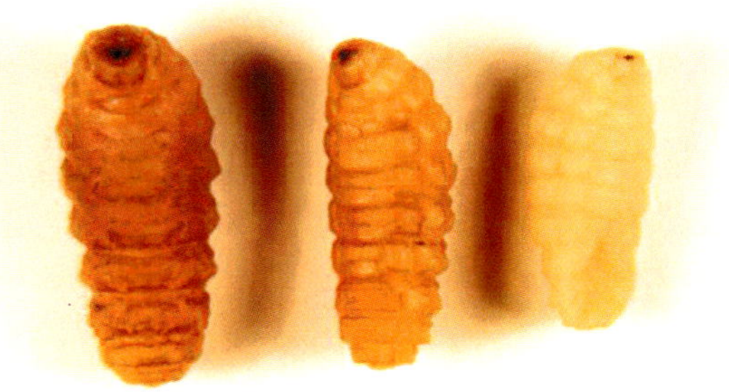

L3 larvae can reach up to 30 mm in length for *H. bovis* and slightly shorter in *H. lineatum*, with a width of 14-17 mm. The colour of the larvae changes as they mature, passing from whitish to dark brown or almost black. The small spines on the ventral face are examined to differentiate between species. *H. lineatum* presents such spines on all segments, whereas *H. bovis* does so on all but the eleventh. *Image courtesy of Dr. P. Morrondo.*

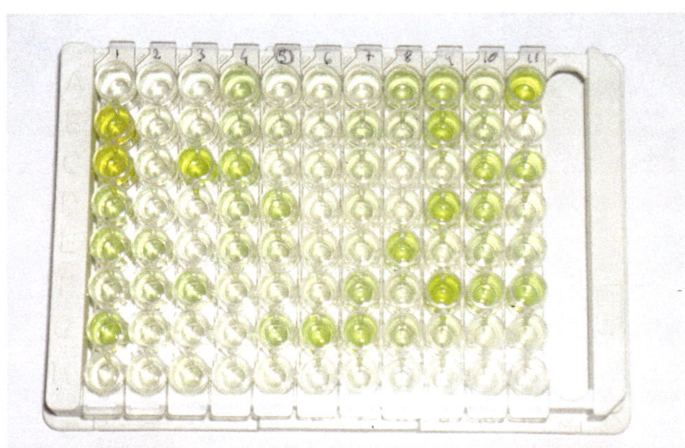

Immunological techniques have the advantage that they allow *Hypoderma* infection to be detected at the onset of larval migration, thereby allowing damage to the animal to be prevented. Current control programs include a monthly nodule count in spring and monitoring of the seroprevalence values in autumn, which indicate the need to apply one or two treatments per year.

54 How can *Hypoderma* species be differentiated?

Crystalline forms around 1.5 cm in length are observed during a routine inspection of carcasses in an abattoir. These forms are almost cylindrical and are located at the ends of the oesophagus in all animals from the same batch. A more careful examination confirms the presence of larvae wrapped in connective tissue, which are always oriented lengthwise along the oesophageal axis. Whitish, opaque and rigid formations that are difficult to separate from the surrounding tissue are also seen. These formations are occasionally calcified and have the same size and appearance as the crystalline formations, although it is impossible to extract a larva from their interior.

1. What species are these larvae from?
2. Where are the lesions caused by *Hypoderma* larvae detected?
3. What measures should be included in a comprehensive hypodermosis control plan?

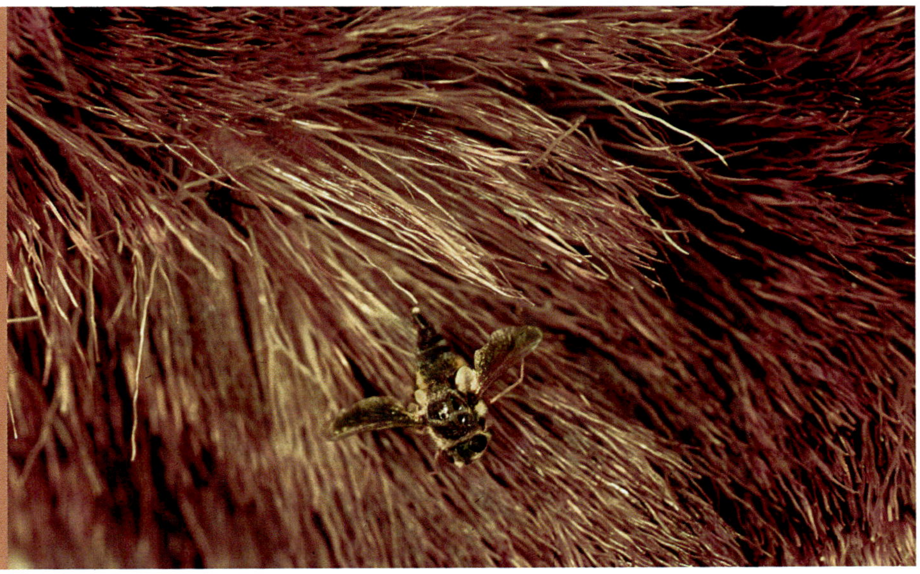

1 What species are these larvae from?

Adult *Hypoderma* parasites start their activity quickly. After fertilisation, the females begin to fly and search for bovines on which to lay their eggs. *H. lineatum* lays its eggs from the base of the hair towards the tip, mainly on the legs and lower parts of the body, whereas *H. bovis* lays its eggs (one by one) at the base of the hair, preferably on the pasterns, abdomen and hind third.

The larvae hatch shortly afterwards (between 4 and 6 days) and pass through the skin to the subcutaneous connective tissue, using their cephalic structure, proteolytic enzymes and the spines covering their body. Once the skin has been perforated migration varies by species. Thus, during migration, *H. lineatum* "rests" in the oesophageal submucosa, where the larvae mature and grow for up to 7 months, a characteristic which is not shared with *H. bovis*. They subsequently continue their journey to the back of the animal, moult twice and transform into L3 larvae after 1-1.5 months. It appears that *H. lineatum* migrates via the diaphragm, caudal edge of the ribs, thoracic cavity and intercostal muscles until it reaches the subcutaneous connective tissue in the dorsal region, where it perforates the skin in order to breathe.

2 Where are the lesions caused by *Hypoderma* larvae detected?

Once the larvae have hatched they penetrate the skin, causing breaks that normally go unnoticed.

The typical lesions associated with hypodermosis are subcutaneous dorsal nodules, which appear as well-defined hemispherical bulges the size of a walnut (or bigger) with regular borders that are hard upon palpation. The apex of each nodule (warble) contains an opening some 2-6 mm in diameter, depending on the development of the parasite, which is

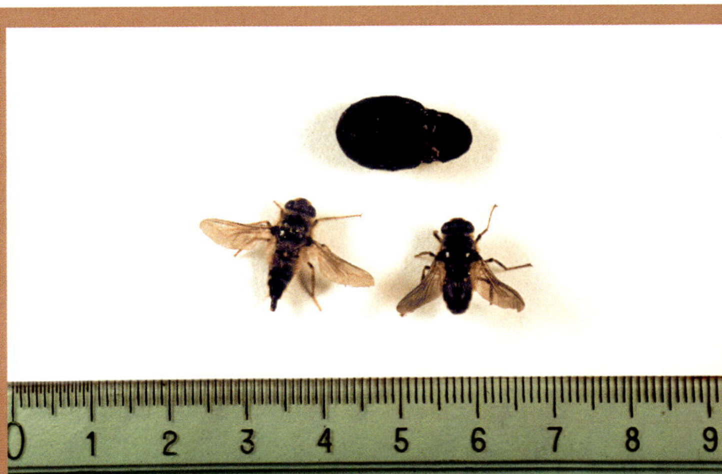

Flies from the genus *Hypoderma* are large and hairy (12 to 15 mm), closely resembling horseflies. The main species affecting cattle are *Hypoderma bovis* and *Hypoderma lineatum*. The mature L3 larva falls to the ground, where it pupates. Once metamorphosis is complete, the adult fly perforates the operculum at its anterior end and exits. Pupae from both species are found buried in the soil and measure 2-3 cm in size, with a stiff black covering and flat dorsal face, at the end of which the operculum is located.

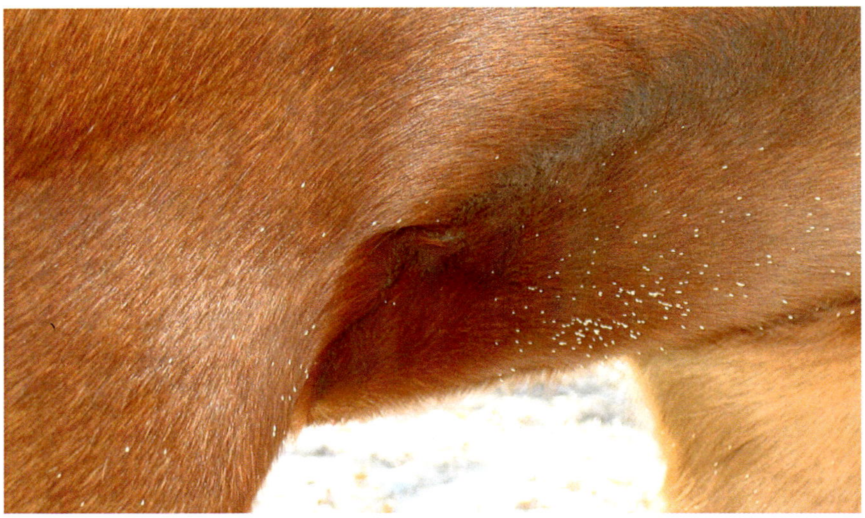

Adult flies do not feed and live for only about two weeks, during which time they lay several hundred eggs.

H. bovis lays its eggs (one by one) at the base of the hair. As it rarely lays more than one egg at a time it must continually fly around the host, which disturbs the animals.

H. lineatum makes very little noise when flying and lays several eggs (around 20) on the same hair without the host noticing.

readily visible, has regular borders and is coated with a whitish or yellowish exudate.

During the resting phase, *H. lineatum* L1 larvae appear as cylindrical, crystalline formations around 1.5 cm in length with rounded ends and enclosed in translucent connective tissue. These formations are oriented lengthwise along the oesophageal axis, causing deformations in the mucosa. Live or dead larvae can be seen in these regions, with the latter occasionally being calcified and difficult to separate from the surrounding tissue. This surrounding tissue is usually oedematous and presents haemorrhagic trajectories.

As far as *H. bovis* is concerned, the lesions in the resting regions may pass unnoticed, although degenerated, oedematous and hyperemic epidural fat, which on occasions may be haemorrhagic or even, rarely, contain clots, is sometimes observed.

3 What measures should be included in a comprehensive hypodermosis control plan?

As with any disease control-related health planning, actions aimed at combating hypodermosis must target one or more key aspects. Satisfactory results cannot be achieved without collaboration from the farmers, who must be informed of, and understand, the peculiarities of the problem to be controlled. In this respect, the animals' owners must be made aware of the repercussions of hypodermosis as regards yields and the likely benefits of controlling this disease. The approximate scale of the problem must be determined before any control program is put into practice.

An estimation of the parasitation rates by way of prior sampling allows the economic losses to be evaluated and the profitability of the control program to be calculated. Determination of the blood antibody levels by indirect ELISA is particularly useful, although the samples taken over the same period vary from one region to the next. For example, the most appropriate sampling period in the north of Spain is autumn. Information such as the size of the farm should be taken into account when planning sampling. If insufficient data are available to reach a definitive conclusion, a prevalence of 50 % with a 95 % confidence interval should be assumed.

The control plan must include all grazing animals or those on a semi-extensive regimen in the region and should last for at least two consecutive years, with actions being scheduled on the basis of the chronobiology of the *Hypoderma* species concerned. It is also clearly vital to select the most appropriate antiparasitic agent and administer it correctly. The period required for *Hypoderma* spp. to complete its biological cycle depends on climate and other factors. As such, the time at which treatment is administered should be scheduled on the basis of these aspects. In general terms, drugs should be administered as soon as possible once the flying period of *Hypoderma* flies has finished, in other words between mid-September and mid-November.

The drugs of choice are currently macrocyclic lactones (avermectins and milbemycins), which are both highly effective and safe, although their main drawback is that they cannot be used in lactating cows. In contrast, eprinomectin does not require a withdrawal period and can be used in such cows.

As is the case for any control program, regular controls must be performed to evaluate the results. One of the actions in this phase involves the detection of any residual foci using appropriate laboratory techniques. This should be complemented by treatment of the animals in both autumn and spring and an awareness of the situation on neighbouring farms and in neighbouring regions.

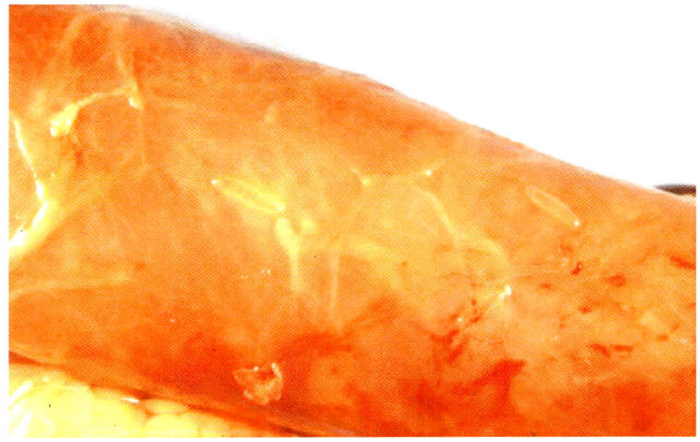

Migratory larvae do not normally cause much damage to their hosts. *H. lineatum* migrates via the diaphragm, caudal edge of the ribs, thoracic cavity and intercostal muscles until it reaches the subcutaneous connective tissue in the dorsal region. *H. bovis* follows a neurotropic migratory route via the ischiatic and radial nerves and the sacral, lumbar and brachial plexi until it finally reaches the epidural fat in the spinal canal, where it rests.
Image courtesy of Dr. P. Morrondo.

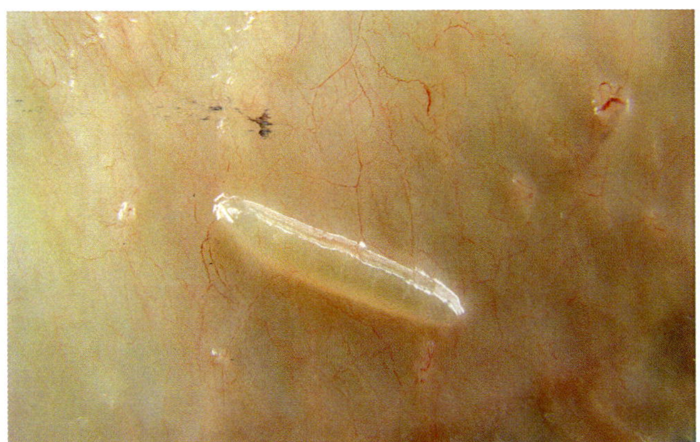

During the resting phase in the oesophagus, *H. lineatum* L1 larvae can be seen as cylindrical, crystalline formations around 15 mm in length with rounded ends and enclosed in translucent connective tissue. These formations are oriented lengthwise along the oesophageal axis. L1 larvae can be extracted by separating the keratinised mucosa from underlying tissue.
Image courtesy of Dr. P Morrondo.

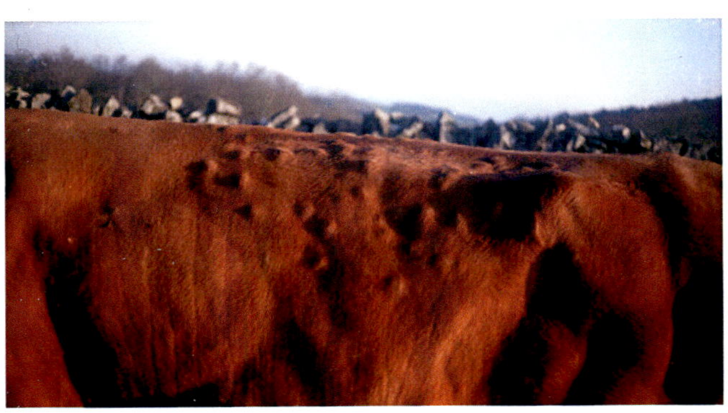

The larvae mature and grow in their resting sites, which differ for each species, for up to 7 months. The presence of nodules, commonly known as warbles, in the dorsolumbar region of cattle can be detected in late winter and spring.
Image courtesy of Dr. P. Morrondo.

Biological cycle of *Hypoderma*

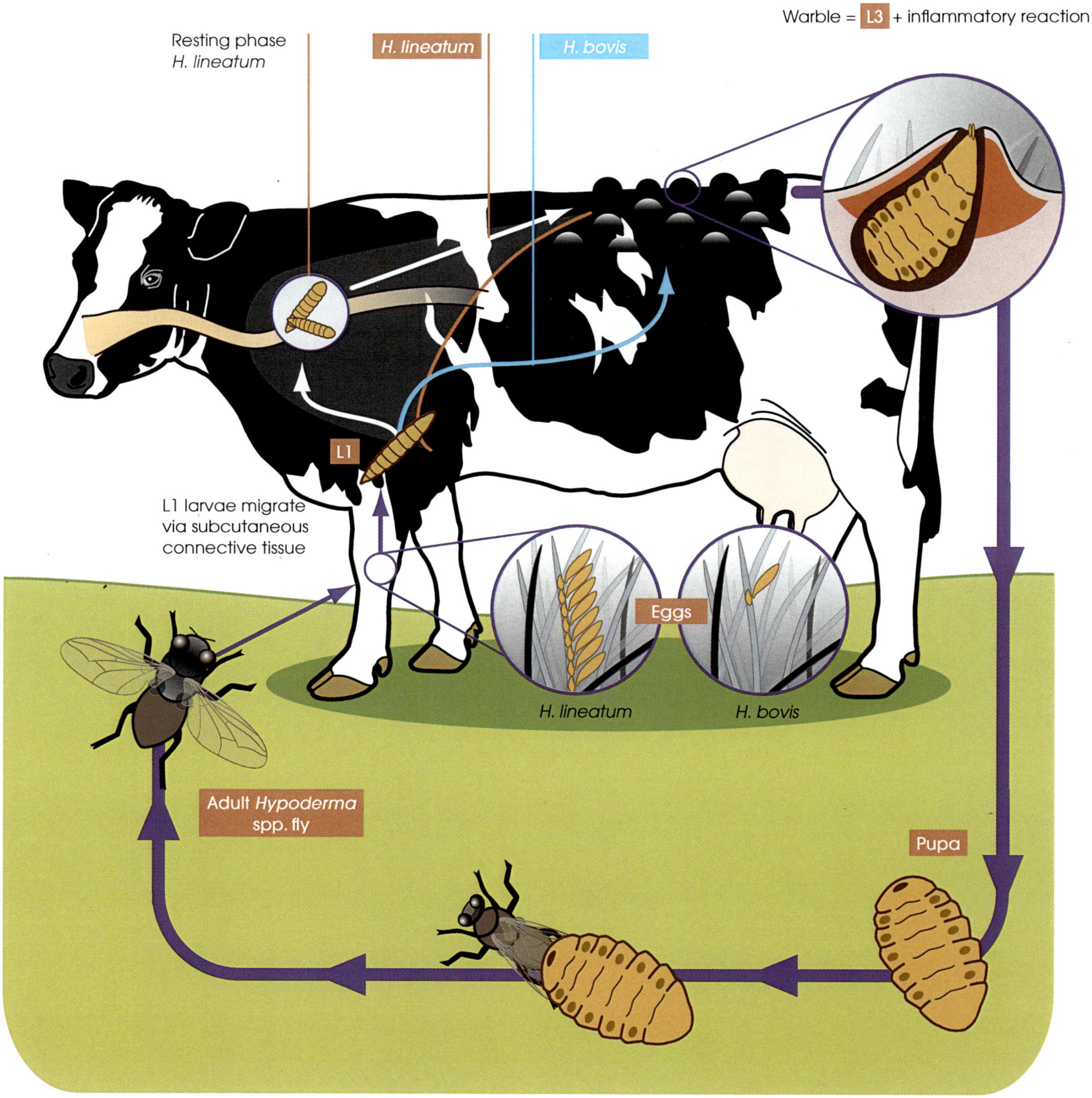

55 Is myiasis common in cattle?

Whitish larvae are observed in lesion-free and previously undamaged regions of skin, specifically around the genitals and on the back of the animals, on a visit to a cattle farm in Costa Rica. This parasite is known as *gusano barrenador* in this part of Costa Rica and comes from the laying of eggs by flies. Both young and adult animals are withdrawn, inactive and present clear signs of pain.

1. What parasite species, which are not found in Europe, cause this process in American cattle?
2. What measures should be taken to prevent them from being imported?
3. Can they affect humans?

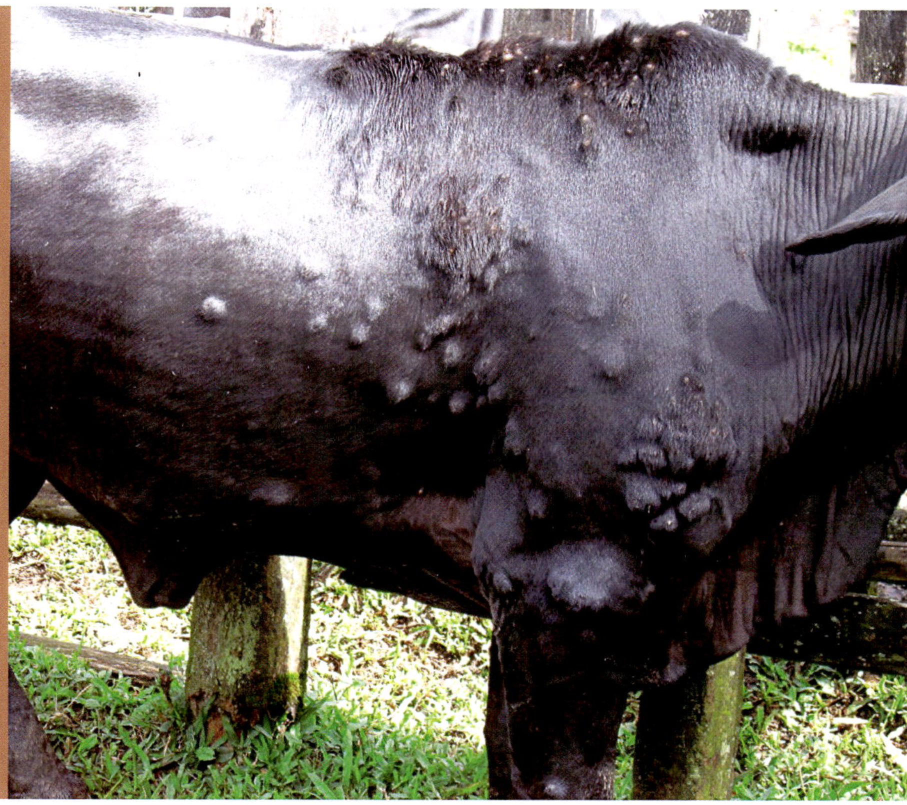

Image courtesy of Dr. G. López.

1 What parasite species, which are not found in Europe, cause this process in American cattle?

This is a woodland diptera whose adult forms are unrelated to humans and other mammals, although its life cycle phases develop in them. This fly belongs to the species *Dermatobia hominis* and is also known as the "human botfly". Its larvae cause a myiasis that affects cattle and other animal species (dogs, cats, sheep, rabbits and other wild animals), including humans. It is a major pest for cattle in some regions of Latin America.

Dermatobia has a very unique biology. After fertilisation the female captures other diptera (haematophagous mosquitoes or flies) or ticks in order to deposit its eggs on their abdomen, where they remain attached. When these diptera land on a warm-blooded animal, the *D. hominis* larvae hatch and penetrate the host's skin, often via the break produced by the bite of the haematophagous insect. As the larvae grow under the skin they form a very painful boil and can also attract myiasis-producing muscids. After around 10 weeks the larvae fall to the ground and pupate.

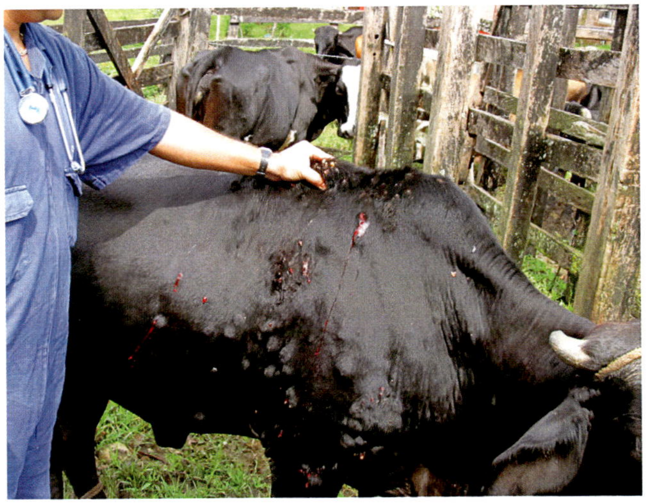

Dermatobia hominis is very common in tropical and subtropical regions. The nodules caused by larvae often become infected with bacteria and other pathogenic microorganisms. They are very painful for the host, causing significant stress and discomfort. Once the parasite has reached the host, the larvae pass through its skin but do not migrate internally. Within three days they appear inside visible cavities in the host, which are noted externally as surface nodules.
Image courtesy of Dr. G. López.

2 What measures should be taken to prevent them from being imported?

The biological characteristics of these flies, which do not come into contact with either humans or animals, mean that measures aimed at controlling the adult forms make little practical sense unless the entire region is to be treated. For the same reason, it is essentially impossible to control the insects that act as vectors as they vary widely. Prevention is therefore limited to the use of repellent substances.

Modern insecticides and other antiparasitic agents used against *Hypoderma* spp. appear to be highly effective against the larvae of this parasite. As such, application of such products should be the first step in controlling the problem in animals infected by *D. hominis*. However, basic quarantine measures should also be put into place to prevent the introduction of this type of parasite into a region currently free from it.

3 Can they affect humans?

Most problems caused by fly larvae in humans are uncommon, at least in some parts of the world. However, the relationship between mosquito bites and the appearance of subcutaneous nodules has been known in Latin America for many years.

Humans are normally infected when they come into contact with domestic animals (farm workers). The larvae can invade the skin via clothing and produce inflammation and painful ulcers. The parasites are usually removed surgically in humans.

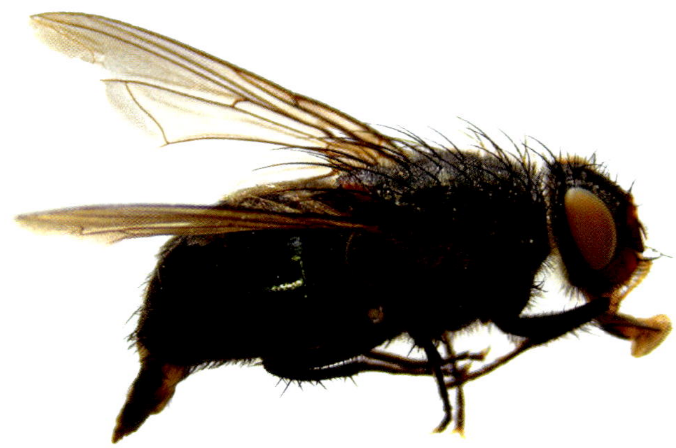

Female *Dermatobia* lay their eggs on other insects (other species of fly, mosquitoes, etc.), which carry them, attached to their abdomen, to the final host. The larvae emerge after 5 days, still on the vector insect, where they remain until this insect visits a suitable host.
Image courtesy of Dr. C. Botias.

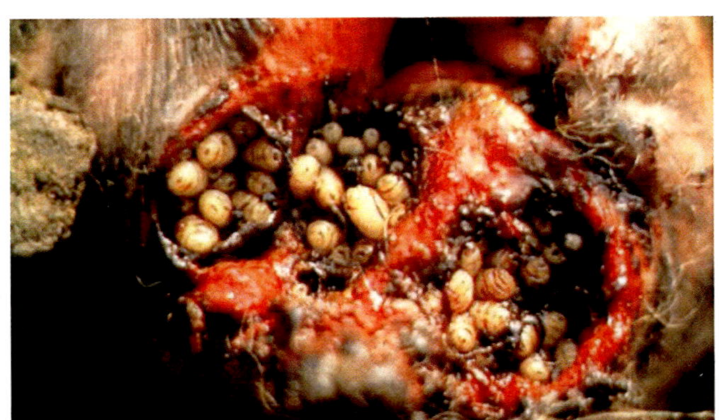

Female calliphoridae, such as *Wohlfahrtia magnifica*, are attracted by rotten smells. They are most common in sheep as they are attracted by the smell of the urine and faeces that soil the wool in the groin region, as well as by the dermatitis caused by moisture and the proliferation of bacteria on the surface of the skin. The larvae "devour) surface tissue, causing large wounds that spread rapidly and can become infected with bacteria.
Image courtesy of Dr. J. Pérez.

56 Can severe allergic reactions be caused by mosquito bites?

The horses used for daily work on a fighting bull farm in Extremadura (Spain) often suffer from a characteristic dermatitis caused by the bites of some types of mosquito. The resulting lesions are highly pruriginous, which causes significant anxiety in the animals, thus meaning that they cannot be used on some days. This behaviour is not common in steers.

1. Are allergic reactions caused by mosquitoes common in cattle?
2. Which insect species can cause lesions and pruritus in cattle?
3. What measures can be taken to prevent these processes?

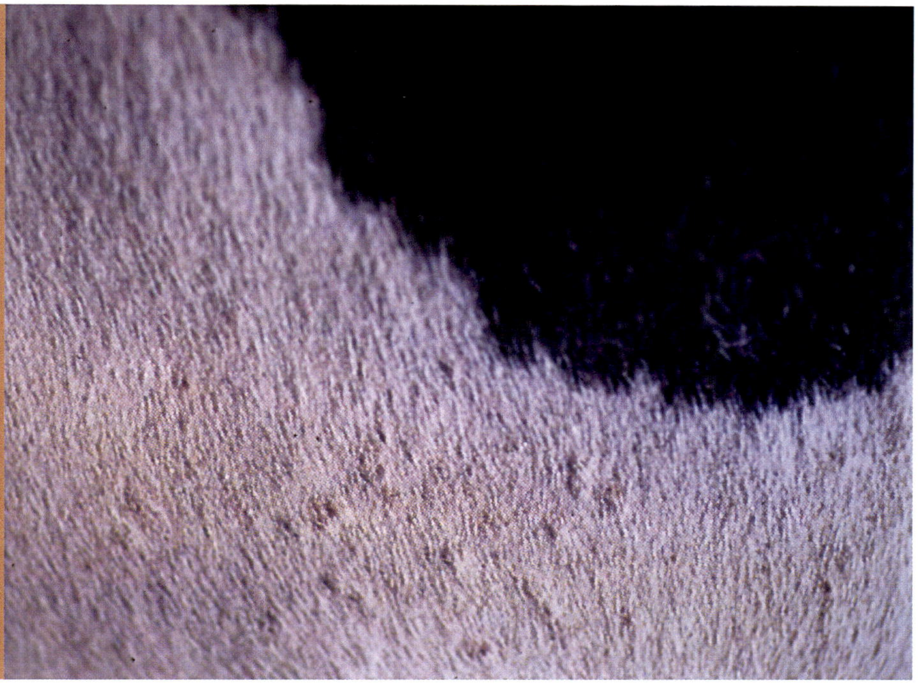

1 Are allergic reactions caused by mosquitoes common in cattle?

The aetiology of allergic dermatitis in cattle varies widely. Although mosquitoes tend not to represent a major problem in this animal species, their bites can trigger allergic reactions, although this is relatively uncommon. If the density of the insect population is not particularly high, the reaction after a bite may go unnoticed. However, at times of higher densities (mainly summer) and in animals kept more or less permanently in pasture, pruriginous signs of some intensity and local inflammation appear, the aetiology of which is not easy to define.

In some regions mosquitoes are not considered to be a problem. For example, a reindeer breeder in Finland considers that the presence of mosquitoes is a positive sign and expects their population to increase in summer. The reason for this is that the more mosquitoes the fewer problems in finding the

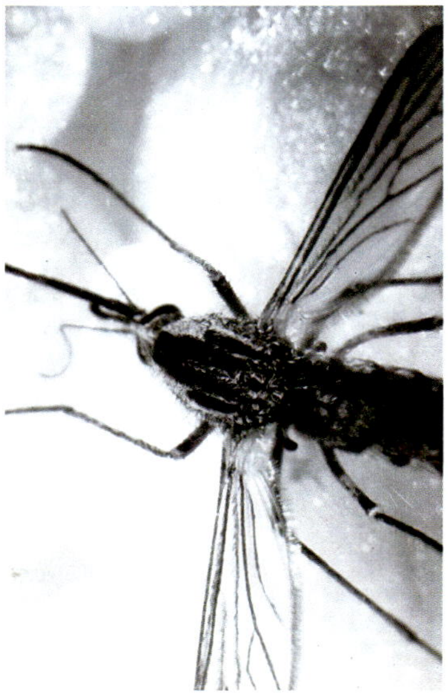

Female mosquitoes possess a very thin and elongated tube (proboscis), which they use like a stiletto to pierce the skin of vertebrates, and extract blood from them. This diptera uses small filaments (palps) at each side of the proboscis to detect the carbon dioxide (CO_2) generated by humans and animals when they breathe. It then bites its victim, using an anticoagulant substance to extract and store blood from its host. *Image courtesy of Dr. A. Encinas*

reindeer will the workers have. The reindeers live in semi-wild conditions in the woods, and thus the animals tend to group together in summers with high mosquito densities, so herding is simplified. This behaviour is a clear reaction of the animals to attacks by these insects.

2 Which insect species can cause lesions and pruritus in cattle?

As far as cattle are concerned, mosquitoes from the sub-order Nematocera, especially those from the families Culicidae (culicids), Simuliidae (simulids or "black fly") and Ceratopogonidae (ceratopogonids), are the most important. Culicids and ceratopogonids are cosmopolitan. All these mosquitoes are haematophagous and can act as vectors for very important pathogens in both animals and humans.

A bite from these insects, especially simulids, can result in petechiae and oedema in various parts of the body (thorax, abdomen, udder, scrotum and perineum). Their bites are very painful and produce severe irritation, thus causing the animals to become restless and present local inflammation. Grazing cattle (extensive farming) tend to be the most affected by these insects. The clinical signs caused by mosquito bites include pruritus, petechiae or local inflammatory skin reactions. The main consequences are weight loss and lower milk production.

3 What measures can be taken to prevent these processes?

Obviously, the best way of controlling the problems caused by mosquitoes is to prevent exposure of the animals to their bites and annoyance. This can be achieved by taking animals to pasture during the day, to prevent culicid and culicoid bites, or at night to prevent simulid bites. However, such measures cannot always be put into practice.

The fight against larval breeding grounds requires a major economic outlay to construct water drainage systems. Chemical methods can also be used, although the environmental problems associated with their use means that great care must be taken.

Another measure, which has been widely used for many years, involves installing metallic screens on the doors and windows of the farms where the animals are kept. Furthermore, the fight against common mosquitoes requires all bodies of water to be controlled and specific actions targeting adults to be undertaken.

These insects have major public health implications as many species can transmit pathogens to humans. Current climate conditions in Europe mean that the greatest impact caused by mosquito bites involves local inflammatory reactions.

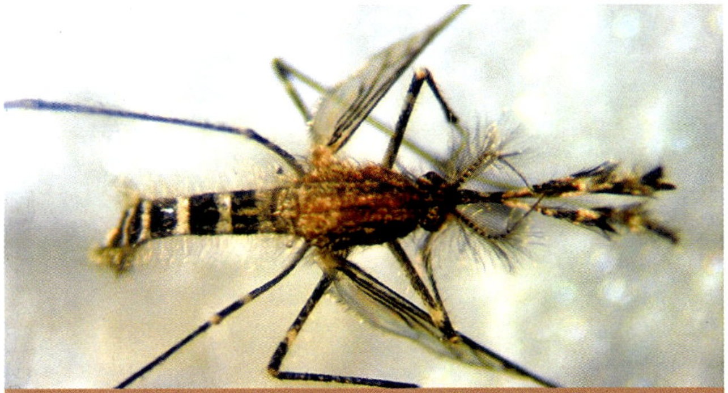

Only females are important from a health viewpoint as they are the only ones able to transmit the pathogens responsible for diseases such as malaria, dengue, yellow fever, encephalitis and filariosis. Adult mosquitoes seek refuge in wet regions with no air currents. Males feed on sugary substances (nectar and fruit exudates), whereas females also need to ingest blood (haematophagy) in order to lay eggs.
Image courtesy of Dr. A. Encinas.

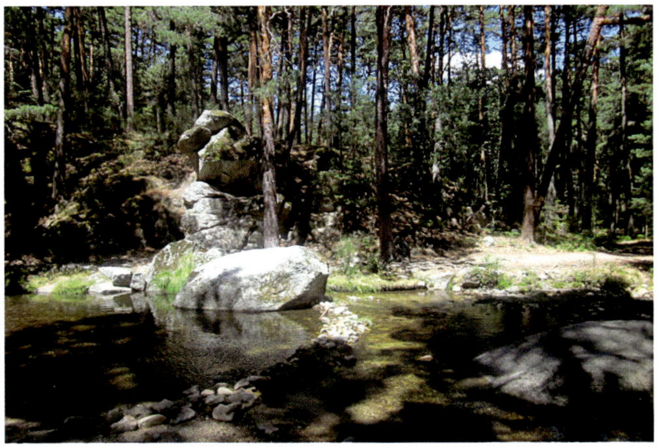

The immature stages of mosquitoes (egg, larva, pupa) are aquatic whereas adults are land-based. Females can lay their eggs on the surface of water, on aquatic vegetation or in wet regions. Preventing the build up of water can prevent the proliferation of these insects as their larvae cannot develop in the absence of water.

57 What control measures can be taken to combat flies?

It is common to observe cattle grazing with a large number of flies on their skin or flying around them in the most northern mountain passes on the Iberian Peninsula. This situation causes the animals to be continually moving their head and tail, to stamp and kick, and to seek refuge in shaded regions or under trees. A careful observation shows difference in terms of the size and location of the flies.

1. Which fly species affect cattle?
2. Which flies are the most annoying?
3. How can the fly population be reduced?

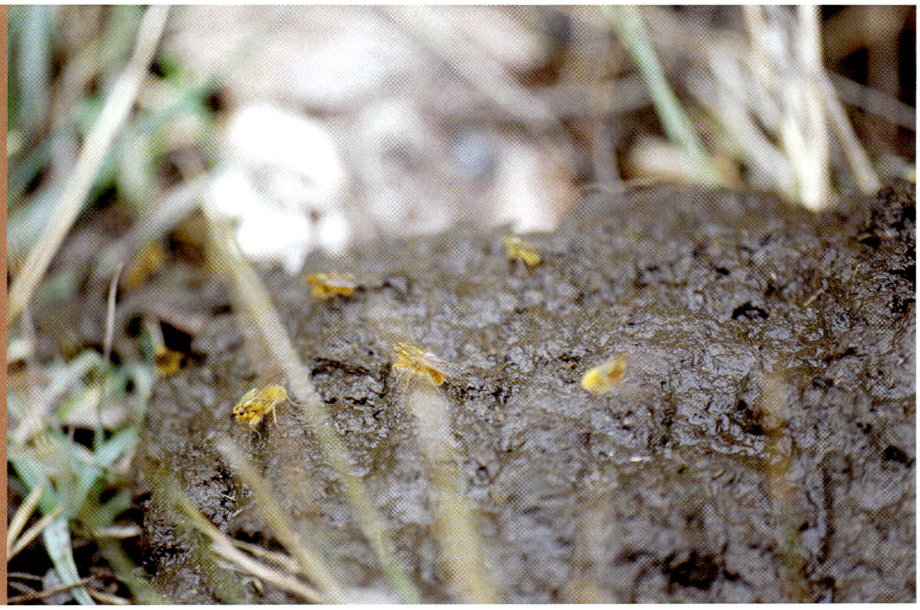

1 Which fly species affect cattle?

Numerous species of fly (as many as 20) can annoy cattle at our latitude and lead to disorders of varying importance. Their mode of feeding, location and other characteristics allow them to be classified as sucking or biting flies.

The first group (sucking flies) included various species from the genus *Musca*. The most common and widespread in both human habitations and on farms is *Musca domestica*. It feeds on secretions from natural orifices (mouth, eyes, nose, anus, teats and genitals) as well as from wounds. Another common species is a type of large fly similar to the housefly, known as *Musca autumnalis*, which is usually found around the eyes. Other species of small flies from the genus *Hydrotaea*, which tend to be found on cows' heads and udders, are common in pastures. The habitats of these flies favour the spread of pathogens of various types between animals to a greater or lesser degree, thereby contributing to the onset of infections, mainly of the bacterial type.

The second group (biting flies) are of greater importance from a pathogenic viewpoint as they are haematophagous. They extract blood up to 20 times a day and only leave the host to lay their eggs on fresh cow pats. The larvae, which overwinter as pupae, develop in the faeces and then transform into imagoes the following spring. Once it has laid its eggs, the female returns to its bovine host.

Some fly species (stomoxys), such as *Stomoxys calcitrans*, are common in cowsheds, whereas others, such as *Haematobia irritans*, prefer to live in pastures. *H. irritans* can produce four or five generations of fly per year. It is a very small insect and its bite is very irritating, hence its specific name. Hundreds of individuals can be seen on the back and flanks of animals. *Haematobosca stimulans*, which differs from the previous species by being larger, are present only during the day (it hides in vegetation at night) and the lower numbers found on animals (up to a maximum of 100 individuals), also lives in pastures.

2 Which flies are the most annoying?

The muscid species affecting animals can vary depending on the farming system used. The problems differ in terms of stabling and grazing over large areas during some or all of the year, as occurs, in the latter case, in the northern mountain passes in Spain.

Both sucking and biting flies are a major nuisance to the animals, causing restlessness and uneasiness. When the number of these arthropods is high, as is the case when climate conditions favour their presence and reproduction, production yields suffer markedly.

However, from a viewpoint of possible disorders, the presence of biting species is much more relevant than that of sucking species as the former also extract blood from their host and can therefore transmit various pathogens. The activity period of flies, which can occasionally last for many months, is also important in this regard, although their presence in one zone or another in the same region varies widely.

Thus, as noted above, whereas some species prefer cowshed and others live better in pastures in the open air, some can be found in both biotopes. According to the altitude at which pastures are located, there is a variation in the most important species, and the seasonal nature of their cycles. Similarly, the sex ratio in populations of each species varies markedly depending on the time of year.

Hydrotaea species, mainly *Hydrotaea irritans* and *H. borussica*, as well as *Musca autumnalis, Haematobosca stimulans* and *Haematobia irritans* predominate in mountain pastures. Although with some differences between the most common species, their activity commences in late spring (June), with populations of *Hydrotaea irritans* increasing markedly in number in August, disappearing again in October. In contrast, *Haematobia irritans* populations develop later (from mid summer until early autumn).

Haematobia irritans, Stomoxys calcitrans and *Musca domestica* predominate in lower zones (valleys and coast) and in stabled dairy cattle, with *Musca autumnalis, Haematobia irritans* and *Hydrotaea* spp. predominating in pastures.

Musca autumnalis is a nuisance to cattle between June and October and the size of its populations varies markedly (a graph with numerous peaks), although the sharp increase in the number of individuals in the second half of September should be noted. These individuals overwinter in a diapausing stage until the following spring, when they recommence their cycle and mature sexually.

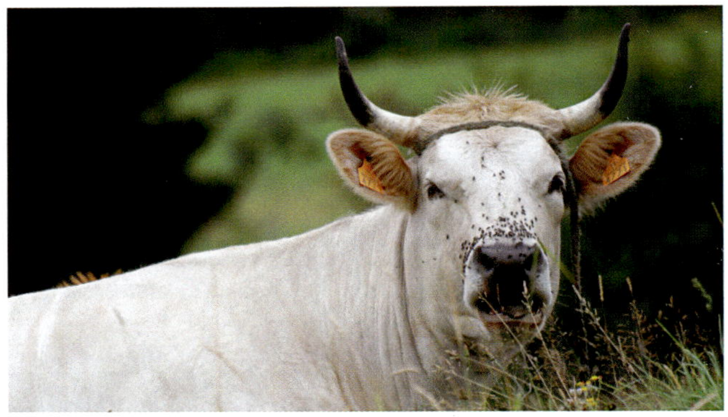

Musca autumnalis, or the face fly, is very common in farming regions. It feeds on secretions from the eyes and facial wounds on animals, which respond by blinking and moving their ears, head and tail. The animals appear irritated and exhibit a higher metabolic spend, thus reducing their food conversion efficiency.

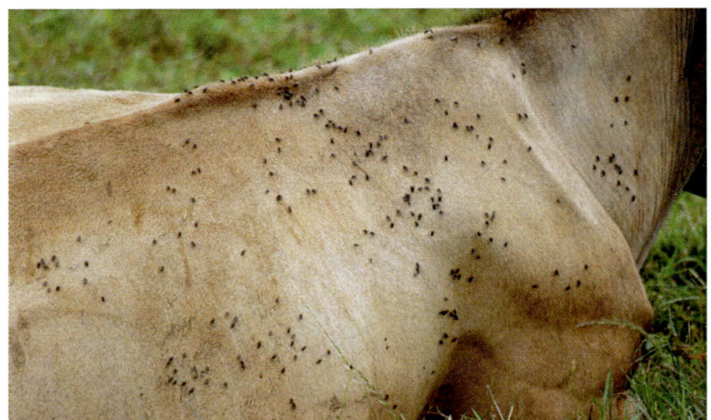

Musca domestica, or the housefly, does not bite and reproduces in animal excrement, dung heaps, decomposing silage, spilt food, bedding and other organic materials. Under favourable conditions, it can complete its biological cycle (from egg to adult) in as little as 10 days in summer.

Haematobosca stimulans has a bicuspid population dynamic with two peaks: one in mid summer and the other in early autumn. Haematophagous males and females are both found on cattle and present a sex ratio of approximately 1:1. Although the proportion of females is highest between June and August and early September (with more than 80 % of individuals being inseminated), and exhibits a marked decrease after this period, the period of maximum aggressiveness for cattle is August and September. It is at that time when similar proportions of males and females are present, with a large number of females not being inseminated. *H. stimulans* is considered to have a reproductive winter diapause.

3 How can the fly population be reduced?

It is very complicated to effectively control the fly population in pastures. However, repellents can be used as a control measure to reduce the number of flies. Pyrethroids in the form of pour-on, spray or tag formulations are used in most cases. Anthelmintic treatment with macrocyclic lactones can also partially reduce the number of flies, especially biting flies. However, other measures, such as stabling during the day and grazing at night, should be adopted in the most serious cases.

Fly control has been based on the use of chemicals such as arsenic-based compounds, chlorinated hydrocarbons, organophosphorus compounds, carbamates, pyrethroids, macrocyclic lactones and, more recently, insect growth regulators, mainly when the animals are stabled. Control in the cowshed itself must be based on strict hygiene measures and the application of insect growth regulators (spinosad, λ–cyhalothrin).

The aim of this is to ensure that the flies do not find suitable conditions in which to reproduce. This can be achieved by removing faeces and other substances on which they lay their eggs and grow and destroying adult individuals in the installations (cowsheds, feeders, etc.) using insecticides or traps. Methods such as artificial castration, which involves releasing sterile flies into the environment, have been used with some success in the fight against flies and the myiasis that some species can cause.

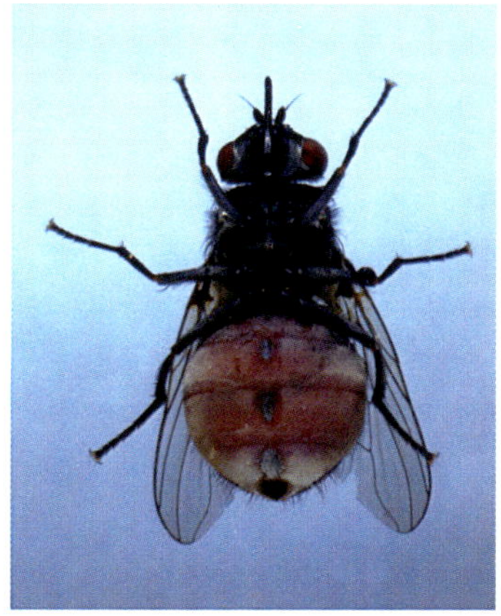

The stable fly (*Stomoxys calcitrans*) is approximately the same size as the housefly but is dark grey in colour. The stable fly mates on wet straw, manure, spilt food, silage, grass cuttings and various type of decomposing vegetation. Each female fly lives for between 20 and 30 days and lays around 200-400 eggs during its life. Under optimal conditions, an egg transforms into an adult in approximately three weeks.
Image courtesy of Dr. J. Butler.

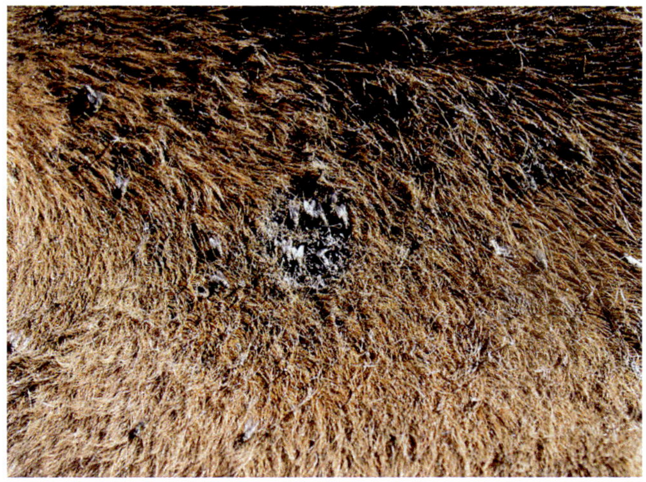

Haematobia irritans (a small and irritating biting fly) is found in pastures. Hundreds of individuals from this species can attack the back and flanks of cattle, where they come to rest with their heads pointing towards the floor and their wings in a delta shape.

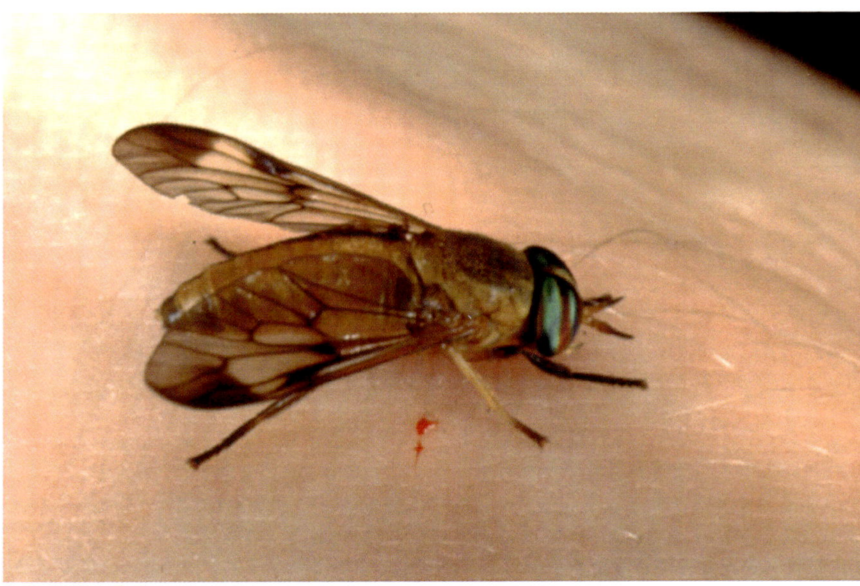

As is the case with *Haematobia irritans*, both sexes feed on blood, although *Stomoxys* is not as selective and its range of common hosts also includes horses, swine, dogs and other mammals, including humans. Its bite is very painful but it does not suck blood, therefore this diptera is not considered to be a good disease vector.
Image courtesy of Dr. J. Butler.

58 Are nematodes present in the skin of bovids?

Several large nodules are observed on the backs of calves on an extensive farm. Each nodule resembles a hard, round or oval, non-hypersensitive and clearly delimited subcutaneous tumour. They are mobile, although on occasions are attached to the periosteum or skin. Some animals present a single nodule whereas others present large conglomerates. After incision, it can be seen that these nodules are formed by a wall of hyalinised fibrous tissue. Moreover, they are vascularised and some contain very long white worms. Outbreaks of sporadic, seasonal, exudative or papular dermatitis have also been reported in the affected animals. The owners link this cutaneous clinical presentation to an allergic reaction to insect bites.

1. Which worm is found in the nodules on the animals' skin?
2. How are the nodules related to the dermatitis?
3. Are these nematodes zoonotic?
4. Can other nematode species be found in the skin?

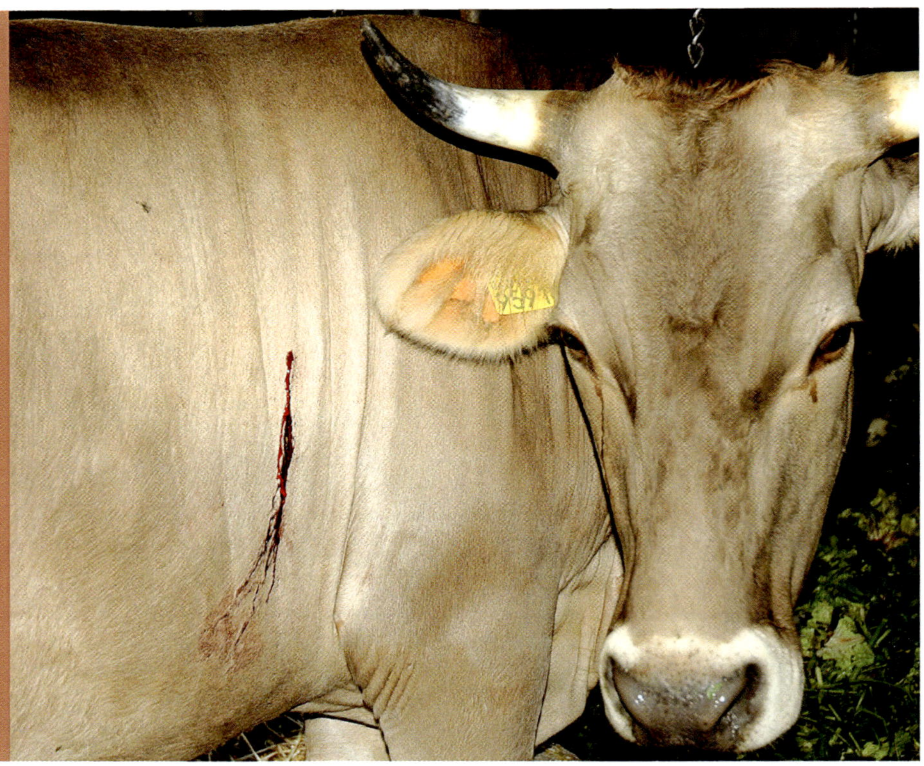

Image courtesy of Dr. A. Gentile.

1 Which worm is found in the nodules on the animals' skin?

The presence of nodules of varying sizes and shapes in the subcutaneous tissue of the neck, back and limbs is common in grazed cattle. These nodules arise due to infection by *Onchocerca* species. Adult worms are quite large (males: 3-5 cm; females: 15-19 cm) and filiform. These parasites enter the connective or subcutaneous tissue or various organs, forming hard nodules in which one or more nematodes can be found. They are transmitted by insects of the Simuliidae and Ceratopogonidae families (*Culicoides* and *Simulium* spp.), which act as intermediate hosts.

Various species that cause onchocercosis are known. In Spain, *Onchocerca gutturosa,* which produces yellowish nodules in the cervical and femorotibial ligament, as well as in other parts of the body, is the most important. Several *Onchocerca* species, for example *O. gibsoni,* which form nodules in the chest and limbs of cattle, are found in some countries. Some onchocerca are found in the aorta, gastrosplenic ligament and splenic capsule.

2 How are the nodules related to the dermatitis?

The subcutaneous nodules (also known as "onchocercomas") host adult parasites, the presence of which is characterised by a fibroblastic reaction. In some cases scar tissue is present throughout the nodule, whereas in others the worms are contained inside a granulation tissue containing precipitated immunocomplexes, neutrophils and eosinophils, macrophages, giant cells, lymphocytes and plasmocytes. If males and females coincide microfilaria may also be present. Indeed, the presence of microfilaria is consistent with a sporadic, seasonal exudative dermatitis. Although this process is related to the presence of numerous microfilaria, in some animals it seems to be associated with an allergic reaction to insect bites. Both these causes may be responsible for symptoms of this type.

3 Are these nematodes zoonotic?

The possibility that humans and animals share these nematode species has not been described to date. Although there are some reports in the literature, these are vague due to lack of identification of some of the parasites isolated from process with these characteristics.

4 Can other nematode species be found in the skin?

In countries in the northern hemisphere, other types of filaria can be found in the skin. One of these, namely *Stephanofilaria stilesi*, causes so-called "bovine premammary eczema". This parasite is transmitted by the diptera *Haematobia irritans* and species from the genera *Stomoxys* and *Lyperosia*, which act as intermediate hosts. Although the exact details of its cycle are unknown, it is thought that adults, which are located in the cutaneous lesions, eliminate the microfilaria, which are then ingested by the intermediate hosts. Once they have reached the infective stage, the intermediate hosts deposit the larvae on other definitive hosts. Lesions tend to affect the abdominal region, preferably being found forward of the breast region and above all, at the base of the teats and in the folds of the chin. They may also appear in the scrotal region in males.

Stephanofilariosis is initially identified by the presence of small papules, which join together to form lesions some 3-15 cm in diameter. A well-defined, oval or rounded inflammatory process with a brick-red colour, smooth surface and serous exudate that attracts flies is observed after 3-4 days. The lesion spreads towards the periphery, then the centre of the nodule hardens and a thick, dry scab that can reach 25 cm in diameter appears. Sick animals exhibit intense

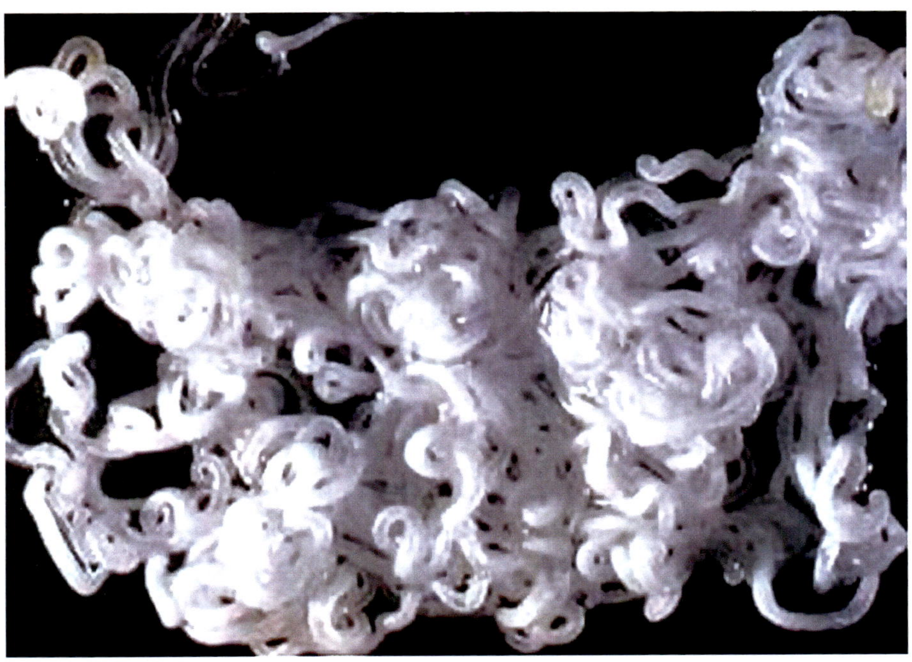

Adult *Onchocerca* are filiform and measure between 3 and 19 cm in length; females are always larger. They present a particularly thick cuticle, especially in the middle part of the body, with transversal striations. Depending on the species, these parasites are firmly inserted into the connective and subcutaneous tissue or in some organs, where they cause hard nodules that can host one or more worms.

Adult *Parafilaria bovicola* are found inside nodules in the skin and subcutaneous connective tissue, especially in the upper part of the body. Those nodules containing adult worms are painful and cause cutaneous oedema. They may even burst as the animal exercises, thereby generating a haemorrhagic dermatitis that can readily become infected with bacteria transmitted by the flies that visit the wound. *Image courtesy of Dr. A. Gentile.*

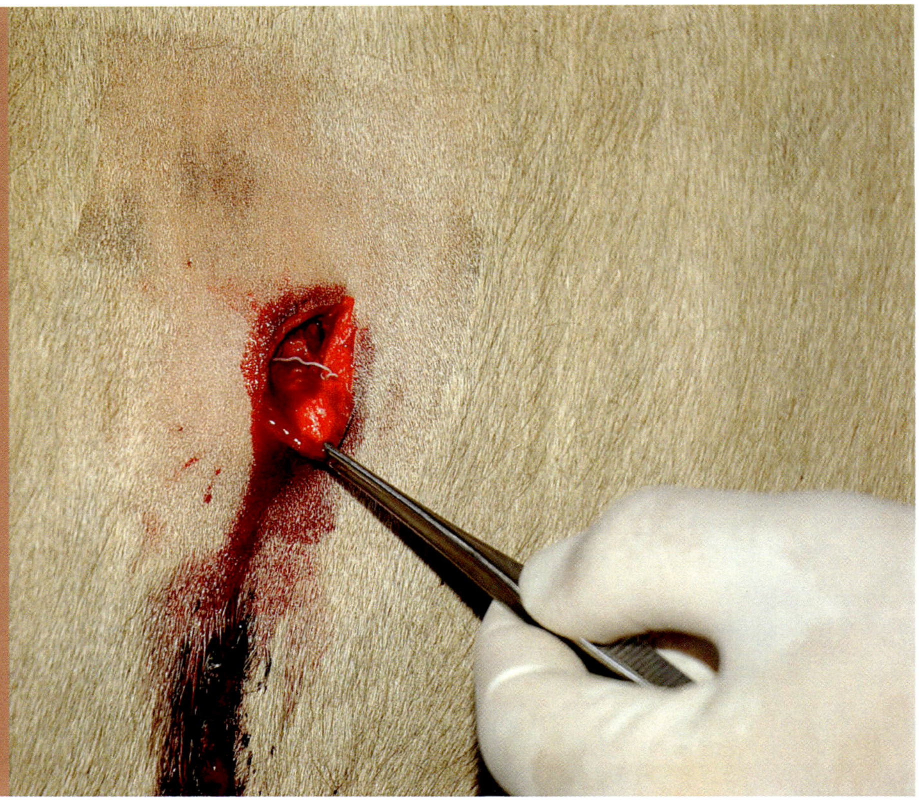

pruritus, which causes them to aggressively scratch and lick the affected area, worsening the symptoms. Milking is difficult or impossible due to the location of the lesions. Cases of refractory ulcerous dermatitis with skin lesions caused by this nematode have been reported in humans.

Parafilariosis is also known as "subcutaneous haemorrhagic nodules" in cattle. The causative agent is *Parafilaria bovicola*, which is found in the subcutaneous tissue throughout the dorsal surface of the animal. Female parasites perforate the skin and lay their eggs in the serous exudate that they excrete.

Musca autumnalis acts as an intermediate host. This fly is markedly seasonal: in the summer months these flies ingest the microfilaria and transmit the third-stage larvae (L3) to other hosts, where they migrate to the subcutaneous tissue and reach sexual maturity in around 7-10 months.

Parafilariosis is characterised by the development of lesions on the neck, back, withers, hindquarters and limbs in the form of prominent nodules around 12-15 cm in diameter. Pregnant females produce irritation, which coincides with an increase in the size of the nodule and the onset of very painful haemorrhages, upon moving inside the dermis to lay their eggs.

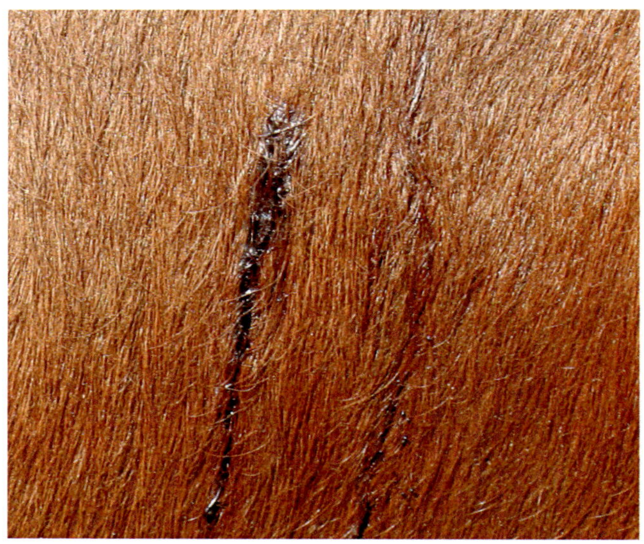

Cutaneous filariosis is caused by nematodes around 8 mm in length which invade the dermis in some parts of the body, such as the midline of the abdomen, udder and scrotum. They destroy the hair follicles and sweat glands.

59 Which parasite causes blindness in grazing cattle?

It is relatively common to detect animals with profuse epiphora and conjunctivitis, as well as severe congestion of the conjunctiva and photophobia, on beef farms in early spring. As the process progresses, a purulent secretion may appear, the pus and tears of which causes the eyelashes to stick together. The animals' eyes are so swollen that they cannot be opened, and animals exhibit clear signs of blindness. Most animals recover almost fully with time. Perforation of the cornea with haemorrhagic iridocyclitis and loss of vision is only observed in the most severe cases. After cleaning the zone and applying a local anaesthetic, the animals affected are carefully examined and nematodes visible to the naked eye are detected in the conjunctival sac.

1. What are these nematodes like and how did they reach the eye?
2. Can they be transmitted to humans?
3. How can this disease be prevented?

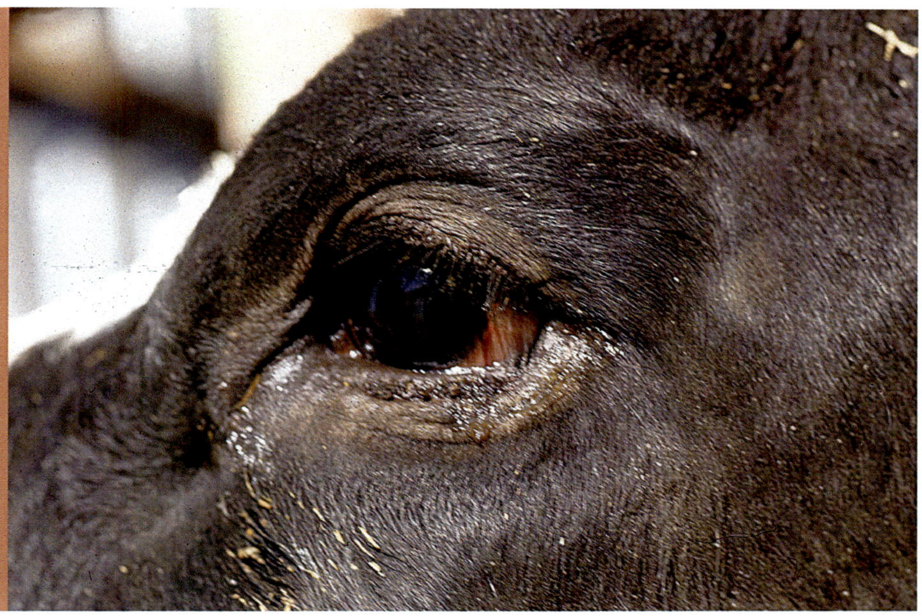

1 What are these nematodes like and how did they reach the eye?

The nematodes responsible for these symptoms are *Thelazia* spp., which are transmitted by flies, infect animals' eyes and trigger a seasonal conjunctivitis known as thelaziosis. Worms can be seen in the conjunctiva or conjunctival sac of infected animals.

Infection is caused by parasites of the genus *Thelazia*. The most important species in Spain is *Thelazia rhodesi*. This is a small parasite (1-2 cm) with prominent transversal striations at its anterior end. Males possess numerous cranial and caudal papillae (around the anus). Other species, such as *Th. gulosa* and *Th. skrjabini*, have also been diagnosed.

Female *Thelazia* give birth to larvae in the lagrimal secretions, from where they are ingested by flies. First stage (L1)

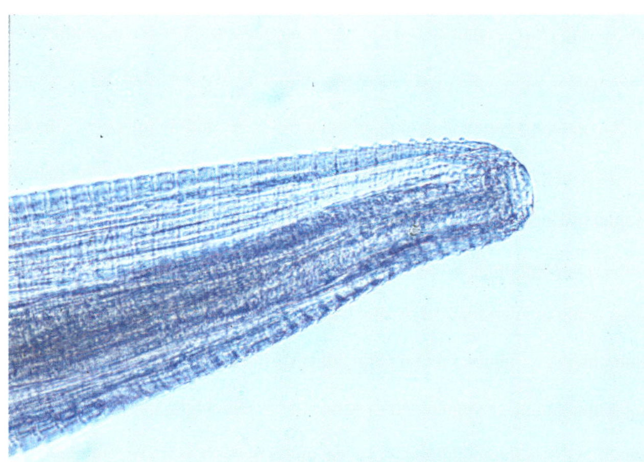

Thelazia rhodesi is a spirurida some 1 to 2 cm in length that lives in the conjunctival sac of cattle. It has prominent transversal striations at its anterior end and the posterior end is coiled.

larvae develop in the ovaries of these diptera until they reach the infective phase (L3). L3 larvae migrate to the buccal parts of the flies, from where they again gain access to cattle. Development of *Thelazia* in the intermediate host lasts between 15 and 20 days. Transmission is seasonal and does not occur in winter due to lack of fly activity.

The lesions are caused by movement of the parasites and contact with their serrated cuticle when it is inserted into the conjunctival sac and under the third eyelid. The animal exhibits profuse epiphora for the first 3-4 days post-infection, even before irritation is first noted. Conjunctivitis with marked congestion and photophobia then appears. As the process worsens, a purulent secretion containing pus and tears that causes the eyelashes to stick together arises.

Setaria cervi is another filaria that can be found in the eyes of cattle. Adults are found in the peritoneal cavity and are not pathogenic, although they may cause mild fibrous peritonitis. On rare occasions they may be observed in the anterior chamber of the eye. *Setaria* causes keratitis, conjunctivitis and ophthalmia in cattle, and the aqueous humour appears cloudy, with abundant inflammatory cells. Preadults and adults can also be found in the pericardium and epicardium, as well as in the wall of the urinary bladder, where they cause haemorrhage and granulomatous foci.

If *Setaria cervi* are inoculated into an unsuitable host (sheep, goat, horse, etc.) by the intermediate host, they migrate erratically through the nervous system. This enzootic cerebrospinal nematodosis is most common in summer and autumn and coincides with the flying period of the flies. Affected animals suffer focal and acute encephalomyelomalacia.

2 Can they be transmitted to humans?

There is no known reference to human infection by *Thelazia* species from cattle in the literature, therefore no natural zoonotic processes involving *Thelazia rhodesi* have been recorded.

However, another species from the same genus, namely *Thelazia callipaeda,* is very common in dogs, cats, foxes and rabbits in Asia. Moreover, infected people can go unnoticed in some parts of the world. In Europe, *Thelazia callipaeda* has been detected in cats and dogs. Several cases have been reported recently in dogs from Italy, south-eastern France, southern Switzerland, southern Germany and some parts of Spain. According to some authors, this is an emerging parasitosis in humans.

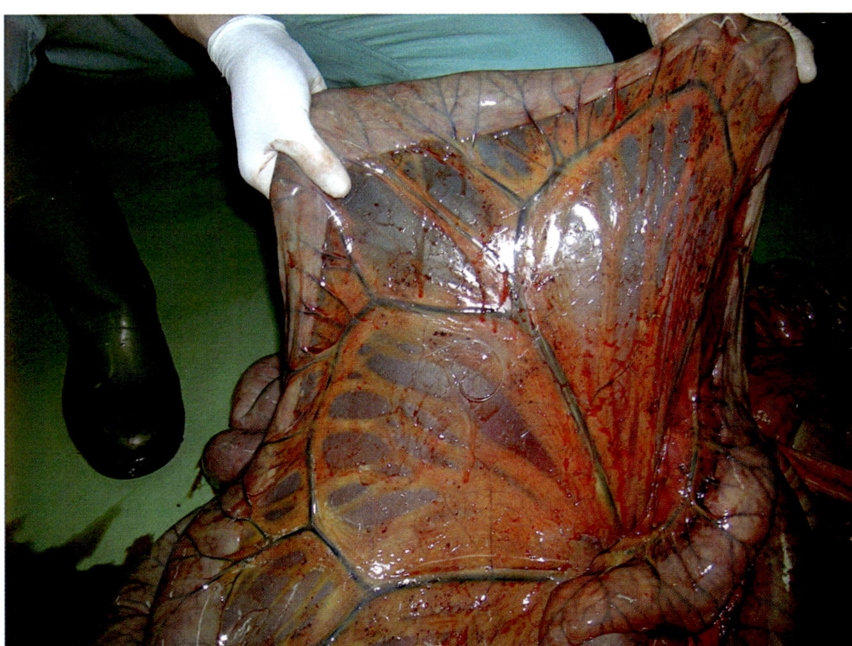

Adult *Setaria cervi* measure between 4 and 15 cm in length, with females being larger than males. They live in the abdominal cavity, although they may occasionally appear in the thoracic cavity (pleura and pericardium) and scrotum. Microfilaria measure between 200 and 250 μm in length and exhibit haematic periodicity, with their number increasing markedly early and late in the day, coinciding with the times when their vectors feed.

3 How can this disease be prevented?

Prevention and control of this type of problem in facilities and sites where the animals live is by no means easy. L1 larvae are found in the lagrimal secretions, from where they are ingested by flies (*Musca autumnalis* and other species). Once inside the diptera the larvae moult to the infective phase (L3), migrate to the buccal apparatus of the fly and then complete the cycle (approximate duration of 15-20 days in total).

In light of the above, prevention is very complicated. Despite this, the biological seasonality of flies corresponds to presentation of the disease it produces (thelaziosis). Thus, some 3-4 weeks after climate conditions begin to favour the presence of flies infected with microfilaria, clinical thelaziosis processes begin to appear in the definitive hosts.

General (levamisole, lactones) or local anthelmintics (levamisole, morantel which are applied to the conjunctival sac) can be applied systematically to the animals during risk periods. Some degree of control is also possible using insecticides, repellents, etc., although in practical terms such measures are very difficult to put into practice. The worms can even be removed from the conjunctival mucosa using forceps and a local anaesthetic, and the eye subsequently washed with saline solution.

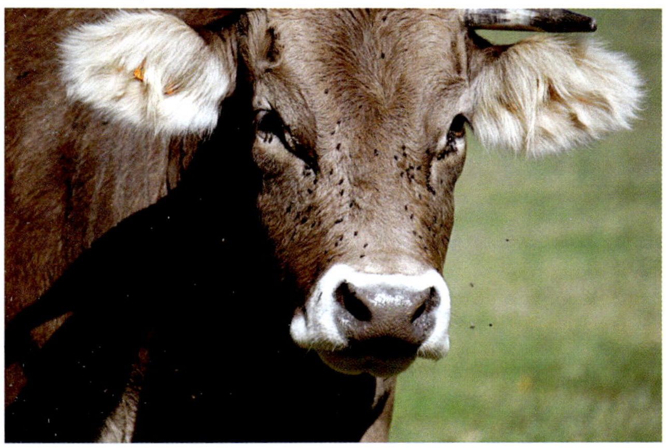

Thelazia larvae are ingested by flies together with ocular secretions, then continue to develop in the ovarian follicles of the fly until they reach the infective L3 stage.
They then migrate to the buccal parts of the fly, from where they are again transmitted to cattle. Transmission is seasonal and does not occur in winter due to lack of fly activity during this period.

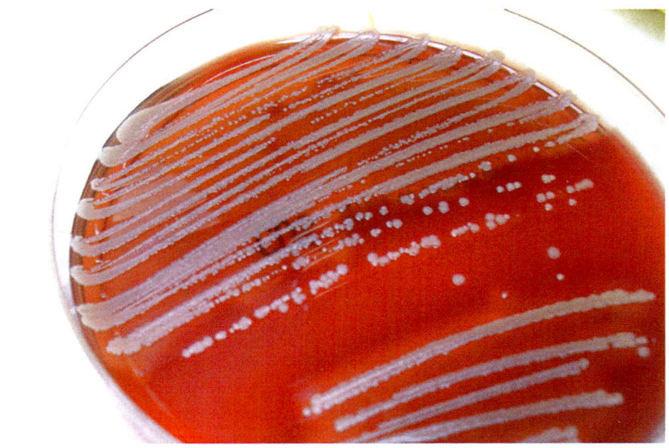

Thelaziosis has also been linked to infection with *Moraxella bovis*, which is responsible for very serious cases of keratoconjunctivitis in cattle (infectious bovine keratoconjunctivitis) and is also transmitted by the same vectors.

60 Which parasite remains in ocular nodules?

In summer time, a non-gestating Charolais cow aged 3-4 years, with uncommon lesions and a temperature of 39.2 °C, is referred to a university college hospital in the north of Spain. The animal comes from a farm with a herd of approximately 200 Charolais and Limousin beef cattle. The herd was formed 12 years ago, and the first animals (both males and females) were obtained from neighbouring countries. Both the farm owner and vet have noted various cases (5 or 6 in total) similar to that described in the past two years. The symptoms start with an increase in temperature (≥ 39.5 °C), swelling of the lower limbs and stiff walking. The animals have less appetite and therefore lose weight. Swelling of the skin, especially around the udder and the distal part of the rear legs, where hypotrichia and erythema can be seen, is observed shortly afterwards. Although small nodules can also be seen in the conjunctiva, no animal exhibits pruritus. Treatment with ivermectin does not improve the symptoms. Moreover, the affected animals are not genetically related.

1. What signs can be seen during the clinical examination of an animal with besnoitiosis?
2. Why do subcutaneous cysts appear in besnoitiosis?
3. From what other cutaneous processes should besnoitiosis be differentiated?
4. What diagnostic tests are used to identify these cysts?
5. How is besnoitiosis transmitted?

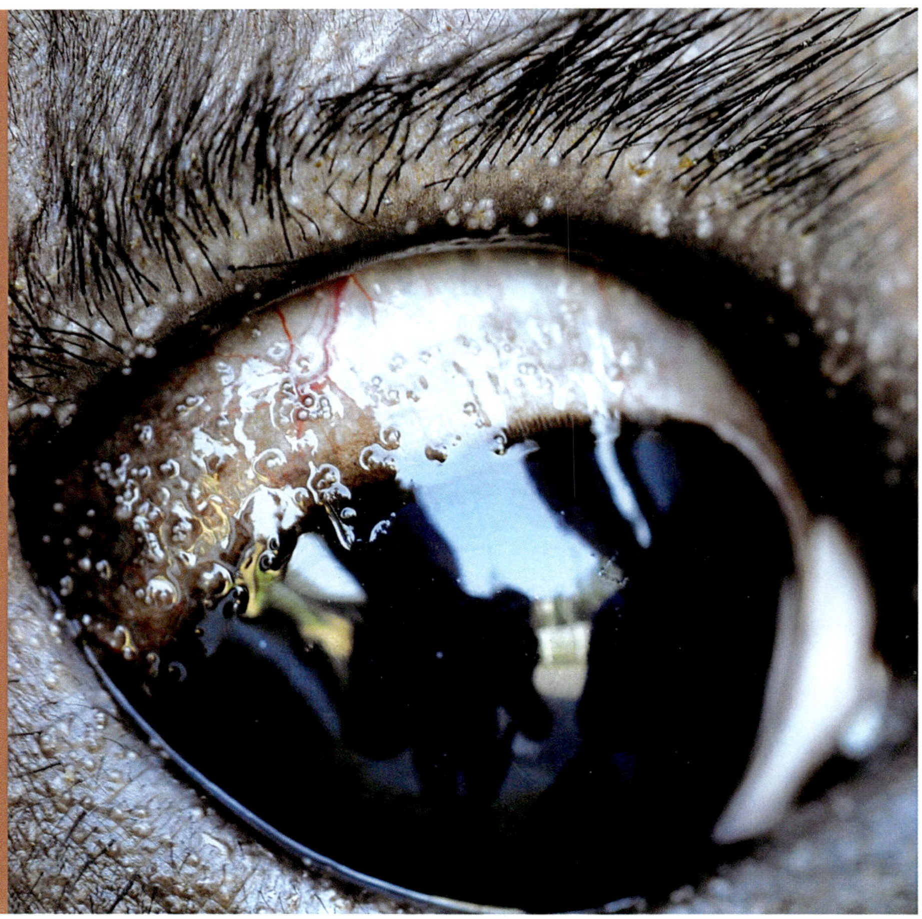

Image courtesy of Dr. A. Gentile.

1 What signs can be seen during the clinical examination of an animal with besnoitiosis?

No major alterations are usually observed during the examination (cardiovascular, respiratory, digestive and urinary apparatus) of an animal with besnoitiosis, although sick animals may sometimes present slight lameness of the rear limbs, where ulcers may be detected. All explorable lymph nodes are usually enlarged, and papules the size of a pinhead are often found in the ocular and vaginal conjunctiva.

The skin on the limbs is usually swelled, with mild hypotrichosis, severe lichenification and erythema on the hind limbs and udder. The end of the tail presents seborrhoeic symptoms. Mild periocular and perinasal hypotrichosis and lichenification can also be seen.

2 Why do subcutaneous cysts appear in besnoitiosis?

Bovine besnoitiosis is a parasitosis produced by a cyst-causing protozoan known as *Besnoitia besnoiti*. This parasite has previously been known as *Sarcocystis besnoiti* and *Globidium besnoiti*, amongst others. Indeed, this disease in bovines (cutaneous globidiosis) was first reported by Besnoit and Robin some 100 years ago. Despite this, the biological cycle of this parasite is still not fully understood, although as is the case for other apicomplex parasites, it involves two types of host: intermediate and definitive.

This thick cystic coat is a characteristic structure of *Besnoitia* and is probably responsible for the high persistence of bradyzoite cysts in tissue. This capsule can isolate the parasite from the host's immune response by limiting the presentation of antigens and even protecting the parasite against the action of antiparasitic agents, which cannot access the inside of the cysts.

Bovines (either domestic or wild) are the intermediate hosts in which the asexual reproduction phase of *Besnoitia* takes place. After infection, and over a period of less than four weeks, the parasite multiplies rapidly in the blood vessel endothelium as well as in other cells of the body, resulting in the appearance of tachyzoites by endodyogeny. This biological phase of the parasite coincides with the acute form of the disease. These tachyzoites are distributed throughout the body via the blood stream, penetrate the fibroblasts in connective tissue and continue to develop, although more slowly than before. Finally, they form thick-walled cysts that host the bradyzoites, which can grow sufficiently large to be seen by the naked eye.

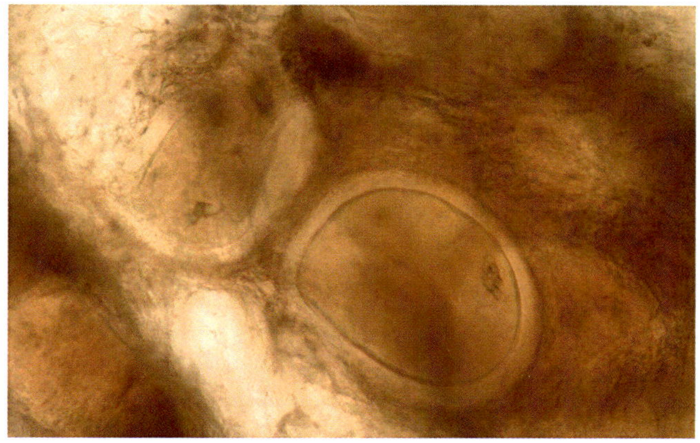

Multiple cysts surrounded by granulomatous inflammatory tissue are observed in the skin and internal organs during moderate or severe infections. Nodules are visible in the ocular, nasal and genital mucosa and in thin-skinned regions such as the breast or carpus.

3 From what other cutaneous processes should besnoitiosis be differentiated?

Besnoitiosis can progress acutely or chronically. The clinical manifestations of the acute (short-lasting) form commence at two weeks post-infection. This disease is characterised by fever with hyperthermia of up to 42 °C, despondency, dyspnoea, general malaise and congestion of the ocular mucosa, which occasionally exhibit petechiae, conjunctivitis, tearing and photophobia. Miscarriages may also occasionally occur at around 5-6 days after the onset of symptoms. In light of the above, it is possible to confuse this parasitosis with any other disease of varying aetiology that presents with such non-specific signs.

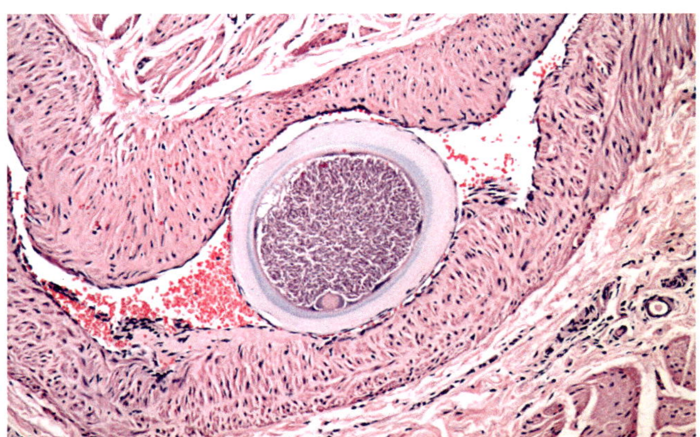

Cysts are rounded structures around 250 to 300 µm in size. They have a thick wall of around 20 µm, which comprises external hyaline, intermediate multinucleated and internal layers, and surrounds an intracytoplasmic parasitophorous vacuole and numerous elongated bradyzoites with a size of around 7-8 µm.
Image courtesy of Drs. G. Militerno and A. Gentile. University of Bolonia.

Fortunately, fewer problems are encountered when it comes to distinguishing chronic besnoitiosis from other diseases. Thus, the chronic form is characterised by dry skin, alopecia, swelling of the dermis and the onset of a tissular exudate that dries rapidly to form scabs. The sick animal goes on to develop furfuraceous sclerodermatitis. This form may be accompanied by a seborrhoeic phase with formation of thick scabs and readily visible cracks on some parts of the body (teats, muzzle). The whitish, pinhead-sized nodules in the ocular and vaginal mucosa that are pathognomonic for this parasitosis are also easy to identify.

Although diagnosis of the chronic form is relatively easy, other skin diseases that also present with hyperkeratotic dermatitis and other common alterations should be ruled out. The pathogens that should be considered during the differential diagnosis include sarcoptic or psoroptic mange, which are highly contagious and readily transmitted.

4 What diagnostic tests are used to identify these cysts?

An *in vivo* diagnosis is normally based on the observation of typical (pathognomonic) clinical signs for the chronic phase, such as swelling of the skin, sclerodermia and whitish granules in the conjunctiva (ocular, palpebral, nasal and genital), which are readily detected upon palpation. However, a suspected diagnosis should always be confirmed by several tests. Skin biopsies performed in the upper and side regions of the neck are particularly useful. The samples obtained can be studied fresh (on compression plates) or using histological methods to check the parasitic structures described.

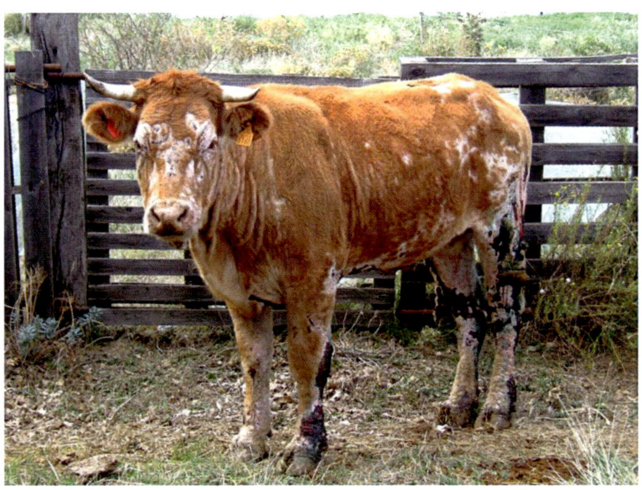

The clinical signs of the chronic phase include generalised lymph node hyperplasia and swelling of the skin (about 2 cm). The most obvious changes are seen around the eyes, muzzle, udder and limbs. It is also characterised by hypotrichosis, lichenification and small, readily recognisable papules.
Image courtesy of Dr. P. Jacquiet.

A serological diagnosis also provides good results. The method of choice is currently indirect immunofluorescence (IIF) using tachyzoites obtained from cell cultures or gerbils as antigen. The safe cut-off point can be established at a dilution of 1/80 for positives as it is very difficult to determine an infestation below this dilution. A correlation between the 1/80 titre and the onset of clinical signs or a positive biopsy is usually very high.

For epidemiological studies, a serological diagnosis using IIF and immunoenzymatic methods (indirect ELISA) is recommended.

5 How is besnoitiosis transmitted?

The biological cycle of *Besnoitia* is heteroxenous and requires two hosts, one of which is clearly defined as intermediate (bovines), whereas the animals that act as definitive hosts are yet to be established. It is suspected that the definitive hosts ought to be carnivores that follow a predator-prey pattern. Direct or indirect transmission between the intermediate hosts themselves is possible as mother-child transmission and the potential role of insects has been demonstrated. The viability of bradyzoites in the tissues of some insect species (for example *Culex* spp.) for more than 50 hours has been confirmed.

The only preventive measures currently known include tightening quarantine on infection-free farms, separating healthy animals from sick ones, increasing insect control, avoiding contact with wild bovines and possible definitive hosts such as cats, as well as other measures that prevent iatrogenic transmission.

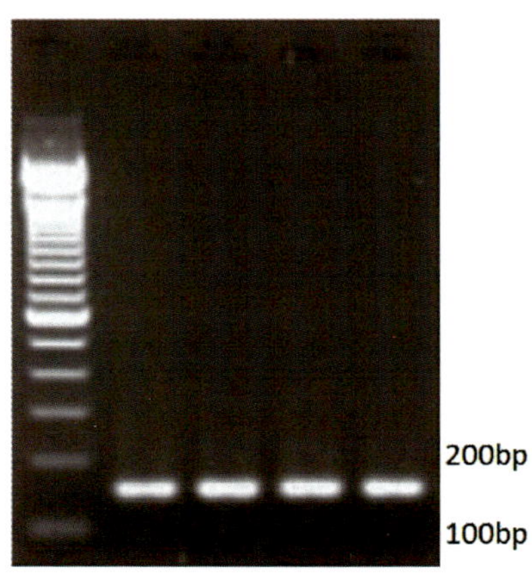

Besnoitiosis can be diagnosed by the clinical signs and by cytology and histopathology. The presence of the parasite can also be specifically confirmed using serological and molecular techniques.